Methods in Molecular Biology

Series Editor
John M. Walker
School of Life and Medical Sciences
University of Hertfordshire
Hatfield, Hertfordshire, AL10 9AB, UK

For further volumes:
http://www.springer.com/series/7651

Prenatal Diagnosis

Second Edition

Edited by

Brynn Levy

Department of Pathology and Cell Biology, Vagelos College of Physicians and Surgeons, Columbia University Irving Medical Center, New York, NY, USA

Humana Press

Editor
Brynn Levy
Department of Pathology and Cell Biology
Vagelos College of Physicians and Surgeons
Columbia University Irving Medical Center
New York, NY, USA

ISSN 1064-3745 ISSN 1940-6029 (electronic)
Methods in Molecular Biology
ISBN 978-1-4939-8887-7 ISBN 978-1-4939-8889-1 (eBook)
https://doi.org/10.1007/978-1-4939-8889-1

Library of Congress Control Number: 2018963827

Cover Illustration: Artist rendering of prenatal diagnosis in the genomics era. By: Allan Mezhibovsky

This Humana Press imprint is published by the registered company Springer Science+Business Media, LLC part of Springer Nature.
The registered company address is: 233 Spring Street, New York, NY 10013, U.S.A.

Preface

It has been ten years since the first edition of this book was published. Over this period, the concept of "genetic testing," which historically conjured up the notion of single assays and pinpoint precision in clinical diagnostics, has evolved to include a broader whole genome testing approach that often leverages big data and complex algorithms. As such, we can now consider ourselves to be deeply entrenched in the genomics era where bioinformatics and terabytes of data are an integral part of analysis and diagnostics. Indeed, the American College of Medical Genetics officially changed their name to the American College of Medical Genetics and Genomics to recognize this paradigm shift.

The biggest change in the field of prenatal diagnosis has been observed in the area of cytogenomics where microarray and next-generation sequencing technologies have become the preferable genomic tool for the assessment of preimplantation embryos and first and second trimester fetuses. The introduction of these newer genomic technologies has had a major effect on the success rates of IVF as demonstrated in recent prospective randomized clinical trials. In traditional prenatal diagnosis, chromosomal microarray analysis (CMA) has been recommended for all pregnancies with a fetal structural anomaly and currently offers the most comprehensive assessment of fetal aneuploidy, aneusomy, and microdeletions and microduplications possible.

While microarray diagnostics currently provides the most complete cytogenomic assessment of the fetus, the appeal of a highly sensitive noninvasive blood test that screens for the common aneuploidies has made noninvasive prenatal testing (NIPT) one of the fastest-adopted genetic tests. In fact, in the United States, the mass adoption of NIPT is believed to be the primary reason for the decline in the number of invasive prenatal diagnosis procedures performed. It is important to emphasize that NIPT, in its current form, is a screening test while CMA is a diagnostic test. As a screening test, NIPT offers superior detection of Down syndrome and the other common aneuploidies compared to traditional biochemical markers and nuchal translucency (NT) measurements. However, as a screening test, it does not cover the vast scope of genomic abnormalities that are detectable by CMA. NIPT has also been developed to predict the fetal RhD gene status in order to guide targeted prenatal anti-D prophylaxis and prevent hemolytic disease of the fetus and the newborn. This approach has been particularly well received in Europe, especially in Scandinavia.

Next-generation sequencing (NGS) entered the prenatal world predominantly for aneuploidy detection in preimplantation embryos and for noninvasive copy number assessment of cell-free DNA. It is now increasingly utilized to evaluate single nucleotide variations (SNVs) in fetuses with structural anomalies as well as assess cryptic complex rearrangements and imbalances in fetuses carrying apparently balanced translocations. It is likely that in the future NGS will serve to assess both SNVs and copy number changes in a single assay. In order to replace CMA, NGS as a single test will need to match the current resolution and accuracy of CMA testing. This will certainly require greater coverage of the genome which will only become a reality for routine testing when whole genome sequencing costs decrease.

Over the past decade, novel technologies have been utilized for the development of new diagnostic tests. However, the newer prenatal tests have not necessarily replaced the older ones. A prime reason pertains to payment/reimbursement of the new and often more expensive tests. Payment/reimbursement in countries with national health systems and even by private health insurance companies is often not approved as the new tests are usually deemed "experimental" with "insufficient evidence" to support clinical utility. In addition, there is often a large time gap before these tests are universally adopted worldwide and even within individual countries. In some instances, the time gap is directly related to the amount of time it takes for the appropriate clinical trials to be performed to support clinical utility. In other cases, there may be a lack of the necessary expertise to interpret the more complex genomic assays. In many cases, the delay in adoption has to do with the economic resources available to purchase the genomic equipment as well as validate and implement the new tests. As such, there remains tremendous utility for many of the old style and less expensive targeted tests like FISH, QF-PCR and MLPA.

This second edition of Prenatal Diagnosis is divided into three major sections; preimplantation genetic testing, traditional prenatal testing and finally non-invasive prenatal testing. The first part of the book begins with a historical introduction to each of the three major sections. Traditional prenatal testing methodologies that have served as the gold standard for decades remain an important aspect of this book as they continue to serve as the primary testing assays in many regions of the world. New to this book are methodologies that employ next generation sequencing techniques and these can be found in each of the three primary sections.

My appreciation and thanks goes to the authors for their individual contributions. Their willingness to share their protocols and experience provides a valuable resource to clinical laboratories around the globe.

New York, NY, USA *Brynn Levy*

Contents

Contributors

AVINASH ABHYANKAR • *Molecular Diagnostics, New York Genome Center, New York, NY, USA*

ADEDOYIN AKINWOLE • *IGENOMIX USA, Torrance, CA, USA*

CAROLINE W. ANTOLIK • *Massachusetts General Hospital, Boston, MA, USA; Broad Institute, Harvard Medical School, Cambridge, MA, USA*

SUE BERUTI • *Illumina, Inc., San Diego, CA, USA*

CHRISTIE M. BUCHOVECKY • *Department of Pathology and Cell Biology, Vagelos College of Physicians and Surgeons, Columbia University Irving Medical Center, New York, NY, USA*

BIRGITTE SUHR BUNDGAARD • *Department of Clinical Immunology, Section 2034, Copenhagen University Hospital, Copenhagen, Denmark*

HONGJIE CHEN • *Mount Sinai Genomics, Inc., DBA Sema 4, New York, NY, USA; Department of Genetics and Genomic Sciences, Icahn School of Medicine at Mount Sinai, New York, NY, USA*

CENGIZ CINNIOGLU • *IGENOMIX USA, Torrance, CA, USA*

FREDERIK BANCH CLAUSEN • *Department of Clinical Immunology, Section 2034, Copenhagen University Hospital, Copenhagen, Denmark*

RYAN L. COLLINS • *Massachusetts General Hospital, Boston, MA, USA; Broad Institute, Harvard Medical School, Cambridge, MA, USA*

KIRSTEN J. CURNOW • *Illumina, Inc., Foster City, CA, USA*

BENJAMIN B. CURRALL • *Massachusetts General Hospital, Boston, MA, USA; Broad Institute, Harvard Medical School, Cambridge, MA, USA*

TRISTAN DARVIN • *IGENOMIX USA, Torrance, CA, USA*

MORTEN HANEFELD DZIEGIEL • *Department of Clinical Immunology, Section 2034, Copenhagen University Hospital, Copenhagen, Denmark; Institute of Clinical Medicine (IKM), Copenhagen University, Copenhagen, Denmark*

BLAKE EBERT • *Department of Pathology and Cell Biology, Vagelos College of Physicians and Surgeons, Columbia University Irving Medical Center, New York, NY, USA*

JENNIFER ECCLES • *Baylor Genetics, Houston, TX, USA*

LISA EDELMANN • *Department of Genetics and Genomic Sciences, Icahn School of Medicine at Mount Sinai, New York, NY, USA; Mount Sinai Genomics, Inc., DBA Sema4 Genomics, New York, NY, USA*

ANASTASIA M. FEDICK • *Department of Genetics and Genomic Sciences, Icahn School of Medicine at Mount Sinai, New York, NY, USA; Mount Sinai Genomics, Inc., DBA Sema4 Genomics, New York, NY, USA*

VANESSA FELICE • *Molecular Diagnostics, New York Genome Center, New York, NY, USA*

ROBERT-JAN GALJAARD • *Department of Clinical Genetics, Erasmus University Medical Center, Rotterdam, The Netherlands*

MYTHILY GANAPATHI • *Department of Pathology and Cell Biology, Vagelos College of Physicians and Surgeons, Columbia University Irving Medical Center, New York, NY, USA*

GARY HARTON • *IGENOMIX USA, Torrance, CA, USA*

LISA HUI • *Department of Perinatal Medicine, Mercy Hospital for Women, Heidelberg, VIC, Australia; Department of Obstetrics and Gynaecology, University of Melbourne, Parkville, VIC, Australia; Reproductive Epidemiology, Murdoch Children's Research Institute, Parkville, VIC, Australia*
MILENA JAKUBOWSKA • *IGENOMIX USA, Torrance, CA, USA*
CHAIM JALAS • *Foundation for Embryonic Competence, Baskign Ridge, NJ, USA*
VAIDEHI JOBANPUTRA • *Molecular Diagnostics, New York Genome Center, New York, NY, USA; Department of Pathology and Cell Biology, Vagelos College of Physicians and Surgeons, Columbia University Irving Medical Center, New York, NY, USA*
EMMANUEL KANAVAKIS • *Department of Medical Genetics, St. Sophia's Children's Hospital, National and Kapodistrian University of Athens, Athens, Greece; Genesis Genoma Lab, Athens, Greece*
REFIK KAYALI • *IGENOMIX USA, Torrance, CA, USA*
RUTH KORNREICH • *Department of Genetics and Genomic Sciences, Icahn School of Medicine at Mount Sinai, New York, NY, USA; Mount Sinai Genomics, Inc., DBA Sema4 Genomics, New York, NY, USA*
GRETHE RISUM KROG • *Department of Clinical Immunology, Section 2034, Copenhagen University Hospital, Copenhagen, Denmark*
ANVER KULIEV • *Florida International University, Miami, FL, USA; Reproductive Genetics Institute, Inc. (RGI), Northbrook, IL, USA*
BRYNN LEVY • *Department of Pathology and Cell Biology, Vagelos College of Physicians and Surgeons, Columbia University Irving Medical Center, New York, NY, USA*
THOMAS LIEHR • *Jena University Hospital, Institute of Human Genetics, Friedrich Schiller University, Jena, Germany*
CARMEN RUBIO LLUESA • *Igenomix, Valencia, Spain*
ALEX K. LYASHCHENKO • *Department of Pathology and Cell Biology, Vagelos College of Physicians and Surgeons, Columbia University Irving Medical Center, New York, NY, USA*
KATHY MANN • *Viapath Analytics, Guy's Hospital, London, UK*
ODELIA NAHUM • *Department of Pathology and Cell Biology, Vagelos College of Physicians and Surgeons, Columbia University Irving Medical Center, New York, NY, USA*
ANKITA PATEL • *Lineagen, Salt Lake City, UT, USA*
BARBARA PERTL • *Prenatal Centre, Ragnitz Hospital, Graz, Austria*
ERWIN PETEK • *Institute of Human Genetics, Medical University of Graz, Graz, Austria*
ALEX J. RAI • *Department of Pathology and Cell Biology, Vagelos College of Physicians and Surgeons, Columbia University Irving Medical Center, New York, NY, USA*
SVETLANA RECHITSKY • *Florida International University, Miami, FL, USA; Reproductive Genetics Institute, Inc. (RGI), Northbrook, IL, USA*
KLAUS RIENECK • *Department of Clinical Immunology, Section 2034, Copenhagen University Hospital, Copenhagen, Denmark*
REBECCA K. SANDERSON • *Illumina, Inc., Foster City, CA, USA*
JAN SCHOUTEN • *Department of Clinical Genetics, Erasmus University Medical Center, Rotterdam, The Netherlands*
RICHARD T. SCOTT JR. • *Thomas Jefferson University, Basking Ridge, NJ, USA; Rutgers-Robert Wood Johnson Medical School, Piscataway Township, NJ, USA*
JOE LEIGH SIMPSON • *March of Dimes Foundation, White Plains, NY, USA; Florida International University, Miami, FL, USA; Reproductive Genetics Institute, Inc. (RGI), Northbrook, IL, USA*

MELISSA STOSIC • *Department of Obstetrics and Gynecology, Vagelos College of Physicians and Surgeons, Columbia University Irving Medical Center, New York, NY, USA*
JAMES STRAY • *Natera Inc., San Carlos, CA, USA*
MICHAEL E. TALKOWSKI • *Massachusetts General Hospital, Boston, MA, USA; Broad Institute, Harvard Medical School, Cambridge, MA, USA*
AWET TECLEAB • *Department of Pathology and Laboratory Medicine, Staten Island University Hospital, Staten Island, NY, USA*
AMANDA THOMAS • *Department of Pathology and Cell Biology, Vagelos College of Physicians and Surgeons, Columbia University Irving Medical Center, New York, NY, USA*
JOANNE TRAEGER-SYNODINOS • *Department of Medical Genetics, St. Sophia's Children's Hospital, National and Kapodistrian University of Athens, Athens, Greece*
NATHAN R. TREFF • *Genomic Prediction, North Brunswick, NJ, USA*
PAUL VAN VUGHT • *Department of Clinical Genetics, Erasmus University Medical Center, Rotterdam, The Netherlands*
LORENA RODRIGO VIVÓ • *Igenomix, Paterna, Valencia, Spain*
CHRISTINA VRETTOU • *Department of Medical Genetics, St. Sophia's Children's Hospital, National and Kapodistrian University of Athens, Athens, Greece*
ANJA WEISE • *Jena University Hospital, Institute of Human Genetics, Friedrich Schiller University, Jena, Germany*
CHUNLI YU • *Mount Sinai Genomics, Inc., DBA Sema 4, New York, NY, USA; Department of Genetics and Genomic Sciences, Icahn School of Medicine at Mount Sinai, New York, NY, USA*
JINGLAN ZHANG • *Department of Molecular and Human Genetics, Baylor College of Medicine, Houston, TX, USA*
BERNHARD ZIMMERMANN • *Natera Inc., San Carlos, CA, USA*
REBEKAH S. ZIMMERMAN • *Sema4, New York, NY, USA; Department of Genetics and Genomic Sciences, The Icahn School of Medicine at Mount Sinai, New York, NY, USA*

Part I

Historical Introduction

Chapter 1

Traditional Prenatal Diagnosis: Past to Present

Brynn Levy and Melissa Stosic

Abstract

In the nearly 60 years since prenatal diagnosis for genetic disease was first offered, the field of prenatal diagnosis has progressed far past rudimentary uterine puncture to provide fetal material to assess gender and interpret risk. Concurrent with the improvements in invasive fetal sampling came technological advances in cytogenetics and molecular biology that widened both the scope of genetic disorders that could be diagnosed and also the resolution at which the human genome could be interrogated. Nowadays, routine blood work available to all pregnant women can determine the risk for common chromosome abnormalities; chorionic villus sampling (CVS) and amniocentesis can be used to diagnose nearly all conditions with a known genetic cause; and the genome and/or exome of a fetus with multiple anomalies can be sequenced in an attempt to determine the underlying etiology. This chapter will discuss some of the major advances in prenatal sampling and prenatal diagnostic laboratory techniques that have occurred over the past six decades.

Key words History of prenatal diagnosis, Chorionic villus sampling, Amniocentesis, Ultrasound

1 Introduction

It was less than a lifetime ago that, in 1956, Tijo and Levan first correctly determined that humans have 46 chromosomes, rather than 48 as was thought for over 30 years [1]. The establishment of the proper number of human chromosomes laid the groundwork for defining the various common chromosomal aneuploidies that were just waiting to be discovered. The association of chromosome abnormalities and specific clinical phenotypes led to a new era in pediatric diagnosis and it was not long before chromosome analysis was applied to prenatal testing. One of the early scientific reports on transabdominal sampling of amniotic fluid dates back to 1897 when Prochownick reported on the chemical components of amniotic fluid [2]. However, it was not until 1955 and 1956 that the first analyses of amniotic fluid for genetic information were performed utilizing Barr bodies to determine fetal sex [3, 4]. Three years later, in 1959, the underlying causes of common aneuploidies

Brynn Levy (ed.), *Prenatal Diagnosis*, Methods in Molecular Biology, vol. 1885, https://doi.org/10.1007/978-1-4939-8889-1_1,

including Down syndrome, Turner syndrome, Klinefelter syndrome, and XXX were identified and shortly thereafter, XYY [5–9].

In 1960, Riis and Fuchs described performing the amniocentesis procedure on two pregnant women who were Hemophilia A carriers [10]. This is the first report of performing prenatal testing on the basis of an inherited risk for genetic disease. These women would have terminated their pregnancies due to the risk of Hemophilia in their sons, but instead, underwent amniocentesis to determine fetal sex with the plan of continuing the pregnancy if a female fetus was identified.

While the idea of culturing amniotic fluid for chromosome analysis was advanced by Fuchs and Riis in 1960 [11], Steele and Breg published the first proof of concept study in 1966 showing that culturing and karyotyping of amniotic fluid cells was indeed possible [12]. The following year, Jacobsen and Barter initiated cultures on amniotic fluid obtained from 85 human cases. They showed a 67% success rate (67/85) for obtaining viable cell cultures and a 38% success rate (33/85) for yielding a final genetic evaluation [13]. Their cohort included 6 cases which presented with "genetic high risk pregnancies" prompting a "diagnostic" amniocentesis. A successful karyotype was obtained on all 6 cases. From that point onward, the vast field of prenatal diagnosis opened up as major efforts were directed at the development of and improvement upon both invasive testing and the laboratory analysis of prenatal samples. Here, we take a brief look at the progress of routine prenatal screening as well as invasive testing techniques including amniocentesis, fetoscopy, chorionic villus sampling (CVS), and percutaneous umbilical blood sampling. In addition, we will review the major milestones in the technologies developed to diagnose genetic disease in prenatal specimens, taking you on a journey from cytogenetics to sequencing.

2 Noninvasive Screening

2.1 Ultrasound

Case reports identifying fetal and pregnancy abnormalities via ultrasonography began to appear in the 1960s [14–17]. Advances in ultrasonography over the next 20 years provided the ability to better date pregnancies, identify twins, locate the placenta, visualize intrauterine growth restriction, and diagnose anomalies such as spina bifida and limb reduction defects. When real time scanners with improved resolution were introduced alongside color Doppler in the mid-1980s, the potential for imaging all pregnancies became a reality and hospitals began to perform anatomy scans at 20 weeks gestation. The detection rate for fetal anomalies at 20 weeks varied by study but was potentially as low as 17% [18]. This rate has steadily increased over time as has the capacity to detect major anomalies in the first trimester. Dane et al. in 2007, performed a large study of 1290 cases and demonstrated a 70% detection rate for major anomalies after the first trimester scan [19]. When a second trimester ultrasound was added, the detection rate increased to 95% [19]. Furthermore, the ability to perform invasive testing with placental localization, and later, under continuous ultrasound monitoring, lead to reduced complication rates [18, 20–23].

2.2 Biochemical Screening

In 1977, Wald et al. published a large multi-center collaborative study to determine the accuracy of maternal serum alpha-fetoprotein (AFP) in screening for open neural tube defects (ONTDs) [24]. The study included nearly 19,000 unaffected pregnancies and 301 pregnancies with ONTDs. They determined that 16–18 weeks is the best window for screening, allowing for 88% of cases of anencephaly and 79% of cases of open spina bifida to be detected at a 3% false positive rate. This has improved with modifications to the AFP measurement and algorithm [25]. In addition, the sensitivity of ultrasound to identify cases of spina bifida and all cases of anencephaly is now reported to be as high as 95%, making AFP less widely utilized [26].

Benacerraf et al. reported on the association of an increased nuchal fold measurement in the second trimester with Down syndrome in 1985 and shortly after, additional markers such as shortened femurs were noted [27–29]. By 1992, the earlier association of increased nuchal translucency in the first trimester and Down syndrome had also been identified by Nicolaides et al. [30].

In the mid to late 1980s, the association between aneuploidy and abnormal amounts of AFP, unconjugated estriol, and human chorionic gonadotropin (HCG) in maternal serum was uncovered [31–35]. This lead to the creation of the triple screen in 1988 which was able to identify 60% of Down syndrome pregnancies at a 5% false positive rate [36]. Several years later, in 1995, 79% of laboratories were using multiple markers to screen for Trisomy 21; the remainder were using AFP alone [37]. In the early 1990s, abnormal levels of free ß-HCG and pregnancy-associated plasma protein A (PAPP-A) in the first trimester were correlated with aneuploidy [38, 39]. By 1997 it was shown that these two markers, when combined with nuchal translucency measurement, provide an 80% detection rate for Down syndrome for a 5% false positive rate [40]. Around the same time, Inhibin A was found to be a fourth marker in the second trimester and was added to the others to create the quad test, replacing the triple screen [41–43]. With both first and second trimester screening possible, the integrated screen was developed in 1999, combining first and second trimester screens for an 85% detection rate and 0.9% false positive rate [44]. Integrated screening requires waiting until the second trimester for results and therefore, the sequential screen was proposed, which provides results for very high risk women in the first trimester, and those with low risk results proceeded to subsequent additional screening in the second trimester [45]. With the availability of multiple options for maternal serum screening, the First and Second Trimester Evaluation of Risk (FASTER) consortium published findings on the reliability of first and second trimester screening as well as combined screening in 2005 [46].

2.3 Noninvasive Prenatal Testing (NIPT) Using Cell-Free Fetal DNA

In 2011, after decades of reports of fetal cells and cell-free fetal DNA in maternal circulation, the first noninvasive prenatal tests using cell-free fetal DNA for the detection of Trisomy 21 became commercially available [47–49]. Now, NIPT is able to screen for the common aneuploidies (13, 18, 21, X & Y), large deletions and duplications, and the common microdeletion syndromes. The sensitivity of NIPT for Down syndrome is >99% for a very low false positive rate (<1% even when screening for multiple conditions). With NIPT clearly showing superiority over traditional biochemical/sonographic markers for aneuploidy screening [50], the American College of Obstetricians and Gynecologists (ACOG) released guidelines in 2016 stating that NIPT is an appropriate screening test for pregnant women. The same year, the American College of Medical Genetics and Genomics (ACMGG) issued a statement strongly suggesting NIPT replaces serum screening for aneuploidy in women of any age [51, 52].

3 Invasive Procedures

3.1 Amniocentesis

Amniocentesis is the technique for withdrawing amniotic fluid transabdominally from the amniotic sac using a needle guided by ultrasound. Amniotic fluid contains cells that have been sloughed off from the amnion and from the fetus. In 1968, Nadler showed that enzyme levels could be measured in amniotic fluid, thus opening the door for diagnosing metabolic conditions in utero [53]. Together, he and his colleague Walsh, would go on to prenatally diagnose the first cases of cystic fibrosis (one of the most common autosomal recessive genetic diseases in Caucasians) using quantitative and qualitative measurements of methylumbelliferyl-guanidinobenzoate (MUGB) reactive proteases in amniotic fluid [54]. The earliest description of an increase in alpha-fetoprotein (AFP) levels in the amniotic fluid of fetuses affected with open neural tube defects was by Brock and Sutcliffe [55]. In 1970 Nadler and Gerbie published an amniocentesis series of 162 high risk women, diagnosing 10 cases of Down syndrome and 3 additional conditions for a total of 13 affected pregnancies with no reported fetal or maternal complications [56]. Several years later, in 1976, the National Institute of Child Health and Human Development (NICHD) published on the safety and accuracy of amniocentesis, with a quoted diagnostic accuracy of 99.4% and a fetal loss rate of well below 1% [57]. Once the results were published, it became standard of care to recommend an amniocentesis during the second trimester to women over the age of 35 in order to detect fetal chromosome abnormalities. Reports of early amniocenteses performed prior to 15 weeks began to appear in 1987 but the fetal loss rate was found to be 2.3% and a discernable increase in congenital abnormalities, particularly talipes, was observed [58]. As such, early amniocentesis was discouraged and is no longer routinely performed [58–61]. It was not until 2007 that ACOG changed the recommendations for invasive testing, no longer limiting it to pregnant women over the age of 35, but rather offering diagnostic testing and screening to all women, regardless of age [62, 63].

3.2 Fetoscopy

Fetoscopy is an endoscopic procedure that provides access (for biopsy and/or surgery) to the fetus, the amniotic sac, the umbilical cord, and the fetal side of the placenta. As early as 1954, Westin was able to visualize three fetuses in utero via hysteroscope [64]. It wasn't until 1973 that Valenti collected fetal blood and skin biopsies with the goal of eventually using the technique to diagnose hemoglobinopathies and ultimately perform intrauterine therapy [65]. The same year, Scrimgeour used an endoamnioscope to identify central nervous system anomalies in three fetuses [66] and a year later, Hobbins and Mahoney reported on fetal blood collection from a small cohort of eight women [67]. Fetoscopy was readily introduced for the diagnosis of inherited blood disorders, beginning with hemoglobinopathies in 1975 and then hemophilia in 1979 [68, 69]. This method was also utilized to identify genetic conditions by visualizing the fetal anatomy, as was shown in 1977 for the case of a fetus with skeletal dysplasia [70]. Incipient examples of obtaining fetal blood and/or skin biopsy for the diagnosis of skin diseases such as ichthyosis and epidermis bullosa as well as metabolic diseases including galactosemia and Tay-sachs were first reported between 1977 and 1980 [70–74]. Given the fetal loss rate of 3–5% and the relative safety of amniocentesis, fetoscopy is no longer utilized for prenatal diagnosis except in rare instances, such as mosaicism [75]. However, it has become a mainstay in the treatment of prenatal anomalies and complications such as twin to twin transfusion syndrome, diaphragmatic hernia, and amniotic band syndrome.

3.3 Chorionic Villus Sampling (CVS)

Chorionic villi are part of the placenta and can be obtained by two different ultrasound guided methods depending upon the uterine position and the location of the placenta. The transcervical method involves inserting a catheter through the vagina and cervix while the transabdominal method involves inserting a thin needle through a sterile area of the abdomen (similar to amniocentesis).

The concept of first trimester transcervical sampling of the placenta was first proposed by Mohr in 1968 [76]. Five years later, in 1973, Sandahl and Kullander biopsied the placenta in 39 patients undergoing termination of pregnancy. Karyotype was successful in half of them and was shown to truly represent the fetal genetic constitution [77]. The following year, Hahnemann developed new equipment and had a 38% biopsy success rate [78]. In 1975, a group in China reported 99 successful procedures for fetal sex determination [79]. In their case series, only six incorrect fetal sex determinations were made and four fetal losses occurred following the procedure [79]. 1982–3 saw groundbreaking work on transcervical CVS resulting in the procedure being offered in many centers around the globe with each center having a slightly varied technique and instrument [80–85]. When tissue culture of chorionic villi was perfected, it became possible to offer routine cytogenetic testing of the fetus from a CVS. In 1983, Pergament and colleagues performed simultaneous enzyme and chromosome testing on a CVS sample from a woman at risk for Tay-Sachs disease [86]. The same year, Brambati and Simoni reported the prenatal diagnosis of trisomy 21 following a first trimester CVS performed on a woman at 50% risk for a male child with Duchenne muscular dystrophy [87]. In the Brambati case report, they utilized a newly developed technique [88] for direct analysis of the villi which resulted in a karyotype within hours of the procedure.

Transabdominal techniques were unsuccessful initially, as they could only be performed in the second trimester, and amniocentesis was the better option at that gestational age [89, 90]. In 1984, the transabdominal route became possible in the first trimester [91]. Today, both transcervical and transabdominal CVS are commonly performed.

The safety and efficacy of CVS was assessed in large studies toward the end of the 1980s and early 1990s with the finding that the rates of miscarriage after CVS were only slightly higher than those associated with amniocentesis [92, 93]. These studies indicated the rates of miscarriage to be around 0.5%–1.0% [92, 93]. Despite the somewhat higher risk for miscarriage, CVS has various emotional and medical advantages over amniocentesis as it provides an opportunity for earlier decision making in the wake of a diagnosis of a chromosome abnormality (almost 6 weeks earlier than amniocentesis). In the early 1990s, there was considerable worry regarding the causal link between CVS and limb-reduction defects. After much debate and several cohort studies, it was determined that CVS performed before 9 weeks was indeed a risk factor for limb-reduction defects [94]. In 1992, a WHO-sponsored committee recommended that CVS be performed at 9–12 weeks after the last menstrual period [94]. CVS is now safely performed in most institutions between 10 and 12 weeks for the diagnosis of a wide range of genetic conditions.

3.4 Percutaneous Umbilical Blood Sampling (PUBS)

Percutaneous Umbilical Blood Sampling (PUBS) involves obtaining a blood sample from the fetus. It was originally developed in conjunction with fetoscopy in mid 1960s and early 1970s as a means to do prenatal diagnosis of hemoglobinopathies [95, 96]. PUBS is also referred to as Fetal Blood Sampling, Cordocentesis, and Umbilical Vein Sampling. PUBS involves the insertion of a thin needle through the abdomen and uterine walls into the umbilical cord at the site where the cord inserts into the placenta.

In 1983 Daffos et al. extracted fetal blood from the umbilical vein near the cord insertion using ultrasound to guide the procedure in 63 pregnancies [97]. Nicolaides perfected the technique he named cordocentesis, and used it in cases of Rhesus disease to determine the severity of anemia in the fetus [98, 99]. PUBS was also performed to assess for amino acid status in fetuses with intrauterine growth restriction [100].

PUBS carries a risk of fetal death or spontaneous abortion which is higher than that of CVS or amniocentesis and is estimated to be around 1–2% when performed by an experienced operator [101–103]. Today, PUBS is mainly reserved for cases in which diagnostic information cannot be obtained through amniocentesis, CVS, or ultrasound, or the results of these tests are inconclusive and further information is required for appropriately interpreting the clinical significance of the prior results. Examples include chromosomal mosaicism discovered after CVS or amniocentesis, the necessity for a rapid fetal karyotype, and the identification of fetal infection or hematologic condition. However, the procedure is also often performed for therapeutic indications such as transfusions in the case of Rhesus isoimmunization or anemia. The procedure is best performed at or after 18–20 weeks.

4 Techniques for Assessing Fetal Genetic Information

4.1 Karyotype

The ability to diagnose chromosome abnormalities from prenatal specimens dates back to end of the 1960s [12, 13]. In these early studies, chromosomes were grouped based on their length and centromere position since not all of them could be individually identified [104]. Starting in 1970, multiple types of fluorescent dyes such as quinocrine and stains such as Giemsa were utilized to stain the chromosomes and display a banding pattern that allowed unique identification of individual chromosomes and structural changes [105–109]. When the safety and accuracy of amniocentesis was established in the mid-1970s [57], the improved karyotype techniques developed during that same decade became a routine tool for the prenatal diagnosis of fetal chromosome abnormalities. This was fueled primarily by the recognition that advanced maternal age is directly related to an increased risk of chromosome abnormalities in pregnancy. As such, advanced maternal age, generally defined in the United States as 35 or older at delivery, became the most common indication for prenatal cytogenetic diagnosis [110, 111]. To this day, karyotyping remains one of the most commonly performed techniques utilized on prenatal specimens.

4.2 Molecular DNA Testing

The first DNA-based genetic tests were developed in the late 1970s and used the principles of Restriction Fragment Length Polymorphisms (RFLP). RFLP analysis for genetic disease relies on a mutation (DNA base changes/small insertion/deletion) that removes, inserts, or rearranges a restriction enzyme site, thus generating a different sized DNA fragment compared to the wild-type fragment. The classic illustration is that of sickle cell disease where the wild-type β-globin gene fragment is 7.7 Kb and the mutant β-globin gene fragment is 13 Kb when cut with the restriction enzyme *Hpa I* [112]. In 1978, Kan and Dozy demonstrated that these RFLP differences could be utilized for prenatal diagnosis of sickle cell disease from DNA isolated from amniotic fluid [112]. This proved to be the first example of a DNA-based prenatal diagnostic test [112]. From 1978 to 1980, the principles of RFLP analysis were applied for prenatal diagnosis of α- and β-Thalassemias [113–115]. Linkage analysis using RFLPs began to emerge around 1983 when investigators began to track the inheritance of multiple restriction fragments that cosegregated with the disease of interest. This required large family studies to identify informative RFLPs that were in linkage disequilibrium with the disease under consideration.

RFLP analysis at that time was a labor intensive and time-consuming technique that required multiple technical processes such as probe labeling, DNA fragmentation, electrophoresis, Southern blotting, hybridization, washing, and autoradiography. In some instances, it could take up to a month to get results back and in a prenatal setting, this was a major disadvantage. When Kary Mullis conceived of the polymerase chain reaction (PCR) technique in 1983 [116], it set the stage for one of the most significant scientific advances of the twentieth century. For his efforts, Mullis became one of the recipients of the 1993 Nobel Prize for Chemistry. PCR allowed for the rapid generation of millions of copies of a particular DNA sequence [117] making it a highly attractive technique for prenatal diagnosis. Indeed, soon thereafter in 1985, Saiki, together with Mullis and colleagues, reported on two new molecular methods that allowed for a rapid and highly sensitive prenatal diagnostic test for sickle cell anemia [118]. The first method utilized PCR to amplify specific β-globin target sequences, resulting in the exponential increase of target DNA copies. The second technique used end-labeled oligonucleotide probes to hybridize to the amplified β-globin DNA fragments that had been digested with a restriction endonuclease [118]. The two methods, coupled together, dramatically increased the speed and sensitivity of the assay and allowed for a result to be generated overnight instead of after several days [118]. In 1987, Kogan et al. improved the PCR method by substituting the Klenow fragment of *Escherichia coli* DNA polymerase I (Klenow) with a heat-stable DNA polymerase from *Thermus aquaticus* (Taq polymerase) [119]. By utilizing the heat-stable Taq polymerase, Kogan and colleagues showed that they could amplify DNA sequences at an elevated temperature resulting in a marked improvement of the specificity of amplification [119]. This specificity generated an enormous surplus of the desired DNA molecule of the appropriate size, which they could then detect by visual inspection after ethidium bromide staining and without the use of radioactive probes [119]. Kogan et al. used their modified PCR technique to perform prenatal diagnosis of hemophilia and fetal sex determination [119]. In 1989, Gasparini and coworkers used Kogan's updated PCR method to perform prenatal diagnosis for cystic fibrosis [120]. In their report, they described their experience using PCR on eight cases for first-trimester prenatal diagnosis of cystic fibrosis, following fetal sampling by transabdominal CVS [120]. Interestingly, at that time, the gene causing cystic fibrosis was unknown and prenatal studies could only be done by linkage analysis. Utilization of the newly developed PCR technique was not limited to the diagnosis of genetic disorders as it was also embraced for the detection of fetal infectious diseases. In 1990, Grover et al. used PCR for rapid prenatal diagnosis in amniotic fluid of congenital toxoplasma infection [121] while Ho-Terry and colleagues used it for prenatal detection of fetal rubella infection [122]. There are now over 30 different variations of the basic PCR technique, two of which play a major role in rapid prenatal diagnosis of the common aneuploidies. The first is quantitative fluorescent PCR (QF-PCR) which calculates chromosome dosage in real time using polymorphic small tandem repeats (STR) markers. It was developed in 1993 by Mansfield who demonstrated that allele dosage for the affected chromosome in patients with trisomy 18 and trisomy 21 could be distinguished from normal individuals [123]. In 1994, Pertile and coworkers used a similar approach to detect aneuploidies in fetal amniotic fluid samples [124]. The second technique, called multiplex ligation-dependent probe amplification (MLPA), was developed by Schouten and colleagues in 2002, and allows relative quantification of chromosome-specific DNA sequences in a single reaction [125]. Both techniques are widely utilized, primarily outside the USA, for quick assessment of aneuploidy of chromosomes 13, 18, 21, X, and Y. In the USA, fluorescence in situ hybridization (FISH) is the primary method for rapid aneuploidy detection (*see* below).

4.3 Fluorescence In Situ Hybridization (FISH)

The combination of traditional cytogenetic and molecular techniques yielded a new area in the field of human genetics which is referred to as molecular cytogenetics. Fluorescence in situ hybridization (FISH) can be considered the hallmark of molecular cytogenetics and its development added a powerful new dimension to the clinical diagnostic testing arena. Molecular cytogenetics really began in the early 1970s when various groups described a technique for detecting highly repetitive nucleic acid sequences in cell preparations [126–128]. The in situ hybridization (ISH) procedures utilized in the 1970s and early 1980s used radioactive probes that were readily substituted for by fluorescence in situ hybridization (FISH) techniques that instead applied non-radioactive probes labeled with haptens or fluorochromes [129–132].

From a clinical perspective, FISH could be performed using both interphase nuclei and metaphase spreads [133–137] and provided a way to detect cryptic and submicroscopic rearrangements that remained undetected or undecipherable by conventional cytogenetic analysis [134, 138–143]. In the prenatal world, it was readily utilized on uncultured cells (interphase nuclei) derived from chorionic villi or amniotic fluid to rapidly screen for the common aneuploidies [144, 145]. The primary advantage of prenatal FISH was the ability to get preliminary results in as little as 1–2 days. In 2001, a 2-year multi-center retrospective study by Tepperberg and colleagues showed an extremely high concordance rate between FISH and standard cytogenetics (99.8%) as well as sensitivity, specificity, and positive and negative predictive values all being greater than 99.5% [146]. In the Tepperberg study, abnormal ultrasound and advanced maternal age (though not mutually exclusive) followed by an abnormal maternal serum analyte screen were the most common indications for performing interphase prenatal FISH [146]. The clinical use of FISH has not changed much over the years and today, it is still utilized for rapid preliminary results after invasive testing and to test for deletions or duplications in specific regions associated with disease. FISH has also proven useful for follow-up studies assessing the suspicion of chromosomal mosaicism.

4.4 Comparative Genomic Hybridization and Microarray Analysis

The development of chromosomal comparative genomic hybridization (cCGH) by Kallioniemi and coworkers in 1992 can be viewed as the next major leap in molecular cytogenetic diagnostic technologies [147]. cCGH was initially utilized as a cancer research tool to uncover novel oncogenes and tumor suppressor genes [147–153] but was quickly adapted, a few years later, for clinical purposes in constitutional genetics [154–156]. The power of cCGH lays in its ability to reveal any DNA sequence copy number change (i.e., gains, amplifications, or losses) in a particular specimen, and map these changes on normal chromosomes [147, 153, 157, 158]. For the first time, clinical cytogeneticists had a tool that could scan the entire genome without having to preselect specific targeted regions. This proved particularly useful in the prenatal setting for identifying chromosomal material of unknown origin such as marker chromosomes and derivative chromosomes [154, 159–162]. While the clinical utility of cCGH was readily apparent, the technique itself was particularly challenging and tedious and did not lend itself to routine clinical testing. In addition, the resolution of the technique was limited to that of the metaphase chromosome which is theoretically around 2–4 Mb when utilizing high resolution prometaphase chromosomes [163]. This meant that cCGH could not readily detect submicroscopic imbalances like those observed in the microdeletion syndromes such as Prader-Willi. In 1997/8, Solinas-Toldo et al. and Pinkel et al. leveraged sequence data from the Human Genome project and built DNA microarrays by spotting multiple cloned DNA fragments onto glass microscope slides [164, 165]. The use of spatially separated DNA clones on glass slides effectively replaced metaphase chromosomes as the hybridization targets and made it possible to detect imbalances ≥ ~100 kilobases in size [164, 165]. As with cCGH, the clinical utility of array comparative genomic hybridization (aCGH) soon became apparent and in the early to mid-2000s, investigators began to use the new technique for clinical purposes [166–172]. One of the first reports of the use of aCGH in a prenatal setting was in 2004 by Tachdjian and coworkers who demonstrated the origin of the extra chromosomal material observed in a fetus with a reported 46,X,Xq + karyotype [168]. In 2005, Le Caignec et al. reported the first large prenatal case series using aCGH [171]. Their cohort comprised 49 fetuses with three or more significant anomalies and normal karyotype. Their report demonstrated that aCGH on fetuses with anomalies could increase the diagnostic yield over karyotype, which in their study was around 8% [171]. In 2007, a Columbia University lead multi-center trial was initiated in the USA to assess the clinical utility of chromosomal microarray analysis (CMA) in prenatal diagnosis [173]. The trial lasted 5 years and was funded by the National Institute of Child Health and Human Development (NICHD) [173]. The NICHD trial demonstrated that CMA could detect all of the abnormalities that karyotype could, plus additional copy number variants, leading to incremental yields of 1.7% in low risk pregnancies and 6% in anomalous fetuses [173].

The mid-2000s also saw evolutionary advances in array technology with DNA clones (typically bacterial artificial chromosomes) being replaced by short oligonucleotide probes, 25–80 bp in size [174, 175]. Around the same time, investigators also began to use oligonucleotide probes that included single nucleotide polymorphisms (SNPs) [176, 177]. The use of oligonucleotide probes improved the resolution of imbalances that could be detected by CMA to far below 100 Kb, essentially only being limited by the number of probes used on a given array. Today, most clinical laboratories prefer to use SNP-based oligonucleotide arrays as it offers the ability to detect uniparental disomy (UPD), consanguinity, maternal cell contamination, and triploidy, in addition to DNA copy number changes [178–180].

4.5 Next Generation Sequencing (NGS)

Traditional Sanger sequencing, developed in 1977, is a reliable way to sequence individual genes or small regions of DNA [181]. Sanger sequencing, while extremely useful, does not lend itself to high throughput of multiple genes. Next Generation Sequencing (NGS) was first developed in 1990 and provided a way to increase the number of genes being sequenced in parallel [182]. The first type of NGS was done by capillary sequencing which parallelized Sanger sequencing into machines that could run 96 or 384 reactions at once in microplate format [182]. NGS platforms are now capable of sequencing millions or even billions of small fragments of DNA at the same time [183]. Whole genome sequencing (WGS) by NGS allows for the discovery of novel mutations and disease causing genes without requiring prior knowledge of the gene or locus being investigated [183]. Since WGS is expensive, strategies for exclusively assessing coding (exon/gene) regions became an attractive proposition, as this requires sequencing of only 1.5% of the genome. This NGS method is referred to as whole exome sequencing (WES) and its role in gene discovery was demonstrated in 2010 when Ng and colleagues uncovered the genes associated with Miller-Dieker [184] and Kabuki syndromes [185]. Other studies quickly followed along with 100's of additional gene discoveries [186]. WGS and WES have recently made their way onto the prenatal scene and are especially useful in identifying the underlying cause of genetic disease when karyotype, microarray, and FISH or Sanger sequencing of known genes is not fruitful [187]. However, WES and WGS are only recommended prenatally in the case of ultrasound anomalies where other diagnostic tests have failed to reveal an answer [188].

5 Concluding Comments

Amidst the progression in both procedural sampling and analysis techniques in prenatal diagnosis, there has been a strong need to support physicians in educating them and their patients about the benefits and limitations of the new technologies. The first genetic counseling program opened in New York in 1969 and began to provide resources to physicians involved in clinical genetics and prenatal diagnosis. In North America, there are currently 45 accredited programs with more than 4000 genetic counselors across the United States and Canada. As the field continues to expand and the available tests become more technically advanced and nuanced, the need for additional geneticists and genetic counselors to interpret data and correlate genotypic and phenotypic information will definitively increase. The prenatal tests available to women 50 years ago were drastically different to what they are today and it is likely that the future holds even more discoveries, options, and answers.

References

1. Tjio JH, Levan A (1956) The chromosome number of man. Hereditas 42:1–6
2. Prochownick L (1897) Beitrage zur Lehre vom Fruchtwasser und seiner Entstehung. Arch Gynakol 11:304
3. Serr DM, Sachs L, Danon M (1955) The diagnosis of sex before birth using cells from the amniotic fluid (a preliminary report). Bull Res Counc Isr 5B(2):137–138
4. Glenister TW (1956) Determination of sex in early human embryos. Nature 177 (4520):1135–1136
5. Lejeune J, Gautier M, Turpin R (1959) Study of somatic chromosomes from 9 mongoloid children. C R Hebd Seances Acad Sci 248 (11):1721–1722
6. Ford CE, Jones KW, Polani PE et al (1959) A sex-chromosome anomaly in a case of gonadal dysgenesis (turner's syndrome). Lancet 1 (7075):711–713
7. Jacobs PA, Strong JA (1959) A case of human intersexuality having a possible XXY sex-determining mechanism. Nature 183 (4657):302–303
8. Jacobs PA, Baikie AG, Brown WM et al (1959) Evidence for the existence of the human "super female". Lancet 2 (7100):423–425
9. Sandberg AA, Koepf GF, Ishihara T et al (1961) An XYY human male. Lancet 2 (7200):488–489
10. Riis P, Fuchs F (1960) Antenatal determination of fœtal sex: in prevention of hereditary diseases. Lancet 276(7143):180–182. https://doi.org/10.1016/S0140-6736(60)91326-X
11. Fuchs F, Riis P (1960) Fetal sex determination before decision on eugenic indications for abortion. Nord Med 64:1481–1483
12. Steele MW, Breg WR Jr (1966) Chromosome analysis of human amniotic-fluid cells. Lancet 1(7434):383–385
13. Jacobson CB, Barter RH (1967) Intrauterine diagnosis and management of genetic defects. Am J Obstet Gynecol 99(6):796–807
14. Donald I, Brown TG (1961) Demonstration of tissue interfaces within the body by ultrasonic echo sounding. Br J Radiol 34:539–546. https://doi.org/10.1259/0007-1285-34-405-539
15. Donald I (1962) Clinical application of ultrasonic techniques in obstetrical and gynaecological diagnosis. J Obstet Gynaecol Br Emp 69:1036
16. Gottesfeld KR, Thompson HE, Holmes JH et al (1966) Ultrasonic placentography—a new method for placental localization. Am J Obstet Gynecol 96(4):538–547
17. MacVicar J, Donald I (1963) Sonar in the diagnosis of early pregnancy and its complications. BJOG Int J Obstet Gynaecol 70 (3):387–395. https://doi.org/10.1111/j.1471-0528.1963.tb04920.x
18. Ewigman BG, Crane JP, Frigoletto FD et al (1993) Effect of prenatal ultrasound screening on perinatal outcome. RADIUS Study Group. N Engl J Med 329(12):821–827
19. Dane B, Dane C, Sivri D et al (2007) Ultrasound screening for fetal major abnormalities at 11-14 weeks. Acta Obstet Gynecol Scand 86(6):666–670. https://doi.org/10.1080/00016340701253405
20. Hofmann D, Mast H, Hollander HJ (1967) The importance of placenta localization by means of ultrasonics for amniocentesis. Geburtshilfe Frauenheilkd 27 (12):1199–1209
21. Bang J, Northeved A (1972) A new ultrasonic method for transabdominal amniocentesis. Am J Obstet Gynecol 114(5):599–601
22. Platt LD, Manning FA, Lemay M (1978) Real-time B-scan-directed amniocentesis. Am J Obstet Gynecol 130(6):700–703
23. Romero R, Jeanty P, Reece EA et al (1985) Sonographically monitored amniocentesis to decrease intraoperative complications. Obstet Gynecol 65(3):426–430
24. Wald NJ, Cuckle H, Brock JH et al (1977) Maternal serum-alpha-fetoprotein measurement in antenatal screening for anencephaly and spina bifida in early pregnancy. Report of U.K. collaborative study on alpha-fetoprotein in relation to neural-tube defects. Lancet 1 (8026):1323–1332

25. Wald NJ, Hackshaw AK, Cuckle HS (2000) Maternal serum alphafetoprotein screening for open neural tube defects: revised statistical parameters. BJOG 107(2):296–298
26. Cuckle H, Thornton J (1995) Antenatal diagnosis and management of neural tube defects. In: Levene M, Lilford R, Bennett M, Punt J (eds) Fetal and neonatal neurology and neurosurgery. Churchill Livingstone, Edinburgh, pp 295–309
27. Benacerraf BR, Barss VA, Laboda LA (1985) A sonographic sign for the detection in the second trimester of the fetus with Down's syndrome. Am J Obstet Gynecol 151 (8):1078–1079
28. Benacerraf BR, Frigoletto FD Jr, Laboda LA (1985) Sonographic diagnosis of down syndrome in the second trimester. Am J Obstet Gynecol 153(1):49–52
29. Lockwood C, Benacerraf B, Krinsky A et al (1987) A sonographic screening method for down syndrome. Am J Obstet Gynecol 157 (4 Pt 1):803–808
30. Nicolaides KH, Azar G, Byrne D et al (1992) Fetal nuchal translucency: ultrasound screening for chromosomal defects in first trimester of pregnancy. BMJ 304(6831):867–869
31. Merkatz IR, Nitowsky HM, Macri JN et al (1984) An association between low maternal serum alpha-fetoprotein and fetal chromosomal abnormalities. Am J Obstet Gynecol 148(7):886–894
32. Cuckle HS, Wald NJ, Lindenbaum RH (1984) Maternal serum alpha-fetoprotein measurement: a screening test for down syndrome. Lancet 1(8383):926–929
33. Bogart MH, Pandian MR, Jones OW (1987) Abnormal maternal serum chorionic gonadotropin levels in pregnancies with fetal chromosome abnormalities. Prenat Diagn 7 (9):623–630
34. Canick JA, Knight GJ, Palomaki GE et al (1988) Low second trimester maternal serum unconjugated oestriol in pregnancies with Down's syndrome. Br J Obstet Gynaecol 95(4):330–333
35. Wald NJ, Cuckle HS, Densem JW et al (1988) Maternal serum unconjugated oestriol as an antenatal screening test for Down's syndrome. Br J Obstet Gynaecol 95(4):334–341
36. Wald NJ, Cuckle HS, Densem JW et al (1988) Maternal serum screening for Down's syndrome in early pregnancy. BMJ 297 (6653):883–887
37. Palomaki GE, Knight GJ, McCarthy JE et al (1997) Maternal serum screening for down syndrome in the United States: a 1995 survey. Am J Obstet Gynecol 176(5):1046–1051
38. Wald N, Stone R, Cuckle HS et al (1992) First trimester concentrations of pregnancy associated plasma protein A and placental protein 14 in Down's syndrome. BMJ 305(6844):28
39. Ozturk M, Milunsky A, Brambati B et al (1990) Abnormal maternal serum levels of human chorionic gonadotropin free subunits in trisomy 18. Am J Med Genet 36 (4):480–483. https://doi.org/10.1002/ajmg.1320360422
40. Wald NJ, Hackshaw AK (1997) Combining ultrasound and biochemistry in first-trimester screening for Down's syndrome. Prenat Diagn 17(9):821–829
41. Van Lith JM, Pratt JJ, Beekhuis JR et al (1992) Second-trimester maternal serum immunoreactive inhibin as a marker for fetal Down's syndrome. Prenat Diagn 12 (10):801–806
42. Wald NJ, Densem JW, George L et al (1996) Prenatal screening for Down's syndrome using inhibin-A as a serum marker. Prenat Diagn 16(2):143–153. https://doi.org/10.1002/(sici)1097-0223(199602)16:2<143::aid-pd825>3.0.co;2-f
43. Wald NJ, Densem JW, George L et al (1997) Inhibin-A in Down's syndrome pregnancies: revised estimate of standard deviation. Prenat Diagn 17(3):285–290
44. Wald NJ, Watt HC, Hackshaw AK (1999) Integrated screening for Down's syndrome based on tests performed during the first and second trimesters. N Engl J Med 341 (7):461–467. https://doi.org/10.1056/nejm199908123410701
45. Wright D, Bradbury I, Benn P et al (2004) Contingent screening for Down syndrome is an efficient alternative to non-disclosure sequential screening. Prenat Diagn 24 (10):762–766. https://doi.org/10.1002/pd.974
46. Malone FD, Canick JA, Ball RH et al (2005) First-trimester or second-trimester screening, or both, for Down's syndrome. N Engl J Med 353(19):2001–2011. https://doi.org/10.1056/NEJMoa043693
47. Herzenberg LA, Bianchi DW, Schroder J et al (1979) Fetal cells in the blood of pregnant women: detection and enrichment by fluorescence-activated cell sorting. Proc Natl Acad Sci U S A 76(3):1453–1455
48. Lo YM, Corbetta N, Chamberlain PF et al (1997) Presence of fetal DNA in maternal plasma and serum. Lancet 350 (9076):485–487

49. Churina SK, Pritykina N, Zhukovskaia NE (1975) Certain characteristics of pathogenesis of ischemic heart disease in women under 50 (before menopause). Ter Arkh 47 (12):43–48
50. Bianchi DW, Parker RL, Wentworth J et al (2014) DNA sequencing versus standard prenatal aneuploidy screening. N Engl J Med 370 (9):799–808. https://doi.org/10.1056/NEJMoa1311037
51. Committee on Practice Bulletins—Obstetrics, Committee on Genetics, and the Society for Maternal-Fetal Medicine (2016) Practice Bulletin No. 163: screening for fetal aneuploidy. Obstet Gynecol 127(5):e123–e137. https://doi.org/10.1097/aog.0000000000001406
52. Gregg AR, Skotko BG, Benkendorf JL et al (2016) Noninvasive prenatal screening for fetal aneuploidy, 2016 update: a position statement of the American College of Medical Genetics and Genomics. Genet Med 18 (10):1056–1065. https://doi.org/10.1038/gim.2016.97
53. Nadler HL (1968) Patterns of enzyme development utilizing cultivated human fetal cells derived from amniotic fluid. Biochem Genet 2 (2):119–126
54. Nadler HL, Walsh MM (1980) Intrauterine detection of cystic fibrosis. Pediatrics 66 (5):690–692
55. Brock DJ, Sutcliffe RG (1972) Alpha-fetoprotein in the antenatal diagnosis of anencephaly and spina bifida. Lancet 2 (7770):197–199
56. Nadler HL, Gerbie AB (1970) Role of amniocentesis in the intrauterine detection of genetic disorders. N Engl J Med 282 (11):596–599
57. NICHD (1976) Midtrimester amniocentesis for prenatal diagnosis. Safety and accuracy. JAMA 236(13):1471–1476
58. Farrell SA, Summers AM, Dallaire L et al (1999) Club foot, an adverse outcome of early amniocentesis: disruption or deformation? CEMAT. Canadian early and mid-trimester amniocentesis trial. J Med Genet 36(11):843–846
59. Benacerraf BR, Greene MF, Saltzman DH et al (1988) Early amniocentesis for prenatal cytogenetic evaluation. Radiology 169 (3):709–710. https://doi.org/10.1148/radiology.169.3.3055033
60. Hanson FW, Zorn EM, Tennant FR et al (1987) Amniocentesis before 15 weeks' gestation: outcome, risks, and technical problems. Am J Obstet Gynecol 156 (6):1524–1531
61. Hanson FW, Happ RL, Tennant FR et al (1990) Ultrasonography-guided early amniocentesis in singleton pregnancies. Am J Obstet Gynecol 162(6):1376–1381 discussion 1381-1373
62. ACOG Committee on Practice Bulletins (2007) ACOG Practice Bulletin No. 77: screening for fetal chromosomal abnormalities. Obstet Gynecol 109(1):217–227
63. American College of Obstetricians and Gynecologists (2007) ACOG Practice Bulletin No. 88, December 2007. Invasive prenatal testing for aneuploidy. Obstet Gynecol 110 (6):1459–1467. https://doi.org/10.1097/01.AOG.0000291570.63450.44
64. Westin B (1954) Hysteroscopy in early pregnancy. Lancet 264(6843):872. https://doi.org/10.1016/S0140-6736(54)91969-8
65. Valenti C (1973) Antenatal detection of hemoglobinopathies. A preliminary report. Am J Obstet Gynecol 115(6):851–853
66. Scrimgeour J (1973) Other techniques for antenatal diagnosis. In: Emery A (ed) Antenatal diagnosis of genetic disease. Churchill Livingstone, New York, p 49
67. Hobbins JC, Mahoney MJ (1974) In utero diagnosis of hemoglobinopathies. Technic for obtaining fetal blood. N Engl J Med 290 (19):1065–1067. https://doi.org/10.1056/nejm197405092901908
68. Kan YW, Golbus MS, Trecartin R (1975) Prenatal diagnosis of homozygous beta-thalassaemia. Lancet 2(7939):790–791
69. Firshein SI, Hoyer LW, Lazarchick J et al (1979) Prenatal diagnosis of classic hemophilia. N Engl J Med 300(17):937–941. https://doi.org/10.1056/nejm197904263001701
70. Mahoney MJ, Hobbins JC (1977) Prenatal diagnosis of chondroectodermal dysplasia (Ellis-van Creveld syndrome) with fetoscopy and ultrasound. N Engl J Med 297 (5):258–260. https://doi.org/10.1056/nejm197708042970507
71. Golbus MS, Sagebiel RW, Filly RA et al (1980) Prenatal diagnosis of congenital bullous ichthyosiform erythroderma (epidermolytic hyperkeratosis) by fetal skin biopsy. N Engl J Med 302(2):93–95. https://doi.org/10.1056/nejm198001103020205
72. Rodeck CH, Eady RA, Gosden CM (1980) Prenatal diagnosis of epidermolysis bullosa letalis. Lancet 1(8175):949–952
73. Fensom AH, Benson PF, Rodeck CH et al (1979) Prenatal diagnosis of a galactosaemia heterozygote by fetal blood enzyme assay. Br Med J 1(6155):21–22

74. Perry TB, Hechtman P, Chow JC (1979) Diagnosis of Tay-Sachs disease on blood obtained at fetoscopy. Lancet 1 (8123):972–973
75. Mahoney M, Hobbins J (1979) Fetoscopy and fetal blood sampling. In: Milunsky A (ed) Genetic disorders and the fetus. Springer, Boston, MA
76. Mohr J (1968) Foetal genetic diagnosis: development of techniques for early sampling of foetal cells. Acta Pathol Microbiol Scand 73 (1):73–77
77. Kullander S, Sandahl B (1973) Fetal chromosome analysis after transcervical placental biopsies during early pregnancy. Acta Obstet Gynecol Scand 52(4):355–359
78. Hahnemann N (1974) Early prenatal diagnosis; a study of biopsy techniques and cell culturing from extraembryonic membranes. Clin Genet 6(4):294–306
79. (1975) Fetal sex pridiction by sex chromatin of chorionic villi cells during early pregnancy. Chin Med J (Engl) 1(2):117–126
80. Ward RH, Modell B, Petrou M et al (1983) Method of sampling chorionic villi in first trimester of pregnancy under guidance of real time ultrasound. Br Med J (Clin Res Ed) 286(6377):1542–1544
81. Williamson R, Eskdale J, Coleman DV et al (1981) Direct gene analysis of chorionic villi: a possible technique for first-trimester antenatal diagnosis of haemoglobinopathies. Lancet 2(8256):1125–1127
82. Old JM, Ward RH, Petrou M et al (1982) First-trimester fetal diagnosis for haemoglobinopathies: three cases. Lancet 2 (8313):1413–1416
83. Goossens M, Dumez Y, Kaplan L et al (1983) Prenatal diagnosis of sickle-cell anemia in the first trimester of pregnancy. N Engl J Med 309(14):831–833. https://doi.org/10.1056/nejm198310063091405
84. Gustavii B (1983) First-trimester chromosomal analysis of chorionic villi obtained by direct vision technique. Lancet 2 (8348):507–508
85. Kazy ZRI, Bakhaev V (1982) Chorion biopsy in early pregnancy: a method of early prenatal diagnosis for inherited disorders. Prenat Diagn 2:39
86. Pergament E, Ginsberg N, Verlinsky Y et al (1983) Prenatal Tay-Sachs diagnosis by chorionic villi sampling. Lancet 322 (8344):286–287. https://doi.org/10.1016/S0140-6736(83)90270-2
87. Brambati B, Simoni G (1983) Diagnosis of fetal trisomy 21 in first trimester. Lancet 1 (8324):586
88. Simoni G, Brambati B, Danesino C et al (1983) Efficient direct chromosome analyses and enzyme determinations from chorionic villi samples in the first trimester of pregnancy. Hum Genet 63(4):349–357
89. Aladjem S (1968) Phase contrast microscopic observations of the human placenta from six weeks to term. An anatomic and clinical correlation. Obstet Gynecol 32(1):28–39
90. Alvarez H (1964) Morphology and physiopathology of the human placenta. i. studies of morphology and development of chorionic villi by phase-contrast microscopy. Obstet Gynecol 23:813–825
91. Smidt-Jensen S, Hahnemann N (1984) Transabdominal fine needle biopsy from chorionic villi in the first trimester. Prenat Diagn 4(3):163–169
92. Rhoads GG, Jackson LG, Schlesselman SE et al (1989) The safety and efficacy of chorionic villus sampling for early prenatal diagnosis of cytogenetic abnormalities. N Engl J Med 320(10):609–617
93. Olney RS et al (1995) Chorionic villus sampling and amniocentesis: recommendations for prenatal counseling. Centers for disease control and prevention. MMWR Recomm Rep 44(RR-9):1–12
94. Risk evaluation of chorionic villus sampling (CVS): report on a meeting (1992) World Health Organization Regional Office for Europe (WHO/EURO), Copenhagen
95. Morris ED, Beard RW (1965) The rationale and technique of foetal blood sampling and amnioscopy. J Obstet Gynaecol Br Commonw 72:489–495
96. Patrick JE, Perry TB, Kinch RA (1974) Fetoscopy and fetal blood sampling: a percutaneous approach. Am J Obstet Gynecol 119 (4):539–542
97. Daffos F, Capella-Pavlovsky M, Forestier F (1983) Fetal blood sampling via the umbilical cord using a needle guided by ultrasound. Report of 66 cases. Prenat Diagn 3 (4):271–277
98. Nicolaides KH, Soothill PW, Rodeck CH et al (1986) Rh disease: intravascular fetal blood transfusion by cordocentesis. Fetal Ther 1 (4):185–192
99. Nicolaides KH (1988) Cordocentesis. Clin Obstet Gynecol 31(1):123–135
100. Pardi G, Buscaglia M, Ferrazzi E et al (1987) Cord sampling for the evaluation of oxygenation and acid-base balance in growth-retarded

human fetuses. Am J Obstet Gynecol 157 (5):1221–1228
101. Hickok DE, Mills M (1992) Percutaneous umbilical blood sampling: results from a multicenter collaborative registry. The Western Collaborative Perinatal Group. Am J Obstet Gynecol 166(6 Pt 1):1614–1617 discussion 1617-1618
102. Duchatel F, Oury JF, Mennesson B et al (1993) Complications of diagnostic ultrasound-guided percutaneous umbilical blood sampling: analysis of a series of 341 cases and review of the literature. Eur J Obstet Gynecol Reprod Biol 52(2):95–104
103. Liao C, Wei J, Li Q et al (2006) Efficacy and safety of cordocentesis for prenatal diagnosis. Int J Gynaecol Obstet 93(1):13–17. https://doi.org/10.1016/j.ijgo.2006.01.005
104. Patau K (1960) The identification of individual chromosomes, especially in man. Am J Hum Genet 12:250–276
105. Caspersson T, Zech L, Johansson C (1970) Differential binding of alkylating fluorochromes in human chromosomes. Exp Cell Res 60(3):315–319
106. Drets ME, Shaw MW (1971) Specific banding patterns of human chromosomes. Proc Natl Acad Sci U S A 68(9):2073–2077
107. Hirschhorn K, Lucas M, Wallace I (1973) Precise identification of various chromosomal abnormalities. Ann Hum Genet 36 (4):375–379
108. Patil SR, Merrick S, Lubs HA (1971) Identification of each human chromosome with a modified Giemsa stain. Science 173 (999):821–822
109. Seabright M (1971) A rapid banding technique for human chromosomes. Lancet 2 (7731):971–972
110. Galjaard H (1976) European experience with prenatal diagnosis of congenital disease: a survey of 6121 cases. Cytogenet Cell Genet 16 (6):453–467. https://doi.org/10.1159/000130663
111. Niermeijer MF, Sachs ES, Jahodova M et al (1976) Prenatal diagnosis of genetic disorders. J Med Genet 13(3):182–194
112. Kan YW, Dozy AM (1978) Antenatal diagnosis of sickle-cell anaemia by D.N.A. analysis of amniotic-fluid cells. Lancet 2 (8096):910–912
113. Dozy AM, Forman EN, Abuelo DN et al (1979) Prenatal diagnosis of homozygous alpha-thalassemia. JAMA 241 (15):1610–1612
114. Kan YW, Lee KY, Furbetta M et al (1980) Polymorphism of DNA sequence in the beta-globin gene region. Application to prenatal diagnosis of beta 0 thalassemia in Sardinia. N Engl J Med 302(4):185–188. https://doi.org/10.1056/NEJM198001243020401
115. Orkin SH, Alter BP, Altay C et al (1978) Application of endonuclease mapping to the analysis and prenatal diagnosis of thalassemias caused by globin-gene deletion. N Engl J Med 299(4):166–172. https://doi.org/10.1056/NEJM197807272990403
116. Mullis KB (2009) Polymerase chain reaction. https://www.karymullis.com/pcr.shtml. Accessed 22 Apr 2018
117. Mullis K, Faloona F, Scharf S et al (1986) Specific enzymatic amplification of DNA in vitro: the polymerase chain reaction. Cold Spring Harb Symp Quant Biol 51 (Pt 1):263–273
118. Saiki RK, Scharf S, Faloona F et al (1985) Enzymatic amplification of beta-globin genomic sequences and restriction site analysis for diagnosis of sickle cell anemia. Science 230 (4732):1350–1354
119. Kogan SC, Doherty M, Gitschier J (1987) An improved method for prenatal diagnosis of genetic diseases by analysis of amplified DNA sequences. Application to hemophilia A. N Engl J Med 317(16):985–990. https://doi.org/10.1056/NEJM198710153171603
120. Gasparini P, Novelli G, Savoia A et al (1989) First-trimester prenatal diagnosis of cystic fibrosis using the polymerase chain reaction: report of eight cases. Prenat Diagn 9 (5):349–355
121. Grover CM, Thulliez P, Remington JS et al (1990) Rapid prenatal diagnosis of congenital Toxoplasma infection by using polymerase chain reaction and amniotic fluid. J Clin Microbiol 28(10):2297–2301
122. Ho-Terry L, Terry GM, Londesborough P (1990) Diagnosis of foetal rubella virus infection by polymerase chain reaction. J Gen Virol 71(Pt 7):1607–1611. https://doi.org/10.1099/0022-1317-71-7-1607
123. Mansfield ES (1993) Diagnosis of Down syndrome and other aneuploidies using quantitative polymerase chain reaction and small tandem repeat polymorphisms. Hum Mol Genet 2(1):43–50
124. Pertl B, Yau SC, Sherlock J et al (1994) Rapid molecular method for prenatal detection of Down's syndrome. Lancet 343 (8907):1197–1198
125. Schouten JP, McElgunn CJ, Waaijer R et al (2002) Relative quantification of 40 nucleic

acid sequences by multiplex ligation-dependent probe amplification. Nucleic Acids Res 30(12):e57

126. Gall JG, Pardue ML (1969) Formation and detection of RNA-DNA hybrid molecules in cytological preparations. Proc Natl Acad Sci U S A 63(2):378–383
127. John HA, Birnstiel ML, Jones KW (1969) RNA-DNA hybrids at the cytological level. Nature 223(206):582–587
128. Buongiorno-Nardelli M, Amaldi F (1970) Autoradiographic detection of molecular hybrids between RNA and DNA in tissue sections. Nature 225(236):946–948
129. Manning JE, Hershey ND, Broker TR et al (1975) A new method of in situ hybridization. Chromosoma 53(2):107–117
130. Cheung SW, Tishler PV, Atkins L et al (1977) Gene mapping by fluorescent in situ hybridization. Cell Biol Int Rep 1(3):255–262
131. Pinkel D, Straume T, Gray JW (1986) Cytogenetic analysis using quantitative, high-sensitivity, fluorescence hybridization. Proc Natl Acad Sci U S A 83(9):2934–2938
132. Landegren U, Kaiser R, Caskey CT et al (1988) DNA diagnostics-molecular techniques and automation. Science 242 (4876):229–237
133. Kuo WL, Tenjin H, Segraves R et al (1991) Detection of aneuploidy involving chromosomes 13, 18, or 21, by fluorescence in situ hybridization (FISH) to interphase and metaphase amniocytes. Am J Hum Genet 49 (1):112–119
134. Carter NP, Ferguson-Smith MA, Perryman MT et al (1992) Reverse chromosome painting: a method for the rapid analysis of aberrant chromosomes in clinical cytogenetics. J Med Genet 29(5):299–307
135. Klever M, Grond-Ginsbach CJ, Hager HD et al (1992) Chorionic villus metaphase chromosomes and interphase nuclei analysed by chromosomal in situ suppression (CISS) hybridization. Prenat Diagn 12(1):53–59
136. Ried T, Baldini A, Rand TC et al (1992) Simultaneous visualization of seven different DNA probes by in situ hybridization using combinatorial fluorescence and digital imaging microscopy. Proc Natl Acad Sci U S A 89 (4):1388–1392
137. Zahed L, Murer-Orlando M, Vekemans M (1992) In situ hybridization studies for the detection of common aneuploidies in CVS. Prenat Diagn 12(6):483–493
138. Kuwano A, Ledbetter SA, Dobyns WB et al (1991) Detection of deletions and cryptic translocations in Miller-Dieker syndrome by in situ hybridization. Am J Hum Genet 49 (4):707–714
139. Leana-Cox J, Levin S, Surana R et al (1993) Characterization of de novo duplications in eight patients by using fluorescence in situ hybridization with chromosome-specific DNA libraries. Am J Hum Genet 52 (6):1067–1073
140. Franke UC, Scambler PJ, Loffler C et al (1994) Interstitial deletion of 22q11 in DiGeorge syndrome detected by high resolution and molecular analysis. Clin Genet 46 (2):187–192
141. Adinolfi M, Davies A (1994) Clinical application of non-isotopic in situ hybridization methods. CRC Press, Boca Raton, FL
142. Blennow E, Bui TH, Kristoffersson U et al (1994) Swedish survey on extra structurally abnormal chromosomes in 39 105 consecutive prenatal diagnoses: prevalence and characterization by fluorescence in situ hybridization. Prenat Diagn 14 (11):1019–1028
143. Blennow E, Nielsen KB, Telenius H et al (1995) Fifty probands with extra structurally abnormal chromosomes characterized by fluorescence in situ hybridization. Am J Med Genet 55(1):85–94
144. Klinger K, Landes G, Shook D et al (1992) Rapid detection of chromosome aneuploidies in uncultured amniocytes by using fluorescence in situ hybridization (FISH). Am J Hum Genet 51(1):55–65
145. Rao PN, Hayworth R, Cox K et al (1993) Rapid detection of aneuploidy in uncultured chorionic villus cells using fluorescence in situ hybridization. Prenat Diagn 13(4):233–238
146. Tepperberg J, Pettenati MJ, Rao PN et al (2001) Prenatal diagnosis using interphase fluorescence in situ hybridization (FISH): 2-year multi-center retrospective study and review of the literature. Prenat Diagn 21 (4):293–301
147. Kallioniemi A, Kallioniemi OP, Sudar D et al (1992) Comparative genomic hybridization for molecular cytogenetic analysis of solid tumors. Science 258(5083):818–821
148. Forus A, Weghuis DO, Smeets D et al (1995) Comparative genomic hybridization analysis of human sarcomas: II. Identification of novel amplicons at 6p and 17p in osteosarcomas. Genes Chromosomes Cancer 14 (1):15–21
149. Forus A, Weghuis DO, Smeets D et al (1995) Comparative genomic hybridization analysis of human sarcomas: I. Occurrence of genomic imbalances and identification of a novel

major amplicon at 1q21-q22 in soft tissue sarcomas. Genes Chromosomes Cancer 14 (1):8–14

150. Isola J, Kallioniemi OP, Chu LW et al (1995) Genetic aberrations detected by comparative genomic hybridization predict outcome in node-negative breast cancer. Am J Pathol 147(4):905–911

151. Joos S, Bergerheim US, Pan Y et al (1995) Mapping of chromosomal gains and losses in prostate cancer by comparative genomic hybridization. Genes Chromosomes Cancer 14(4):267–276

152. Kallioniemi A, Kallioniemi OP, Citro G et al (1995) Identification of gains and losses of DNA sequences in primary bladder cancer by comparative genomic hybridization. Genes Chromosomes Cancer 12(3):213–219

153. du Manoir S, Speicher MR, Joos S et al (1993) Detection of complete and partial chromosome gains and losses by comparative genomic in situ hybridization. Hum Genet 90 (6):590–610

154. Bryndorf T, Kirchhoff M, Rose H et al (1995) Comparative genomic hybridization in clinical cytogenetics. Am J Hum Genet 57 (5):1211–1220

155. Lapierre JM, Cacheux V, Collot N et al (1998) Comparison of comparative genomic hybridization with conventional karyotype and classical fluorescence in situ hybridization for prenatal and postnatal diagnosis of unbalanced chromosome abnormalities. Ann Genet 41(3):133–140

156. Levy B, Dunn TM, Kaffe S et al (1998) Clinical applications of comparative genomic hybridization. Genet Med 1(1):4–12

157. Kallioniemi OP, Kallioniemi A, Sudar D et al (1993) Comparative genomic hybridization: a rapid new method for detecting and mapping DNA amplification in tumors. Semin Cancer Biol 4(1):41–46

158. Kallioniemi OP, Kallioniemi A, Piper J et al (1994) Optimizing comparative genomic hybridization for analysis of DNA sequence copy number changes in solid tumors. Genes Chromosomes Cancer 10(4):231–243

159. Boceno M, Rival JM, Nomballais MF et al (1998) Characterization of two add(4qter) chromosomes by comparative genomic hybridization. Ann Genet 41(2):83–86

160. Lapierre JM, Cacheux V, Luton D et al (2000) Analysis of uncultured amniocytes by comparative genomic hybridization: a prospective prenatal study. Prenat Diagn 20 (2):123–131

161. Levy B, Papenhausen PR, Tepperberg JH et al (2000) Prenatal molecular cytogenetic diagnosis of partial tetrasomy 10p due to neocentromere formation in an inversion duplication analphoid marker chromosome. Cytogenet Cell Genet 91(1–4):165–170

162. Wang BB, Yu LC, Peng W et al (1995) Prenatal identification of i(Yp) by molecular cytogenetic analysis. Prenat Diagn 15 (12):1115–1119

163. Kirchhoff M, Rose H, Lundsteen C (2001) High resolution comparative genomic hybridisation in clinical cytogenetics. J Med Genet 38(11):740–744

164. Solinas-Toldo S, Lampel S, Stilgenbauer S et al (1997) Matrix-based comparative genomic hybridization: biochips to screen for genomic imbalances. Genes Chromosomes Cancer 20(4):399–407

165. Pinkel D, Segraves R, Sudar D et al (1998) High resolution analysis of DNA copy number variation using comparative genomic hybridization to microarrays. Nat Genet 20 (2):207–211

166. Yu W, Ballif BC, Kashork CD et al (2003) Development of a comparative genomic hybridization microarray and demonstration of its utility with 25 well-characterized 1p36 deletions. Hum Mol Genet 12 (17):2145–2152. https://doi.org/10.1093/hmg/ddg230

167. Vissers LE, de Vries BB, Osoegawa K et al (2003) Array-based comparative genomic hybridization for the genomewide detection of submicroscopic chromosomal abnormalities. Am J Hum Genet 73(6):1261–1270

168. Tachdjian G, Aboura A, Benkhalifa M et al (2004) De novo interstitial direct duplication of Xq21.1q25 associated with skewed X-inactivation pattern. Am J Med Genet A 131(3):273–280. https://doi.org/10.1002/ajmg.a.30359

169. Bejjani BA, Saleki R, Ballif BC et al (2005) Use of targeted array-based CGH for the clinical diagnosis of chromosomal imbalance: is less more? Am J Med Genet A 134 (3):259–267. https://doi.org/10.1002/ajmg.a.30621

170. Cheung SW, Shaw CA, Yu W et al (2005) Development and validation of a CGH microarray for clinical cytogenetic diagnosis. Genet Med 7(6):422–432 https://doi.org/10.109701.GIM.0000170992.63691.32

171. Le Caignec C, Boceno M, Saugier-Veber P et al (2005) Detection of genomic imbalances by array based comparative genomic

hybridisation in fetuses with multiple malformations. J Med Genet 42(2):121–128
172. Schoumans J, Ruivenkamp C, Holmberg E et al (2005) Detection of chromosomal imbalances in children with idiopathic mental retardation by array based comparative genomic hybridisation (array-CGH). J Med Genet 42(9):699–705
173. Wapner RJ, Martin CL, Levy B et al (2012) Chromosomal microarray versus karyotyping for prenatal diagnosis. N Engl J Med 367 (23):2175–2184. https://doi.org/10.1056/NEJMoa1203382
174. Friedman JM, Baross A, Delaney AD et al (2006) Oligonucleotide microarray analysis of genomic imbalance in children with mental retardation. Am J Hum Genet 79 (3):500–513. https://doi.org/10.1086/507471
175. Toruner GA, Streck DL, Schwalb MN et al (2007) An oligonucleotide based array-CGH system for detection of genome wide copy number changes including subtelomeric regions for genetic evaluation of mental retardation. Am J Med Genet A 143A (8):824–829. https://doi.org/10.1002/ajmg.a.31656
176. Huang J, Wei W, Zhang J et al (2004) Whole genome DNA copy number changes identified by high density oligonucleotide arrays. Hum Genomics 1(4):287–299
177. Mei R, Galipeau PC, Prass C et al (2000) Genome-wide detection of allelic imbalance using human SNPs and high-density DNA arrays. Genome Res 10(8):1126–1137
178. Faas BH, van der Burgt I, Kooper AJ et al (2010) Identification of clinically significant, submicroscopic chromosome alterations and UPD in fetuses with ultrasound anomalies using genome-wide 250k SNP array analysis. J Med Genet 47(9):586–594. https://doi.org/10.1136/jmg.2009.075853
179. Srebniak M, Boter M, Oudesluijs G et al (2011) Application of SNP array for rapid prenatal diagnosis: implementation, genetic counselling and diagnostic flow. Eur J Hum Genet 19(12):1230–1237. https://doi.org/10.1038/ejhg.2011.119
180. Tyreman M, Abbott KM, Willatt LR et al (2009) High resolution array analysis: diagnosing pregnancies with abnormal ultrasound findings. J Med Genet 46(8):531–541. https://doi.org/10.1136/jmg.2008.065482
181. Sanger F, Nicklen S, Coulson AR (1977) DNA sequencing with chain-terminating inhibitors. Proc Natl Acad Sci U S A 74 (12):5463–5467
182. Swerdlow H, Gesteland R (1990) Capillary gel electrophoresis for rapid, high resolution DNA sequencing. Nucleic Acids Res 18 (6):1415–1419
183. Behjati S, Tarpey PS (2013) What is next generation sequencing? Arch Dis Child Educ Pract Ed 98(6):236–238. https://doi.org/10.1136/archdischild-2013-304340
184. Ng SB, Buckingham KJ, Lee C et al (2010) Exome sequencing identifies the cause of a mendelian disorder. Nat Genet 42(1):30–35. https://doi.org/10.1038/ng.499
185. Ng SB, Bigham AW, Buckingham KJ et al (2010) Exome sequencing identifies MLL2 mutations as a cause of Kabuki syndrome. Nat Genet 42(9):790–793. https://doi.org/10.1038/ng.646
186. Kaiser J (2010) Human genetics. Affordable 'exomes' fill gaps in a catalog of rare diseases. Science 330(6006):903. https://doi.org/10.1126/science.330.6006.903
187. Rabbani B, Tekin M, Mahdieh N (2014) The promise of whole-exome sequencing in medical genetics. J Hum Genet 59(1):5–15. https://doi.org/10.1038/jhg.2013.114
188. Henson M (2018) Joint Position Statement from the International Society of Prenatal Diagnosis (ISPD), the Society of Maternal Fetal Medicine (SMFM) and the Perinatal Quality Foundation (PQF) on the use of genome-wide sequencing for fetal diagnosis. Prenat Diagn 38(1):6–9. https://doi.org/10.1002/pd.5195

Chapter 2

Overview of Preimplantation Genetic Diagnosis (PGD): Historical Perspective and Future Direction

Joe Leigh Simpson, Anver Kuliev, and Svetlana Rechitsky

Abstract

Preimplantation genetic diagnosis (PGD) can be considered the earliest form of prenatal testing. It was first used in humans over 26 years ago. At its inception, PGD could only be performed for a limited number of genetic disorders. Technological advances in molecular biology and cytogenomics have been utilized in the field of PGD to greatly expand the spectrum of genetic disorders that can now be detected in early human embryos.

Key words Preimplantation genetic diagnosis, PGD, PGT, PGT-A, PGT-M, PGT-SR, PGT-HLA, Single gene disorder, Biopsy, Blastomere, Trophectoderm, Mosaicism

1 Introduction

Preimplantation genetic diagnosis (PGD)[1] was first accomplished in humans over 26 years ago. The first 1000 PGD births were not reached until 2004 [2], but since then cases have progressively increased. PGD is now accepted as not simply an earlier extension of traditional prenatal genetic diagnosis, but also offering novel indications. This chapter will review the history of PGD in humans, describing some of the key events and major breakthroughs that have occurred over the past three decades.

[1] Preimplantation genetic diagnosis (PGD) is the term traditionally applied. For aneuploidy, preimplantation genetic screening (PGS) is often used. However, preimplantation genetic testing (PGT) is now considered by WHO to be more appropriate [1]. The reason is that rarely does a confirmatory "test" follow PGD, and especially after interrogation for aneuploidy testing to increase pregnancy rates. That "screening" is a misnomer is increasingly recognized. Here we use the terms interchangeably given historical literature but accept that PGT is the term to be used going forward.

Brynn Levy (ed.), *Prenatal Diagnosis*, Methods in Molecular Biology, vol. 1885, https://doi.org/10.1007/978-1-4939-8889-1_2,

2 Pioneers in Detection of Single Gene Disorders and Chromosomal Abnormalities

PGD can be said to have begun in 1968 when Gardner and Edwards [3] biopsied a rabbit blastocyst and performed X-chromatin analysis. The application to X-linked recessive traits was noted. This was then followed by Modlinsky and McLaren's [4] work on the visualization of the mouse second polar body chromosomes, which, however, did not result in a sufficiently reliable method for practical application [4]. Over the next decade, mouse geneticists demonstrated occasional success in generating metaphase chromosomes from blastomeres [5]. Human in vitro fertilization (IVF) was finally achieved in 1978 [6], and thereafter animal studies in the preparation of human PGD accelerated. Biopsy and analysis of mouse blastomeres soon showed feasibility for detecting single gene disorders [7].

Pioneering animal work was performed in the United Kingdom by Marilyn Monk and, Alan Handyside; in Australia by Leanda Wilton and Alan Trounson; in Brussels by Andre Van Steirteghem and colleagues; and in the United States by Yury Verlinsky and colleagues.

Development of polymerase chain reaction (PCR) in the 1980s had made human PGD feasible. This allowed molecular analysis of a single cell (6 pg of DNA). In Europe, emphasis in the late 1980s focused on blastomere biopsy. Handyside, Braude, and Winston pursued blastomere biopsy and analysis, determining in 1990 sex in two couples known to be at risk of transmitting adrenoleukodystrophy and X-linked mental retardation. Two female embryos were transferred after in vitro fertilization (IVF), biopsy of a single cell at the six- to eight-cell stage, and sexing by DNA [8]. Soon cystic fibrosis was detected, using PCR [9].

In the United States, Verlinsky and colleagues preferred polar body biopsy, reporting their first clinical case at the 1987 International Congress on IVF in Kyoto [10].The first peer publication of that case (α 1-antitrypsin deficiency) was delayed until 1990 [11]. In 1990, PGD for cystic fibrosis was also reported by this same group [12].

PGD for chromosomal abnormalities had to await development of chromosome-specific fluorescence in situ hybridization (FISH) probes. In the United Kingdom, Darrel Griffin successfully performed FISH on blastomeres [13], whereas in the United States Grifo [14, 15] working with Cohen reported a pregnancy following embryo biopsy subjected to both X and Y FISH [16]. Munné and this same group later applied multicolor FISH on blastomeres [17], setting the stage for modern PGD aneuploidy testing. In 1998, Munné used FISH to identify unbalanced chromosomal translocations [18, 19], using breakpoint-specific probes. In the United Kingdom, Delhanty and Harper performed rapid FISH [20] and observed mosaicism in cleavage stage embryo; Munné also recognized this problem, but considered it manageable with optimal diagnostics. Verlinsky et al. [21] likewise applied FISH but to polar bodies.

3 Professional and Scientific Organizations

Scientific presentations and clinical application of preimplantation genetic diagnosis (PGD)—now properly called preimplantation genetic testing (PGT)—has progressively become more organized. Early cooperation was demonstrated by yearly international meetings arranged by Verlinsky [22]. Beginning in 1990, an annual "International Working Group on PGD" held in sites around the world, often in conjunction with other major international meetings. Materials of First International Conference on Preimplantation Genetics in Chicago in 1990 yielded a 1991 volume by Verlinsky and Kuliev that exercised traction for the broader scientific community [23].These meetings focused early PGT investigators on technology development until clinical application caught up with their vision. In a few years, PGD had evolved from a boutique component of prenatal genetic diagnosis to mainstream, having its own distinct indications [24]. This set the stage for rapid progress that followed [25–27].

In 2003, the Preimplantation Genetic Diagnosis International Society (PGDIS) was incorporated in the United States (Illinois), de facto the direct continuation of the yearly International Working Group on PGD. The first meeting after incorporation was in London in 2005. Annual meetings have been also held in Chicago, Bologna, Cyprus, Antalya, Miami, Montpellier, Bergenz, Istanbul, and Canterbury. The membership elected Yury Verlinsky as a founding President of PGDIS. Terms of offices were set for 2 years. Subsequent Presidents have been Luca Gianaroli, Joe Leigh Simpson, Robert G. Edwards, Renée Martin, Semra Kahraman, and Svetlana Rechitsky. Anver Kuliev serves as the Executive Director (www.pgdis.org).PGDIS meetings are robust, with pre-congress workshops. PGDIS now serves as the largest aggregation of dedicated PGD investigators globally.

In Europe, PGD workshops and formal communication are organized through the European Society for Human Reproduction and Embryology (ESHRE). PGD activities exist under aegis of the ESHRE Special Interest Group (SIG) in Genetics, which in 1997 formed the ESHRE PGD Consortium. This Consortium collates clinical results annually, and places data on the ESHRE web site and in peer review publications [1, 28, 29]. Founding leaders were Karen Sermon, Joep Geraedts, and Joyce Harper.

The American Society for Reproductive Medicine (ASRM) formed its own SIG on PGD in 2005. Participation is open to all

ASRM members. Presidents (currently Chairmen) serve 2 year terms and to date have been Yury Verlinsky, Jacques Cohen, Marcus Hughes, Santiago Munné, Luca Gianaroli, and Anver Kuliev, with Semra Kahraman Chairman Elect, and Svetlana Rechitsky Vice Chairman. ASRM PGD SIG members provide recommendations for PGD activities at the annual ASRM meeting. This includes postgraduate courses, abstract review, and other educational and scientific events.

The Reproductive Health and Research Program of the WHO recently codified terms used to designate diagnosis of preimplantation embryos. This was undertaken through WHO NGOs ICMART and as well as ASRM, IFFS, FIGO. In particular, the term preimplantation genetic screening (PGS) to connote aneuploidy testing was considered inappropriate because not screening but "testing" was performed (*see* the footnote 1 to this Chapter). The concept of a "screen" has long been accepted (National Academy of Science, 1975) as implying follow-up with a definite test (T). That is, screening merely identifies individuals in the general population or in at-risk population who could benefit from a definitive test not offered otherwise. In prenatal genetic diagnosis, of which preimplantation genetics is a component, the "test" is an invasive test, e.g., amniocentesis. The term preimplantation genetic screening thus implies that it will be followed by an invasive "test." The 2016 ICMART and WHO Glossary for reproductive has codified these terms [30]:

Preimplantation Genetic Testing (PGT)
PGT-A: Aneuploidy.
PGT-M: Monogenic (Single Gene).
PGT-SR: Structural (Chromosomal) Rearrangement.
PGT-HLA: Human Leukocyte Antigen.

4 Selecting the Stage for Analysis of Gamete or Embryonic Stage for Analysis

PGD requires access to DNA from gametes or embryos within 6 days of conception, when implantation occurs. DNA can be obtained at three stages: (1) polar body I or II or both; (2) cleavage stage, a single blastomere from the 3 day six- to eight-cell embryos; and (3) blastocyst, trophectoderm from the 5- to 6-day embryo. All three are still used, but preferences have changed with respect to stages preferentially utilized.

4.1 Polar Body Biopsy

Polar body biopsy received the most focus in early human PGD, being espoused by the pioneer Yury Verlinsky. Genotype of the oocyte can be deduced by the analysis of the first or second polar biopsy. The underlying principle is fully explained elsewhere [31]. Briefly, let us suppose the first polar body from a heterozygous individual shows a mutant maternal allele; the complementary primary oocyte should have the normal allele. Oocytes deduced to be genetically normal can then be fertilized in vitro to be transferred for potential implantation. Conversely, a normal polar body indicates an abnormal oocyte having the mutant allele; thus, fertilization would not proceed. Similarly, if the first polar body showed no chromosome 21, the oocyte would be presumed to have two 21 chromosomes and, hence, lead to a trisomic zygote. The above assumes lack of recombination, which if present requires delaying definitive diagnosis until assessment of the second polar body.

As additional laboratories embarked upon PGD in the late 1990s and early 2000s, relatively few chose polar body biopsy as their preferred biopsy method. Cleavage stage was more often utilized. One reason was the obvious disadvantage of being unable to assess paternal genotype, precluding in part application if the father had an autosomal dominant disorder, thus making analysis less efficient in managing couples at risk for autosomal recessive traits. Another reason seems to be technical difficulty.

Still, polar biopsy retains an indispensable role. Information can be obtained on genotype of potential offspring from the first polar body, which is present before fertilization. Only biopsy of the first polar body allows normal oocytes to be deduced to be fertilized as normal for single gene diagnosis. Polar body is the only viable option if regulatory statutes require a provider to inseminate every oocyte that can be fertilized or restrict the number and preclude cryopreservation. Identifying and fertilizing only euploid oocytes allows pregnancy rates to be maintained despite onerous legislation [32].

Centers experienced in polar body biopsy appear to have pregnancy rates comparable to those achieved using blastomere biopsy. However, no attempts have been made to compare relative safety of blastomere or trophectoderm biopsy versus polar body biopsy. Given relatively few centers performing polar body biopsy, any RTC conducted at present might be misleading if technical expertise were not comparable for both techniques.

4.2 Cleavage Stage Embryo

Until approximately 2010, most PGT-A cases were performed by blastomere biopsy of the cleavage state embryo. The zona pellucida—the glycoprotein layer that surrounds a cleavage stage embryo—is breached by mechanical, laser, or chemical means to extract a cell containing DNA (blastomere). Typically, only a single cell is removed because even one fewer cell at this stage is believed to reduce embryo survival. Actually, the frequently cited 10% reduction in survival after blastomere biopsy was initially deduced by correlating pregnancy rates as a function of numbers of blastomeres remaining after thawed cryopreserved embryos [33] were transformed. Loss of one cell after thawing was correlated with10% reduced pregnancy rates, and loss of two cells even more [34]. In a later direct study, one experienced center reported livebirth rates of 22.4% and 37.4% after removal of one versus two cells, respectively [35].

A notable decrease in number of cleavage stage biopsies performed in the 2007–2010 interval occurred following concerns related to safety and accuracy. During this interval, fluorescence in situ hybridization (FISH) using 5–9 chromosome-specific probes was used for diagnosis. This was at that time the only diagnostic approach possible for detecting of chromosomal abnormalities; however, so few chromosomes were obviously not optimal. At present, 24 chromosome array CGH and NGS-based technologies are being performed with considerable increase in pregnancy rates. However, the embryonic stage selected for biopsy is now more often trophectoderm biopsy.

4.3 Blastocyst Biopsy

Biopsy of trophectoderm in the 5- to 6-day approximately 120-cell blastocyst as stated above is increasingly the approach used at present. More cells (DNA) can be removed at this stage, potentially facilitating diagnosis. Trophectoderm forms the placenta; thus, embryonic cells per se are not removed. In fact, blastocyst was initially envisioned as *the* approach for PGD. Gardner and Edwards recovered blastocysts for PGD in rabbits [3], and in humans Buster et al. [36] recovered human blastocysts by uterine lavage. Lavage to recover blastocysts was envisioned to be an approach by which cells removed by trophectoderm biopsy could allow genetic diagnosis [37]. Prior to PCR, no other approach seemed feasible. Ultimately, lavage for PGT was not pursued because of fear of retained, undiagnosed embryos.

By 2005 McArthur, Jansen, and their Australian team demonstrated feasibility of blastocyst biopsy for PGT-A [38, 39], as did Schoolcraft (2010)** and others in the USA [40]. Usually 5–10 cells are obtained, facilitating diagnosis by next generation sequencing. The additional 2 to 3 days in vitro beyond that required for the 8-cell cleavage stage embryo allows self-selection against non-thriving embryos. Approximately one third of embryos with chromosomal abnormalities do not survive the day 3 to 5 transition. Still, PGT-A remains necessary to exclude remaining aneuploidies, the frequency of which depends upon maternal age.

4.4 Embryo Biopsy and Cryopreservation

Cryopreservation of biopsied embryos was once not considered possible. Biopsied embryos thus had to be transferred by day 6; all diagnostic results had to be completed by that time.

With development of cryopreservation by vitrification, biopsied embryos could be thawed and transferred with considerable success [41–43]. In fact, a viable approach is blastocyst biopsy and vitrification of all embryos ("freeze all"). In the intervening time, 24 chromosome and other diagnostic applications can be performed. One may then thaw and transfer normal embryos one or more months later. "Freeze-all" approaches with later transfer may even result in higher pregnancy rates than "same-cycle" transfer. The presumptive explanation is a more hospitable endometrium, no longer perturbed by ovarian hyperstimulation.

5 Single Gene Disorders (PGT-M)

PGT-M was the original intent of PGD. Perhaps 20% or more of all PGT cases currently still involve couples at risk for one or more single gene disorders. PGT-M can be performed whenever the chromosomal location of the gene causing a given disorder is known. The causative mutation need not be known so long as affected and unaffected family members are available to determine phase (cis/trans) of markers linked to a mutant allele. This allows one to deduce whether a given embryo has or has not inherited the gamete containing the mutation. Close to 500 different conditions have now been tested worldwide.

By 2009, Reproductive Genetic Innovations (Chicago) had tested over 202 different conditions [44], the most frequent being hemoglobinopathies, cystic fibrosis and fragile X syndrome; in 2010 Verlinsky and Kuliev [45] enumerated disorders tested by that time. The latest tabulation from this group came from Rechitsky et al. [46], 2982 cycles involving 1685 patients. These yielded 1095 pregnancies and 1118 live births; 47 pregnancies were still ongoing at the time of publication [47].

In Europe, the ESHRE PGD Consortium [29] reported that in 2005 cycles the most common single gene indications to be myotonic dystrophy ($N = 76$ of 500), Huntington disease ($N = 56$), cystic fibrosis ($N = 55$), fragile X syndrome ($N = 51$), spinal muscular atrophy ($N = 27$), tuberous sclerosis ($N = 15$), and Marfan syndrome ($N = 13$); β-thalassemia/sickle cell anemia ($N = 61$). A total of 110 other conditions had by that time been interrogated. Several disorders seem more common in this cohort than in the ESHRE PGD consortium than RGI, examples being neurofibromatosis and familial dysautonomia; however, the spectrum of disorders tested was overall similar.

Gutierrez-Mateo et al. reported the Reprogenetics experience over a 51-month period ending March 2008 [48]. A total of 162 couples in 224 cycles were at risk for 46 different single gene disorders. Biopsy was performed in 59 different ART centers, blastomeres being sent from IVF center to Reprogenetics labs for laboratory analysis. By far the most common indication was cystic fibrosis ($N = 73$ cycles).

5.1 Unique Indications for Single Gene Disorder

5.1.1 Avoiding Clinical Termination (PGT)

As already discussed, only PGT allows information to be obtained prior to implantation, thus obviating necessity for pregnancy termination. In the 2001 ESHRE PGD Consortium, 36% of 1561 couples stated that their reason for undergoing PGD was avoiding clinical pregnancy termination [49]. Some were in their initial pregnancy, but others probably reflected the disquiet expected of any couple having previously undergone pregnancy termination. In the 2001 report, 21% of the absolute number of women undergoing PGD had a previous termination and wished to avoid another. Since 2001, PGT-A has increased considerably in frequency and, hence, the proportion (but probably not absolute number) of women undergoing PGT-M to avoid clinical pregnancy termination has decreased.

Increasing number of PGT-M is presently performed for conditioned determined by de novo mutations (DNM). Development of special PGD designs is always required for DNM, detected in a parent or affected children, as neither origin, nor relevant haplotypes are available for tracing the inheritance of DNM in single cells biopsied from embryos or oocytes. With the improved awareness of PGT, increasing number of couples request PGT, without any family history of the genetic disease that has been first diagnosed in one of the parents or in their affected children. The first systematic PGD for DNM was reported by RGI, describing a large series of 38 different genetic disorders, determined by dominant, recessive, and X-linked DNM, of both maternal and paternal origin [50]. PGD strategies for these families depend on the origin of DNM, and included an extensive DNA analysis of the parents and affected children prior to PGT, with the mutation verification, polymorphic marker evaluation, whole and single sperm testing and PB analysis in order to establish the normal and mutant haplotypes, without which PGT-M cannot be performed. In cases of DNM of paternal origin, the DNM is first confirmed on the paternal DNA from blood and total sperm, followed by single sperm typing to determine the proportion of sperm with DNM and relevant normal and mutant haplotypes. For a higher reliability of testing, the relevant maternal linked markers are also detected, to be able to trace for possible shared maternal and paternal markers. In cases of DNM of maternal origin, DNM is first confirmed in maternal blood, and PGD was performed, when possible, by PB analysis, to identify the normal and mutant maternal haplotypes. Also, in order to trace the relevant paternal haplotypes, single sperm typing is performed, whenever possible, for avoiding misdiagnosis caused by possible shared paternal and maternal markers. In cases of DNM detected first in children, the mutation is verified in their whole blood DNA, followed by testing for the mutation in paternal DNA from blood, total and single sperm, if the DNM appears of paternal origin. In DNM of maternal origin, PGD is performed by PB approach, with confirmation of the diagnosis by embryo biopsy, if necessary. So despite the complexity of PGT-M for DNM, the applied strategies are highly accurate, representing an important addition to the practice of PGT-M for Mendelian diseases, as it makes now possible to offer PGD to any couple at risk for producing the offspring with genetic disease, despite the traditional requirement of family data.

5.1.2 Non-Disclosure of Parental Genotype (PGT-M)

PGT-M is the only practical approach if a person at risk for an adult-onset disorder wishes to avoid transmitting to his/her offspring a mutant gene he/she may (or may not) [51]. In addition, they wish to remain unaware of his/her own genotype. Such an individual can still avoid transmitting a mutant allele to offspring without learning their own genotype. The prototypic example is the son or daughter of a parent known to be affected with an autosomal dominant disorder, for example Huntington disease or autosomal dominant Alzheimer disease.

All this PGT-M and transfer of a genetically normal embryo without knowledge of parental genotype can thus be accomplished. The caveat is that the couple needs to remain clueless as to details on their own ART cycle—number of embryos, number available for transfer, certainly diagnosis per embryo. In subsequent cycles, the protocol must then be repeated even if the person in question has proved unaffected. Otherwise, the at-risk patient would readily deduce his or her genotype.

The number of PGT-M cases performed for non-disclosure is about 5 to 10% of single gene disorders in the ESHRE PGD Consortium and in large U.S. centers. Not significantly different proportion of cases has been at RGI, mainly for HD (61 HD of a total 1685 patients) [47].

5.1.3 Cancer and Adult-Onset Disorders (PGT-M)

Performing prenatal genetic diagnosis for any adult-onset Mendelian conditions was once considered highly arguable [52]. In the United States, little controversy now exists, but there remains reticence in much of Europe. The first PGT case for inherited adult onset cancer was performed by Verlinsky et al. [53] to avoid transmitting an adult-onset autosomal dominant cancer involved Li-Fraumeni syndrome, caused by a p53 perturbation. Diagnosis of other disorders soon followed and by 2002 the RGI group [54] had performed 337 cycles for 169 patients, resulting in 113 births free of predisposition to cancer. PGT-M for BRCA1 and BRCA 2, multiple endocrine neoplasia, familial adenomatous polyposis (FAP), Li-Fraumeni syndrome, Fanconi anemia, retinoblastoma and Von Hippel-Lindau (VHL) syndrome, neurofibromatosis 1 (NF1) and neurofibromatosis 2 (NF2), and Gorlin syndrome are now well accepted indications. Given diagnosis of cancer is usually known in a person to be at risk or under active clinical surveillance, non-disclosure PGT-M protocol is usually unnecessary; however, this could be applicable if only a less closely related relative were affected. PGT-M to exclude transmission of any adult onset autosomal trait potentially affecting offspring a prospective parent now seems well accepted worldwide.

PGD-M also provides a relief for the at-risk couples for inherited cardiac disease, another group of late onset disorders which may manifest despite pre-symptomatic diagnosis and follow-up. The majority of inherited cardiac disorders are dominant, for which no cure may be administered, because their first and only clinical occurrence may be a premature or sudden death. One of such conditions is the familiar hypertrophic cardiomyopathy (HCM), which clinically manifests at different ages, with no symptoms observed for years until provoked by different factors, such as excessive exercise. PGD-M was applied to different conditions leading to HCM, including HCM4 and HCM7, which may cause an asymmetric ventricular hypertrophy and defect in interventricular septum, with high risk of cardiac failure and sudden death.The other condition for which PGD is strongly indicated is dilated cardiomyopathy (CMD), which is an autosomal dominant disease caused by different mutations in LMNA gene located on chromosomes 1. This cardiac disease is characterized by ventricular dilation and impaired systolic function, resulting in a heart failure and arrhythmia, which causes premature or sudden death. While the large phenotypic variability of patients may be determined by different mutations in LMNA gene, differences from one family to another may be observed within the same mutation, with possible involvement of skeletal muscles that leads to the muscles weakness.

At RGI, 51 PGD cycles were performed for 14 cardiac diseases, determined by 23 different gene mutations. This resulted in the embryo transfer in 44 of 51 PGD cycles, yielding 29 (66%) unaffected pregnancies and birth of 27 healthy, disease predisposition-free children [55, 56]. Results show that PGD may be a realistic option for couples at risk for producing offspring with cardiac disease, determined by inherited predisposition. Inheritance of such susceptibility factors places the individual at risk of serious cardiac disease, clinically manifested from as early as the first year of life such as in cardioencephalopathy, to as late as later in life, with the only clinical realization of premature or sudden death, as in CMD and CMH.

Among the conditions in the family history of the couples at risk that may indicate to a possible need of PGD may be a heart attack and sudden death at young ages, family members with pacemakers or internal cardiac defibrillators, arrhythmia, and heart surgery. The chances that the offspring of these patients will develop the same heart disease will differ depending on the mode of inheritance, but their penetrance is difficult to predict, because many inherited cardiac conditions are difficult to diagnose and will develop with age and may be induced by certain medications or activities, such as excessive exercise, which may lead to cardiac arrest or sudden death, justifying the parents' requests for PGD-M.

5.1.4 HLA-Compatible Embryos (PGT-HLA)

Among sibs, one in four is HLA compatible (identical). HLA-compatibility among siblings becomes attractive if there exists an older, moribund sibling with a lethal disease who could benefit from stem cell transplantation to repopulate his or her bone marrow. PGT-HLA is the only practical way to identify the few embryos that are HLA compatible with an affected individual [57, 58]. Sometimes, the affected individual is a child of a couple of reproductive age. Given this, one attractive strategy is using umbilical cord blood from a neonate to repopulate the bone marrow of an older, affected sibling. Odds that a couple can both avoid another genetically abnormal child for an autosomal recessive disorder (3/4) and also utilize HLA compatible umbilical cord stem cells to repopulate a bone marrow is 3 in 16 (1 in 4 HLA-compatible embryos multiplied by the 3 in 4 likelihood of also being affected = 3/16). Actually, the likelihood is less because recombination can occur within the HLA locus, established by RGI to be 4.3% [57]; thus a 100% HLA match is not possible for the affected child because the exact recombination event cannot be expected to recur. A similar proportion of embryos recovered in any cycle will not be HLA identical.

PGT-H for the transferring HLA-compatible embryos was first performed by Verlinsky and colleagues in a couple of at risk for Fanconi anemia [58]. Like inherited PGT-HLA for autosomal disorders like cancer, this generated considerable controversy at the time (2001). By 2004, however, the RGI group reported 45 cycles for HLA typing had been performed [2, 59]; 17.5% embryos were genetically suitable for transfer, very near the expected (3/16) (16%). The most common genetic indication is β-thalassemia; however, the strategy is applicable for any bone marrow infiltrative disorder [60].

Testing for HLA-compatible embryos *without* risk of genetic disease is now also widely accepted in United States and Turkey, with the prime indication being an older sib with sporadic Blackfan–Diamond anemia or leukemia, first performed in 2004 [61]. In the United States, this now accounts for approximately one third of PGD-HLA cases. A 2004 compilation by RGI showed 11% of their single cell PGD cases involved HLA testing. By 2009, 15% of 1666 single gene PGD cases were performed for HLA typing [44]. In Istanbul, 261 HLA cases had been performed by 2009, all but 61 for β-thalassemia [61]. In Europe, however, PGT-HLA for this indication has remained uncommon [28]. Because the majority of patient requesting PGT-HLA are of an advanced reproductive age, PGT-HLA is now increasingly performed concurrently with PGT-A, and it was demonstrated that PGT-M or PGT-H concurrent with PGT-A increases pregnancy rates by 20% or more compared to age-matched cases (<35 years) not concurrently undergoing PGT-A [46].

By the present time, the list of disorders for which PGT-HLA has been applied with successful stem cell transplantation treatment includes thalassaemia, Wiscott–Aldrich syndrome, X-linked hyper IgM syndrome, X-linked hypohidrotic ectodermal dysplasia with immune deficiency and incontinentia pigmenti, and Blackfan–Diamond anemia, with the list continuously expanding [2, 57–60, 62–65]. The accumulated experience of approximately one thousand cases of PGT-HLA shows that this represents an important prospect for radical treatment of the affected members of the families with congenital and acquired bone marrow failures and immunodeficiencies. Still the majority of PGT-HLA was performed for thalassemia, with over 400 cases performed in Istanbul and Chicago, resulting in birth of dozens unaffected HLA matched children, who served as donors for stem cell transplantation to their affected sibling, resulting in a complete recovery in almost all the cases.

6 Chromosomal Rearrangements (PGT-SR)

Chromosomal rearrangements (translocation or inversion) are well recognized as leading to unbalanced gametes and, hence, an unbalanced zygote. Couples with rearrangements are often detected after repeated spontaneous abortions, reflecting lethality conferred by unbalanced gametes. Not long after FISH became available and PGT possible, PGT-SR was predictably performed, initially using chromosome-specific probes [19, 66]. This was recognized to be an attractive approach for assuring transfer of only cytogenetically normal embryos. Euploid embryos not only precluded another miscarriage and avoided abnormal liveborn, but increased reproductive efficiency. Relatively few gametes/embryos of any translocation heterozygote are normal or balanced. PGT-SR can identify and transfer only the relative few embryos that are normal.

Breakpoint-specific probes were initially devised unique to each case [18]. PGD-SR translocation analysis using this approach was accurate, but costs prohibitive [18]. Thus, commercially available probes are now used. A limitation is that usually one cannot distinguish an embryo with a balanced translocation from an embryo without a translocation.

No RCTs have been conducted to determine whether PGT-SR increases pregnancy rates in couples having a balanced translocation who present with repeated pregnancies losses. However, surrogate evidence is ample. Otani et al. [67] observed only 5.3% miscarriages after PGT-SR for translocations, much less than expected even in the general population. Second, pregnancy can be achieved more rapidly. Otani et al. reported the lifetime cumulative pregnancy rate using PGT-SR to be 57.6% [67]. This is per se not remarkable, but that this was achieved with an average of 1.24 cycles is unexpected for translocation heterozygotes. The short time-frame before which translocation couples undergoing PGD can achieve pregnancy contrasts with the mean 4–6 years necessary for translocation couples who do *not* use PGD [68–70]. In 2008, the Society for Assisted Reproductive Technology (SART) guidelines thus recommended PGD for this indication [71].

7 PGT-Aneuploidy (PGT-A) to Improve Pregnancy Rates

PGT aneuploidy testing is increasingly performed solely to improve pregnancy rates in women who require ART and have no other indication. The logic is irrefutable. Pregnancy rates in ART decline precipitously beginning late in the fourth decade; the primary reason is high embryonic loss due to aneuploidy; thus, transferring only euploid embryos is attractive, and capable of being assured by PGT-A. That endometrial factors were not paramount had, moreover, been shown by successful pregnancies following transfer of donor embryos from younger women to recipients in their late fifth and sixth decades. From the late 1990s onward, favorable results for PGT-A were reported frequently from experienced centers worldwide [31, 72–77]. Most reports compared outcome to historical expectations for age-matched women not undergoing PGD. Two small RCTs showing favorable results were conducted in the United States [78, 79], both showing increased pregnancy rates although neither sufficiently powered.

During 2000–2007, larger PGD and ART centers in the United States and Europe increasingly offered PGD to improve pregnancy rates in older women. However, these large centers were not able to complete an RCT. Patients were not willing, and in the U.S. embryo research could not be funded federally (National Institutes of Health). Other centers, with less volume and experience, did conduct RCTs. Results showed no significant improvement in pregnancy rates [80–83], and at least one [81] showed harmful effects. Questionable technical prowess, diagnostic difficulties, and arguable indications were widely criticized by this author and others [84–87]. Not surprisingly however, the increasing trajectory of increasing PGT-aneuploidy cycles to improve ART pregnancy rates was blunted. Perhaps a 20% drop in PGT-A cycles occurred during the years 2007–2010.

Two explanations were commonly accepted as explanations for the disappointing RTC results. One is the technical difficulty in performing cleavage stage embryo. Some embryologists appear more skilled than others, not surprisingly for any surgical procedure. (If so, this explanation would not refute proof of principle for the value of PGT-A but would impede generalizability). Similarly, diagnostic methods available at the time were less than optimal.

Using FISH with chromosome-specific probes, only 5–7 chromosomes or at best 9–12 could be interrogated.

The single RCT generating the most publicity concerning harmful effects of aneuploidy testing was conducted by Mastenbroek et al. [81]. This well-cited report warrants a few comments. One major problem was applying an intent to treat statistical design. When PGT-A was successful (defined as seven chromosomes tested and at least one euploid embryo transferred), the pregnancy rate was 16.8% per embryo. When no biopsy was performed (true control), the pregnancy rate was 14.7% per embryo, 13% lower than with PGT-A. In some 20% of embryos, however, there were no diagnostic results, a rate higher than in other centers at the time [85, 86, 88]. Given lack of results in these 20%, a third (unintended) group evolved: biopsy performed, no diagnostic result, transfer nonetheless. In this group, the pregnancy rate was only 6%. Intent-to-treat statistical analysis dictated that all cases remain assigned to their original group even if the assigned protocol (i.e., PGD) was not completed or even reversed. Insisting on this, the true PGD group (16.8% pregnancy per embryo) was merged with the de facto sham group (6%). This yielded a merged "PGD" live birth rate of 24% per cycle, compared to the statistically higher 35% in the non-biopsied, non-PGD group.

Given this situation, efforts were directed in the cytogenetic community to increase diagnostic robustness and accuracy. Technologies introduced included multiple hybridization cycles to test all 24 chromosomes, testing 11–12 chromosomes tailored expressly per age group, orre-testing to minimize "no result" cases. Still, the obvious need was reliable 24 chromosome testing. Actually, genome-wide molecular approaches for 24 chromosome analysis had begun earlier with metaphase CGH [88–90]. Later, Wells et al. [91, 92] used metaphase (CGH) to interrogate all chromosomes in a small series of blastocysts: 90% gave informative results, and 36 to 42 cycles (86%) resulted in a clinical pregnancy. By contrast, non-PGD blastocysts in the same series showed a 60% pregnancy rate. Single cell genome-wide SNPs (in 2000–2010) were also used reliably on a single blastomere [93–95]. Results were available quickly enough for normal embryos to be transferred in the same cycle: using SNPs. Treff et al. [96] accomplished this in 4 h.

The technique that ultimately became used most commonly for 24 chromosome interrogation proved to be array CGH, using a BAC-platform (BlueGnome). BlueGnome utilized selected sequences from all 24 chromosomes, placed on the proverbial "chip." Reference sequences were derived from bacterial artificial chromosomes (BACs), which cover very large chromosomal regions. This method provides less sensitivity than arrays that utilize smaller sequences and thus broader "coverage." That PGT-A used BAC arrays paradoxically proved advantageous clinically. Results on a single blastomere could be stratified simply into euploid, aneuploid, or no result bins. Of course, it was realized that some aneuploidy embryos were actually mosaic and containing an unrecognized euploid cell line, yet undetectable given analysis restricted to a single blastomere. The single cell tested could have been trisomic whereas the remaining 7–8 cells unknowingly euploid, (i.e., mosaicism). Still, clinical utility was pragmatically achieved with BlueGnome. Based on data from disaggregated cleavage stage embryos, the frequency of mosaicism was concluded to 1–2% [97].

By the 2010s there had been further transformative movement in expanding use of PGT-A [40, 98]. One advance is moving from cleavage stage biopsy to trophectoderm biopsy. Improved embryo culture, facile laser trophectoderm biopsy, and vitrification were combined to make this feasible. By 2012 several different groups had conducted RCTs with salutary results. These RCTs observed improved ART pregnancy rates by transferring euploid embryos vs. simply morphologically normal embryos. Harton et al. definitely showed that with euploid embryos the "take home baby" rates did not begin to decrease until age 42 years [99]. Multiple gestations could be avoided because transfer of a single euploid embryo protected livebirth rates (without twins) equal to transfer of two morphologically normal non-PGD embryos [100, 101].

BAC Array CGH by next generation sequencing (NGS) technologies had encompassed SNPs, copy number variants (CNVs), and quantitative PCR. With NGS, greater laboratory productivity is possible; however, mosaicism is detected more often. Increased detection of mosaicism thus occurs, presumably reflecting both greater sensitivity of NGS and greater amounts of DNA. In the six-day embryo the number of cells biopsied is 5–15; in cleavage stage blastomere biopsy only one cell was available. Not surprisingly, mosaicism was detected more often in trophectoderm biopsy. Mosaicism can be detected at level of 20% [97]. The frequency of mosaicism in trophectoderm is 20–25% using validated NGS technologies; the frequency on reanalyzed cleavage stage embryos was <2% [97]. Although some mosaic embryos may also be mosaic as well in this inner cell mass (to be developing embryo), other embryos could have normal cells only in their ICM and thus would be suitable for transfer.

It follows that trophectoderm biopsy results characterized by a normal and a monosomic line could be candidates for transfer, given that the monosomic line is probably lethal and would not persist [102]. Greco et al. reported livebirths in four mosaic monosomy cases but none in mosaic trisomies [102]. At present, 7% mosaic aneuploid embryos by Munné et al. [97] are estimated as leading to a livebirth [102]. If a couple lacks non-mosaic euploid embryos, one might thus perform transfer of a mosaic aneuploid embryo with patient consent. The need for clarity is recognized by Commentaries [99, 103–105].

2016 Guidelines by PGDIS (http://www.pgdis.org/docs/newsletter_071816.html) provide recommendations on significance of a given level of mosaicism, on transferring mosaic monosomy embryos, and on priority of transferring mosaic trisomy embryos for a specific chromosome.

8 Repeated Pregnancy Loss (Recurrent Aneuploidy)

Observational studies utilizing PGT-A have long been accepted as decreasing miscarriage rates [31, 72–77]. No RCTs exist, but only surrogate data exist. One can compare results to objective criteria, such as the Brigham formula [106]. This formula takes into account maternal age and the number of prior abortions to derive the priori likelihood of a pregnancy loss. Using this comparison, Munné et al. [107] observed losses in 13% of couples who used PGT-A, compared to the Brigham-expected rate of 33%. Benefit was, not surprisingly, greatest for women older than 35 (39 vs. expected 13%; $P > 0.001$). Thus, using array CGH, and transferring euploid embryos, the miscarriage rate is now 10% [99].

Recurrent miscarriage has multiple etiologies—genetic and nongenetic. How might the above data apply to couples having experienced recurrent miscarriage, but not actually infertile? Non-random distribution appears to exist with respect to successive miscarriages. That is, abortuses tend to be either successively aneuploid or successively euploid [108]. Non-random distribution also occurs in preimplantation embryos in successive cycles [109].

Given all the above, the rationale for performing PGT aneuploidy testing in women having repeated miscarriages is strong if the goal is preventing recurrent miscarriage. Less clear is whether the livebirth rate is improved and if so whether this justifies ART with PGT-A. Successive aneuploidy carries implications for diagnostic testing and management. However, there is not consensus [110]. If recurrent aneuploidy is an indication for PGT aneuploidy, at least one loss should have documented aneuploidy if one is to perform PGT-A solely for this purpose.

References

1. Goossens V, Harton G, Moutou C et al (2009) ESHRE PGD consortium data collection IX: cycles from January to December 2006 with pregnancy follow-up to October 2007. Hum Reprod 24(8):1786–1810. https://doi.org/10.1093/humrep/dep059
2. Verlinsky Y, Cohen J, Munne S et al (2004) Over a decade of experience with preimplantation genetic diagnosis: a multicenter report. Fertil Steril 82(2):292–294. https://doi.org/10.1016/j.fertnstert.2003.09.082
3. Gardner RL, Edwards RG (1968) Control of the sex ratio at full term in the rabbit by transferring sexed blastocysts. Nature 218(5139):346–349
4. Modlinski J, Mclaren A (1980) A method for visualizing the chromosomes of the 2nd Polar body of the mouse egg. J Embryol Exp Morphol 60(Dec):93–97
5. Dyban AP (1991) Experimental cytogenetics of preimplantation development. In:

Verlinsky Y, Kuliev A (eds) Preimplantation genetics. Plenum Press, New York, pp 15–23
6. Steptoe PC, Edwards RG (1978) Birth after the reimplantation of a human embryo. Lancet 2(8085):366
7. Monk M, Handyside AH (1988) Sexing of preimplantation mouse embryos by measurement of X-linked gene dosage in a single blastomere. J Reprod Fertil 82(1):365–368
8. Handyside AH, Kontogianni EH, Hardy K et al (1990) Pregnancies from biopsied human preimplantation embryos sexed by Y-specific DNA amplification. Nature 344 (6268):768–770. https://doi.org/10.1038/344768a0
9. Handyside AH, Lesko JG, Tarin JJ et al (1992) Birth of a normal girl after in vitro fertilization and preimplantation diagnostic testing for cystic fibrosis. N Engl J Med 327 (13):905–909
10. Verlinsky Y, Pergament E, Binor Z et al (1987) Genetic analysis of human embryos prior to implantation: future applications of in-vitro fertilization in treatment and prevention of human genetic diseases. In: Feichtinger W, Kemeter P (eds) Future aspects in human in-vitro fertilization. Springer-Verlag, Berlin, pp 262–266
11. Verlinsky Y, Ginsberg N, Lifchez A et al (1990) Analysis of the first polar body: preconception genetic diagnosis. Hum Reprod 5 (7):826–829
12. Strom CM, Verlinsky Y, Milayeva S et al (1990) Preconception genetic diagnosis of cystic fibrosis. Lancet 336(8710):306–307
13. Griffin DK, Handyside AH, Penketh RJ et al (1991) Fluorescent in-situ hybridization to interphase nuclei of human preimplantation embryos with X and Y chromosome specific probes. Hum Reprod 6(1):101–105
14. Grifo JA, Boyle A, Fischer E et al (1990) Preembryo biopsy and analysis of blastomeres by in situ hybridization. Am J Obstet Gynecol 163(6 Pt 1):2013–2019
15. Grifo JA, Boyle A, Tang YX et al (1992) Preimplantation genetic diagnosis. In situ hybridization as a tool for analysis. Arch Pathol Lab Med 116(4):393–397
16. Grifo JA, Tang YX, Cohen J et al (1992) Pregnancy after embryo biopsy and coamplification of DNA from X and Y chromosomes. JAMA 268(6):727–729
17. Munne S, Lee A, Rosenwaks Z et al (1993) Diagnosis of major chromosome aneuploidies in human preimplantation embryos. Hum Reprod 8(12):2185–2191
18. Munne S, Fung J, Cassel MJ et al (1998) Preimplantation genetic analysis of translocations: case-specific probes for interphase cell analysis. Hum Genet 102(6):663–674
19. Munne S, Sandalinas M, Escudero T et al (2000) Outcome of preimplantation genetic diagnosis of translocations. Fertil Steril 73 (6):1209–1218
20. Harper JC, Coonen E, Ramaekers FC et al (1994) Identification of the sex of human preimplantation embryos in two hours using an improved spreading method and fluorescent in-situ hybridization (FISH) using directly labelled probes. Hum Reprod 9 (4):721–724
21. Verlinsky Y, Cieslak J, Freidine M et al (1995) Pregnancies following pre-conception diagnosis of common aneuploidies by fluorescent in-situ hybridization. Hum Reprod 10 (7):1923–1927
22. Edwards RG, Cohen JA, Gianaroli L et al (2009) Yury Verlinsky (01/09/1943–16/07/2009): pioneer in CVS, PGD and hESC. Reprod Biomed Online 19(3):298–299. https://doi.org/10.1016/S1472-6483(10)60162-9
23. Verlinsky Y, Kuliev A (1991) Preimplantation genetics. Plenum Press, New York
24. Simpson JL, Carson SA, Buster JE et al (1994) Preimplantation genetic diagnosis: indications and pitfalls. In: Mori T, Tominaga T, Aono T, Horoi M (eds) Frontiers in endocrinology: perspectives on assisted reproduction. Ares-Serono Symposia Publications, Rome, pp 689–696
25. Harper JC (2009) Preimplantation genetic diagnosis, 2nd edn. Cambridge University Press, Cambridge
26. Kuliev A, Verlinsky Y (2004) Preimplantation HLA typing and stem cell transplantation: report of International Meeting, Cyprus, 27-8 March, 2004. Reprod Biomed Online 9(2):205–209
27. Simpson JL (2001) Changing indications for preimplantation genetic diagnosis (PGD). Mol Cell Endocrinol 183(Suppl 1):S69–S75
28. Goossens V, Harton G, Moutou C et al (2008) ESHRE PGD consortium data collection VIII: cycles from January to December 2005 with pregnancy follow-up to October 2006. Hum Reprod 23(12):2629–2645. https://doi.org/10.1093/humrep/den238
29. Harper JC, de Die-Smulders C, Goossens V et al (2008) ESHRE PGD consortium data collection VII: cycles from January to December 2004 with pregnancy follow-up to October 2005. Hum Reprod 23

(4):741–755. https://doi.org/10.1093/humrep/dem354
30. Zegers-Hochschild F, Adamson GD, de Mouzon J et al (in press) International Committee for Monitoring Assisted Reproductive Technology (ICMART) and the World Health Organization (WHO) revised glossary of ART terminology. Human Reproduction
31. Verlinsky Y, Kuliev A (2005) Practical preimplantation genetic diagnosis. Springer-Verlag, London
32. Gianaroli L, Magli MC, Lappi M et al (2009) Preconception diagnosis. Reprod Biomed Online 18(Supplement 3):S-5
33. Cohen J, Wells D, Munne S (2007) Removal of 2 cells from cleavage stage embryos is likely to reduce the efficacy of chromosomal tests that are used to enhance implantation rates. Fertil Steril 87(3):496–503. https://doi.org/10.1016/j.fertnstert.2006.07.1516
34. De Vos A, Staessen C, De Rycke M et al (2009) Impact of cleavage-stage embryo biopsy in view of PGD on human blastocyst implantation: a prospective cohort of single embryo transfers. Hum Reprod 24 (12):2988–2996. https://doi.org/10.1093/humrep/dep251
35. Goossens V, De Rycke M, De Vos A et al (2008) Diagnostic efficiency, embryonic development and clinical outcome after the biopsy of one or two blastomeres for preimplantation genetic diagnosis. Hum Reprod 23 (3):481–492. https://doi.org/10.1093/humrep/dem327
36. Buster JE, Bustillo M, Rodi IA et al (1985) Biologic and morphologic development of donated human ova recovered by nonsurgical uterine lavage. Am J Obstet Gynecol 153 (2):211–217
37. Carson S (1991) Biopsy of blastocysts. In: Verlinsky Y, Kuliev A (eds) Preimplantation genetics. Plenum Press, New York
38. McArthur SJ, Leigh D, Marshall JT et al (2005) Pregnancies and live births after trophectoderm biopsy and preimplantation genetic testing of human blastocysts. Fertil Steril 84(6):1628–1636. https://doi.org/10.1016/j.fertnstert.2005.05.063
39. McArthur SJ, Leigh D, Marshall JT et al (2008) Blastocyst trophectoderm biopsy and preimplantation genetic diagnosis for familial monogenic disorders and chromosomal translocations. Prenat Diagn 28(5):434–442. https://doi.org/10.1002/pd.1924
40. Schoolcraft WB, Fragouli E, Stevens J et al (2010) Clinical application of comprehensive chromosomal screening at the blastocyst stage. Fertil Steril 94(5):1700–1706. https://doi.org/10.1016/j.fertnstert.2009.10.015
41. Kuwayama M (2007) Highly efficient vitrification for cryopreservation of human oocytes and embryos: the cryotop method. Theriogenology 67(1):73–80. https://doi.org/10.1016/j.theriogenology.2006.09.014
42. Schlenker T, Stevens J, Rawlins M et al (2009) Clinical success with vitrification following trophectoderm biopsy for comprehensive chromosomal screening. Fertil Steril 92(3): S71
43. Zheng WT, Zhuang GL, Zhou CQ et al (2005) Comparison of the survival of human biopsied embryos after cryopreservation with four different methods using non-transferable embryos. Hum Reprod 20(6):1615–1618. https://doi.org/10.1093/humrep/deh808
44. Rechitsky S, Kuliev A, Sharapova T et al (2009) PGD impact on stem cell transplantation. Reprod Biomed Online 18(Supplement 3):S-2
45. Verlinsky Y, Kuliev A (2010) Preimplantation genetic diagnosis. In: Milunsky A, Mulinsky JM (eds) Genetic disorders and the fetus, 6th edn. Blackwell Publishing, Sussex, pp 950–977
46. Rechitsky S, Pakhalchuk T, San RG et al (2015) First systematic experience of preimplantation genetic diagnosis for single-gene disorders, and/or preimplantation human leukocyte antigen typing, combined with 24-chromosome aneuploidy testing. Fertil Steril 103(2):503–512. https://doi.org/10.1016/j.fertnstert.2014.11.007
47. Kuliev A, Rechitsky S, Verlinsky Y (2014) Atlas of preimplantation genetic diagnosis. CRS Press, Taylor and Francis, London
48. Gutierrez-Mateo C, Sanchez-Garcia JF, Fischer J et al (2009) Preimplantation genetic diagnosis of single-gene disorders: experience with more than 200 cycles conducted by a reference laboratory in the United States. Fertil Steril 92(5):1544–1556. https://doi.org/10.1016/j.fertnstert.2008.08.111
49. Committee EPCS (2002) ESHRE preimplantation genetic diagnosis consortium: data collection III (May 2001). Hum Reprod 17 (1):233–246
50. Rechitsky S, Pomerantseva E, Pakhalchuk T et al (2011) First systematic experience of preimplantation genetic diagnosis for de-novo mutations. Reprod Biomed Online 22(4):350–361. https://doi.org/10.1016/j.rbmo.2011.01.005

51. Braude PR, De Wert GM, Evers-Kiebooms G et al (1998) Non-disclosure preimplantation genetic diagnosis for Huntington's disease: practical and ethical dilemmas. Prenat Diagn 18(13):1422–1426
52. Simpson JL (2001) Celebrating preimplantation genetic diagnosis of p53 mutations in Li-Fraumeni syndrome. Reprod Biomed Online 3(1):2–3
53. Verlinsky Y, Rechitsky S, Verlinsky O et al (2001) Preimplantation diagnosis for p53 tumour suppressor gene mutations. Reprod Biomed Online 2(2):102–105
54. Rechitsky S, Verlinsky O, Chistokhina A et al (2002) Preimplantation genetic diagnosis for cancer predisposition. Reprod Biomed Online 5(2):148–155
55. Kuliev A, Pakhalchuk T, Rechitsky S (2015) Preimplantation genetic diagnosis (PGD) for heart disease determined by genetic factors. Arrhythm Open Access 1(1):103–106. https://doi.org/10.4172/atoa.1000103
56. Kuliev A, Pomerantseva E, Polling D et al (2012) PGD for inherited cardiac diseases. Reprod Biomed Online 24(4):443–453. https://doi.org/10.1016/j.rbmo.2011.12.009
57. Rechitsky S, Kuliev A, Tur-Kaspa I et al (2004) Preimplantation genetic diagnosis with HLA matching. Reprod Biomed Online 9(2):210–221
58. Verlinsky Y, Rechitsky S, Schoolcraft W et al (2001) Preimplantation diagnosis for Fanconi anemia combined with HLA matching. JAMA 285(24):3130–3133
59. Kuliev A, Verlinsky Y (2004) Thirteen years' experience of preimplantation diagnosis: report of the Fifth International Symposium on Preimplantation Genetics. Reprod Biomed Online 8(2):229–235
60. Kuliev A, Verlinsky Y (2006) The future of preimplantation genetic diagnosis. Expert Review of Obstetrics & Gynecolog 1 (1):65–72
61. Verlinsky Y, Rechitsky S, Sharapova T et al (2004) Preimplantation HLA testing. JAMA 291(17):2079–2085. https://doi.org/10.1001/jama.291.17.2079
62. Kahraman S (2013) PGD for HLA: clinical outcomes of HLA compatible transplantation following PGD. Reprod Biomed Online 26 (Supplement 1):S9–S10
63. Kahraman S, Beyazyurek C, Ekmekci CG (2011) Seven years of experience of preimplantation HLA typing: a clinical overview of 327 cycles. Reprod Biomed Online 23 (3):363–371. https://doi.org/10.1016/j.rbmo.2011.05.016
64. Kuliev A, Verlinsky O, Rechitsky S (2014) Preimplantation HLA typing for stem cell transplantation treatment of hemoglobinopathies. Thalassemia Reports 4(2):1853
65. Kuliev A (2013) Practical preimplantation genetic diagnosis. Springer, London, Heidelberg, New York
66. Munne S, Morrison L, Fung J et al (1998) Spontaneous abortions are reduced after preconception diagnosis of translocations. J Assist Reprod Genet 15(5):290–296
67. Otani T, Roche M, Mizuike M et al (2006) Preimplantation genetic diagnosis significantly improves the pregnancy outcome of translocation carriers with a history of recurrent miscarriage and unsuccessful pregnancies. Reprod Biomed Online 13(6):869–874
68. Goddijn M, Joosten JH, Knegt AC et al (2004) Clinical relevance of diagnosing structural chromosome abnormalities in couples with repeated miscarriage. Hum Reprod 19 (4):1013–1017. https://doi.org/10.1093/humrep/deh172
69. Stephenson MD, Sierra S (2006) Reproductive outcomes in recurrent pregnancy loss associated with a parental carrier of a structural chromosome rearrangement. Hum Reprod 21(4):1076–1082. https://doi.org/10.1093/humrep/dei417
70. Sugiura-Ogasawara M, Ozaki Y, Sato T et al (2004) Poor prognosis of recurrent aborters with either maternal or paternal reciprocal translocations. Fertil Steril 81(2):367–373. https://doi.org/10.1016/j.fertnstert.2003.07.014
71. Fritz MA, Schattman G (2008) Reply of the Committee: parental translocations and need for preimplantation genetic diagnosis? Distorting effects of ascertainment bias and the need for information-rich families. Fertil Steril 90(3):892–893
72. Gianaroli L, Magli MC, Ferraretti AP et al (1999) Preimplantation diagnosis for aneuploidies in patients undergoing in vitro fertilization with a poor prognosis: identification of the categories for which it should be proposed. Fertil Steril 72(5):837–844
73. Gianaroli L, Magli MC, Ferraretti AP et al (2005) The beneficial effects of preimplantation genetic diagnosis for aneuploidy support extensive clinical application. Reprod Biomed Online 10(5):633–640
74. Munne S, Magli C, Cohen J et al (1999) Positive outcome after preimplantation

diagnosis of aneuploidy in human embryos. Hum Reprod 14(9):2191–2199
75. Munne S, Sandalinas M, Escudero T et al (2003) Improved implantation after preimplantation genetic diagnosis of aneuploidy. Reprod Biomed Online 7(1):91–97
76. Verlinsky Y, Kuliev A (2005) PGD and it role in ART. In: Brisden P (ed) Textbook of IVF and assisted preproduction. Parthenon Publishing Group, London
77. Verlinsky Y, Tur-Kaspa I, Cieslak J et al (2005) Preimplantation testing for chromosomal disorders improves reproductive outcome of poor-prognosis patients. Reprod Biomed Online 11(2):219–225
78. Mersereau JE, Pergament E, Zhang X et al (2008) Preimplantation genetic screening to improve in vitro fertilization pregnancy rates: a prospective randomized controlled trial. Fertil Steril 90(4):1287–1289. https://doi.org/10.1016/j.fertnstert.2007.08.010
79. Werlin L, Rodi I, DeCherney A et al (2003) Preimplantation genetic diagnosis as both a therapeutic and diagnostic tool in assisted reproductive technology. Fertil Steril 80 (2):467–468
80. Hardarson T, Hanson C, Lundin K et al (2008) Preimplantation genetic screening in women of advanced maternal age caused a decrease in clinical pregnancy rate: a randomized controlled trial. Hum Reprod 23 (12):2806–2812. https://doi.org/10.1093/humrep/den217
81. Mastenbroek S, Twisk M, van Echten-Arends J et al (2007) In vitro fertilization with preimplantation genetic screening. N Engl J Med 357(1):9–17. https://doi.org/10.1056/NEJMoa067744
82. Staessen C, Platteau P, Van Assche E et al (2004) Comparison of blastocyst transfer with or without preimplantation genetic diagnosis for aneuploidy screening in couples with advanced maternal age: a prospective randomized controlled trial. Hum Reprod 19 (12):2849–2858. https://doi.org/10.1093/humrep/deh536
83. Staessen C, Verpoest W, Donoso P et al (2008) Preimplantation genetic screening does not improve delivery rate in women under the age of 36 following single-embryo transfer. Hum Reprod 23(12):2818–2825. https://doi.org/10.1093/humrep/den367
84. Cohen J, Grifo JA (2007) Multicentre trial of preimplantation genetic screening reported in the New England Journal of Medicine: an in-depth look at the findings. Reprod Biomed Online 15(4):365–366
85. Munne S, Cohen J, Simpson JL (2007) In vitro fertilization with preimplantation genetic screening. N Engl J Med 357 (17):1769–1770.; author reply 1770-1761. https://doi.org/10.1056/NEJMc076314
86. Munne S, Gianaroli L, Tur-Kaspa I et al (2007) Substandard application of preimplantation genetic screening may interfere with its clinical success. Fertil Steril 88(4):781–784. https://doi.org/10.1016/j.fertnstert.2007.08.002
87. Simpson JL (2008) What next for preimplantation genetic screening? Randomized clinical trial in assessing PGS: necessary but not sufficient. Hum Reprod 23(10):2179–2181. https://doi.org/10.1093/humrep/den250
88. Voullaire L, Slater H, Williamson R et al (2000) Chromosome analysis of blastomeres from human embryos by using comparative genomic hybridization. Hum Genet 106 (2):210–217
89. Wells D, Delhanty JD (2000) Comprehensive chromosomal analysis of human preimplantation embryos using whole genome amplification and single cell comparative genomic hybridization. Mol Hum Reprod 6 (11):1055–1062
90. Wilton L, Williamson R, McBain J et al (2001) Birth of a healthy infant after preimplantation confirmation of euploidy by comparative genomic hybridization. N Engl J Med 345(21):1537–1541. https://doi.org/10.1056/NEJMoa011052
91. Wells D, Alfarawati S, Fragouli E (2008) Use of comprehensive chromosomal screening for embryo assessment: microarrays and CGH. Mol Hum Reprod 14(12):703–710. https://doi.org/10.1093/molehr/gan062
92. Wells D, Fragouli E, Alfarawaty S et al (2009) Highly significant improvement in embryo implantation and increased live birth rate achieved after comprehensive chromosomal screening: implications for single embryo transfer. Fertility and Sterility 92(3 (Supplement)):S79
93. Handyside AH, Harton GL, Mariani B et al (2010) Karyomapping: a universal method for genome wide analysis of genetic disease based on mapping crossovers between parental haplotypes. J Med Genet 47(10):651–658. https://doi.org/10.1136/jmg.2009.069971
94. Johnson DS, Gemelos G, Baner J et al (2010) Preclinical validation of a microarray method for full molecular karyotyping of blastomeres in a 24-h protocol. Hum Reprod 25 (4):1066–1075. https://doi.org/10.1093/humrep/dep452

95. Vanneste E, Voet T, Le Caignec C et al (2009) Chromosome instability is common in human cleavage-stage embryos. Nat Med 15 (5):577–583. https://doi.org/10.1038/nm.1924
96. Treff N, Tao X, Su J et al (2009) Four hour 24 chromosome aneuploidy screening using high throughput PCR SNP allele ratio analyses. Fertility and Sterility 92(3 (Supplement)):S49–S50
97. Munne S, Grifo J, Wells D (2016) Mosaicism: "survival of the fittest" versus "no embryo left behind". Fertil Steril 105(5):1146–1149. https://doi.org/10.1016/j.fertnstert.2016.01.016
98. Debrock S, Melotte C, Spiessens C et al (2010) Preimplantation genetic screening for aneuploidy of embryos after in vitro fertilization in women aged at least 35 years: a prospective randomized trial. Fertil Steril 93 (2):364–373. https://doi.org/10.1016/j.fertnstert.2008.10.072
99. Harton GL, Munne S, Surrey M et al (2013) Diminished effect of maternal age on implantation after preimplantation genetic diagnosis with array comparative genomic hybridization. Fertil Steril 100(6):1695–1703. https://doi.org/10.1016/j.fertnstert.2013.07.2002
100. Forman EJ, Hong KH, Franasiak JM et al (2014) Obstetrical and neonatal outcomes from the BEST Trial: single embryo transfer with aneuploidy screening improves outcomes after in vitro fertilization without compromising delivery rates. Am J Obstet Gynecol 210(2):157 e151–157 e156. https://doi.org/10.1016/j.ajog.2013.10.016
101. Franasiak JM, Scott RT Jr (2014) Embryonic aneuploidy: overcoming molecular genetics challenges improves outcomes and changes practice patterns. Trends Mol Med 20 (9):499–508. https://doi.org/10.1016/j.molmed.2014.06.006
102. Greco E, Minasi MG, Fiorentino F (2015) Healthy babies after intrauterine transfer of mosaic aneuploid blastocysts. N Engl J Med 373(21):2089–2090. https://doi.org/10.1056/NEJMc1500421
103. Chang J, Boulet SL, Jeng G et al (2016) Outcomes of in vitro fertilization with preimplantation genetic diagnosis: an analysis of the United States Assisted Reproductive Technology Surveillance Data, 2011-2012. Fertil Steril 105(2):394–400. https://doi.org/10.1016/j.fertnstert.2015.10.018
104. Scott RT Jr, Galliano D (2016) The challenge of embryonic mosaicism in preimplantation genetic screening. Fertil Steril 105 (5):1150–1152. https://doi.org/10.1016/j.fertnstert.2016.01.007
105. Simpson JL, Kuliev A (2016) Commentary re: causes and estimated incidences of sex-chromosome misdiagnosis in preimplantation genetic diagnosis of aneuploidy. Reprod Biomed Online 33(5):585–586. https://doi.org/10.1016/j.rbmo.2016.08.018
106. Brigham SA, Conlon C, Farquharson RG (1999) A longitudinal study of pregnancy outcome following idiopathic recurrent miscarriage. Hum Reprod 14(11):2868–2871
107. Munne S, Chen S, Fischer J et al (2005) Preimplantation genetic diagnosis reduces pregnancy loss in women aged 35 years and older with a history of recurrent miscarriages. Fertil Steril 84(2):331–335. https://doi.org/10.1016/j.fertnstert.2005.02.027
108. Warburton D, Dallaire L, Thangavelu M et al (2004) Trisomy recurrence: a reconsideration based on North American data. Am J Hum Genet 75(3):376–385
109. Rubio C, Simon C, Vidal F et al (2003) Chromosomal abnormalities and embryo development in recurrent miscarriage couples. Hum Reprod 18(1):182–188
110. Murugappan G, Shahine LK, Perfetto CO et al (2016) Intent to treat analysis of in vitro fertilization and preimplantation genetic screening versus expectant management in patients with recurrent pregnancy loss. Hum Reprod 31(8):1668–1674. https://doi.org/10.1093/humrep/dew135

Chapter 3

Noninvasive Approaches to Prenatal Diagnosis: Historical Perspective and Future Directions

Lisa Hui

Abstract

The field of prenatal screening and diagnosis has undergone enormous progress over the past four decades. Most of this period has been characterized by gradual improvements in the technical and public health aspects of prenatal screening for Down syndrome. Compared to the direct analysis of fetal cells from amniocentesis or chorionic villus sampling, noninvasive approaches using maternal blood or ultrasound have the great advantage of posing no risk of miscarriage to the pregnancy. Recent advances in molecular genetics and DNA sequencing have revolutionized both the accuracy and the range of noninvasive testing for genetic abnormalities using cell-free DNA in maternal plasma. Many of these advances have already been incorporated into clinical care, including diagnosis of fetal blood group and aneuploidy screening. The accelerated pace of these recent developments is creating not just technical and logistical challenges, but is also magnifying the ethical and public policy issues traditionally associated with this field.

Key words Noninvasive prenatal testing, Noninvasive prenatal diagnosis, Cell-free DNA, Fetal cells, Nuchal translucency, Serum screening, Next-generation sequencing

1 Historical Perspective of Noninvasive Prenatal Diagnosis

The field of noninvasive prenatal screening and diagnosis has undergone enormous progress over the past four decades (Fig. 1). Compared to the direct analysis of fetal cells from amniocentesis or chorionic villus sampling, noninvasive approaches using maternal blood or ultrasound have the great advantage of posing no risk of miscarriage to the pregnancy.

1.1 Screening for Chromosome Abnormalities by Maternal Age

Prenatal screening for fetal anomalies has traditionally focused on chromosome abnormalities because they are major causes of perinatal morbidity and mortality. Aneuploidies are also amenable to invasive prenatal diagnosis from fetal cells using standard cytogenetic techniques, allowing a definitive diagnosis before 20 weeks gestation. The first fetal diagnosis of Down syndrome was performed using cultured amniotic fluid cells in 1968 [1].

Brynn Levy (ed.), *Prenatal Diagnosis*, Methods in Molecular Biology, vol. 1885, https://doi.org/10.1007/978-1-4939-8889-1_3,

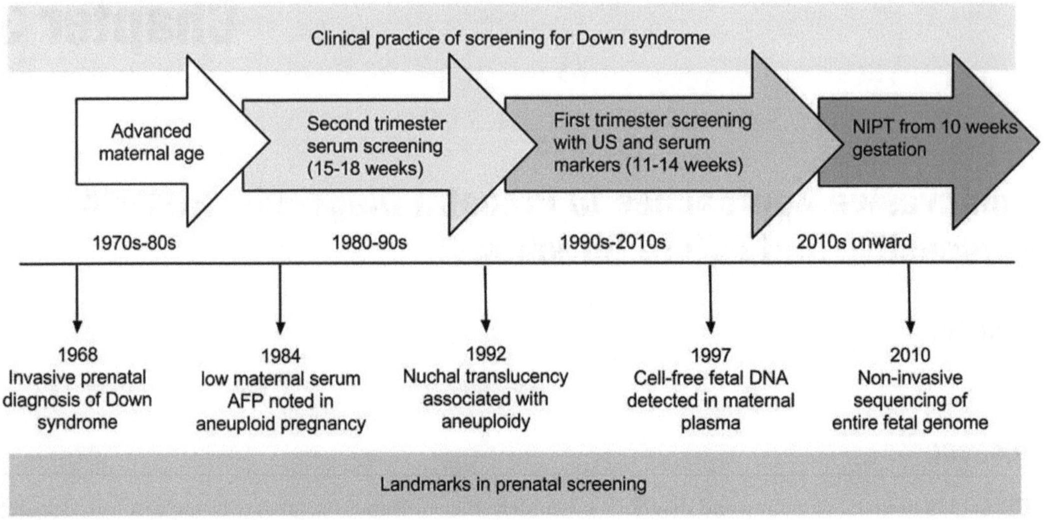

Fig. 1 Timeline of prenatal testing for fetal aneuploidy *AFP* alphafetoprotein, *US* ultrasound, *NIPT* noninvasive DNA-based prenatal testing

Down syndrome, or trisomy 21, is the most common autosomal aneuploidy leading to live birth and consequently is the most important genetic cause of intellectual disability. As invasive testing with amniocentesis or chorionic villus sampling (CVS) carries an appreciable risk of miscarriage, estimated at 0.5 to 1.0% [2], it has been a long-standing goal of prenatal diagnosis to develop a noninvasive test for trisomy 21.

The most important risk factor for trisomy 21 is maternal age. The risk of an affected newborn at term is approximately 1 in 300 for a woman aged 35 years, increasing to 1 in 100 by the maternal age of 40 years [3]. Consequently, the prevalence of trisomy 21 has increased due to trends to later childbearing in most developed counties. The estimated birth prevalence of trisomy 21 is now around 1.4 to 1.7 per 1000 births [4, 5].

For several decades, screening for Down syndrome was based on maternal age alone, with women at increased risk (typically using an age threshold of 35 years or more) being offered invasive prenatal testing. This method only detects 30–40% of all fetuses with trisomy 21 as the majority of affected pregnancies occur in women less than 35 years old. This aged-based approach also exposes older women to high rates of invasive testing (about 50% uptake) for a relatively low diagnostic yield.

1.2 Second Trimester Screening for Aneuploidy Using Maternal Serum Biochemical Markers

In the late 1970s, maternal serum screening for neural tube defects was introduced into clinical practice [6]. From this screening program arose the observation that maternal serum alpha fetoprotein (AFP) was reduced in pregnancies affected by chromosome abnormalities [7]. This serendipitous discovery represented a landmark in prenatal screening for aneuploidy [8]. Subsequently, other serum markers of aneuploidy were discovered and combined with AFP to improve the performance of serum screening for both trisomy 21 and 18. The addition of human chorionic gonadotropin (hCG) [9] and unconjugated estriol [10] to AFP measurement created the "triple test" [11]. This could identify approximately 70% of pregnancies affected by trisomy 21 for a 5% screen-positive rate [12, 13]. The later addition of inhibin-A created the "quadruple test," increasing detection rates to approximately 80% [12]. Second trimester serum screening thus allowed women of all ages to have a risk assessment for aneuploidy, not just those women of advanced maternal age. Screening was confined to a specific gestational age window (ideally 15–18 weeks), and those who received a high risk result (arbitrarily set at around 1/300 risk or higher) were offered a definitive diagnosis with an invasive test.

1.3 Second Trimester Ultrasound Screening for Aneuploidy

The field of prenatal ultrasound underwent major developments in parallel to those of serum screening in the 1980s. A second trimester morphology ultrasound for fetal structural abnormalities became a routine part of prenatal care, enabling the detection of aneuploid fetuses with structural malformations. Major structural malformations that are strongly associated with Down syndrome include atrioventricular septal defects, tetralogy of Fallot, duodenal atresia, cystic hygroma, and hydrops fetalis [14]. The presence of a major anomaly is an indication for invasive testing, however the utility of second trimester ultrasound as a stand-alone screening test for trisomy 21 is limited by its relatively low sensitivity [15].

The second trimester morphology scan also can detect anatomical variants known as "soft markers" that are present in increased frequency in aneuploid fetuses. The sonographic "soft markers" of Down syndrome include increased nuchal fold, hypoplastic nasal bone, echogenic bowel, and short femur. Individually, these markers have poor sensitivity and specificity for Down syndrome, but their predictive value increases if multiple markers are present [16]. These markers have been used to calculate likelihood ratios for an affected pregnancy [17], but the use of this approach is now being questioned in the era of widespread first trimester screening for aneuploidy [18].

1.4 First Trimester Screening with Biochemical and Ultrasound Markers

In the early 1990s an important observation that first trimester fetuses with excessive fluid accumulation in the neck were more likely to be aneuploid was reported [19]. The measurement of the fetal nuchal translucency thickness at 11–13 weeks gestation was subsequently established as the single most powerful sonographic marker of trisomy 21 [20]. For a fixed screen positive rate of 5%, and a risk cutoff of 1 in 300, up to 80% of affected pregnancies could be detected by the combination of nuchal translucency measurement and maternal age. The added attraction of this test was the earlier stage of diagnosis compared with second trimester serum screening.

The performance of the first trimester ultrasound was improved by the addition of first trimester serum markers. In combination with maternal serum measurement of free β-hCG and pregnancy-associated protein-A (PAPP-A), detection rates of 85–90% could be achieved for a false positive rate of 5% [12, 13]. Risk results for trisomy 13 and 18 were also incorporated into the first trimester combined screening algorithm. This first trimester combined test has now largely replaced second trimester maternal serum screening as the standard of care in most developed countries, due to its dual advantages of improved accuracy and earlier diagnosis.

Other first trimester sonographic markers of aneuploidy have been developed, including assessment of the nasal bone [21], ductus venosus waveform [22], and tricuspid valve flow [23]. The addition of these markers to the first trimester combined test increases detection rates to 96% and lowers the false positive rate to 2.5% [24]. However, the practical barriers to universal implementation of these advanced ultrasound markers are even greater than those faced by nuchal translucency measurement alone and as such they have not been uniformly adopted outside of specialist centers [25].

1.5 Combined First and Second Trimester Screening Strategies

Many models have been investigated to determine the utility of combining first and second trimester screening strategies. These include the integrated, stepwise, and contingent screening approaches [12, 13, 26]. However, serial testing with independent risk results in first and second trimesters is not generally recommended due to the higher cumulative false positive rate.

2 DNA-Based Tests Using Maternal Blood

Fetal cells and cell-free nucleic acids derived from the placenta are consistently detectable in maternal blood. This phenomenon provides the opportunity to directly sample fetal genetic material in maternal blood for noninvasive DNA-based testing. It is in this area that the most exciting recent advances in noninvasive testing have taken place.

2.1 Fetal Cells in Maternal Blood

The presence of fetal cells in maternal tissues is a long-recognized phenomenon, first described in 1893 when syncytiotrophoblastic cells were documented in the lungs of women who had died from eclampsia [27]. Fetal lymphocytes were detected in maternal blood many years later in 1969 and their potential for prenatal diagnosis was immediately recognized [28]. However, it was several decades until technology could capitalize on this fetomaternal cell trafficking for the purposes of prenatal diagnosis. In 1990 DNA was successfully isolated from circulating fetal cells in maternal blood to diagnose fetal sex [29]. It was also discovered that some fetal cells, namely lymphocytes, could remain in the maternal body for decades postpartum [30], potentially confounding prenatal testing results from subsequent pregnancies. Fetal erythroblasts, or nucleated red cells, were therefore considered the most suitable for noninvasive prenatal diagnosis (NIPD) because they are detectable from early pregnancy, have short life spans, and can be distinguished from maternal cells using embryonic hemoglobin markers. However, fetal cells are only present in very small numbers in maternal blood despite enrichment protocols [31] and they are difficult to culture without maternal cell contamination [32]. The first major attempt to ascertain the clinical feasibility of using fetal cells for prenatal diagnosis was the NIFTY study [33]. This study reported a sensitivity rate for aneuploidy of 74.4% with a false positive rate 0.6–4.1% and a fetal gender detection rate of 41.4%. The investigators concluded that significant technical challenges needed to be overcome before it was a feasible method for clinical practice. A variety of enrichment methods have continued to be explored, including fluorescence-activated cell sorting, magnetic-activated cell sorting, density gradient centrifugation, and more recently, nuclear reprogramming of fetal erythrocytes [34].

2.2 Cell-Free DNA in Maternal Plasma

The detection of cell-free fetal DNA in maternal plasma in 1997 was a watershed moment in noninvasive prenatal testing [35]. The major source of circulating cell-free fetal DNA is the trophoblast, which releases DNA into the circulation as a result of apoptosis [36–38]. Cell-free DNA of placental origin is detectable as early as 5 weeks of gestation, prior to the establishment of the fetal circulation [39], and it is clearly rapidly after delivery [40, 41]. These circulating nucleic acids have been the subject of remarkable achievements in the past decade.

2.2.1 Obstetric Outcomes Using Quantitative Analysis of Cell-Free Fetal DNA

Obstetric complications due to abnormal placentation may be accompanied by altered levels of circulating nucleic acids of placental origin due to increased trophoblast microparticle release [42]. Quantitative changes in total cell-free fetal DNA in maternal plasma are potential predictors of adverse obstetric complications such as preeclampsia and intrauterine growth restriction [43–45]. Early studies quantifying circulating fetal DNA were based on the detection of Y chromosome-specific sequences, but this approach was limited to pregnancies in which the fetus was male. The lack of a gender-independent, fetus-specific DNA marker was a major barrier to clinical translation. Sequences that are differentially methylated in the fetus compared with the mother, such as MASPIN [46] or the promoter region of RASSF1A [47], have been successfully used as universal fetal DNA markers; however, the technical challenges of studying differential methylation are considerable. An alternative approach to study obstetric disorders using cell-free nucleic acids is to use RNA markers of placental origin [48–50], but this appears some way from application in a clinical setting [45]. More recently, mechanisms involving the TLR9 receptor that link alterations in cell-free DNA levels and parturition have been postulated [51]. This suggests future avenues for non-genetic obstetric disorders such as preterm birth to be investigated using cell-free fetal DNA.

2.2.2 Noninvasive Prenatal Diagnosis Using Cell-Free Fetal DNA

The term noninvasive prenatal diagnosis (NIPD) is generally used to refer to DNA-based tests of fetal health that do not require direct access into the uterus and that are sufficiently accurate not to require follow-up confirmation with amniocentesis or CVS. The earliest successful clinical applications of cell-free fetal DNA were for the noninvasive diagnosis of fetal Rhesus D antigen status and fetal sex.

The detection of a paternally inherited allele in the fetus is a relatively simple problem of detecting the unique sequence in maternal blood. The detection of Y-chromosome-specific sequences in maternal plasma using real-time qPCR was used to first demonstrate the presence of cell-free fetal DNA in maternal blood [35]. Medical indications for early prenatal diagnosis of fetal sex include pregnancies at risk of X-linked disease, or in utero virilization from congenital adrenal hyperplasia. NIPD using qPCR for the male-specific SRY or DYS 14 loci is reliable for fetal sex from 7 weeks gestation, much earlier than is possible for either invasive testing or ultrasound. The accuracy of NIPD for fetal sex is very high [52] and can achieve sensitivity >99.5% with stringent quality control [53]. NIPD for diagnosis of fetal sex has been clinically available in the UK for over 8 years and has substantially reduced the number of women undergoing invasive procedures [53].

NIPD for fetal Rhesus blood group is the other major successful application of cell-free fetal DNA. The basis of this test is the amplification of the RHD gene in Rhesus D negative pregnant women to allow early identification of fetuses at risk of hemolytic disease. NIPD for fetal D antigen status became widely available more than 10 years ago in the United Kingdom through the International Blood Group Reference Laboratory [54]. Other countries in Europe quickly adopted this technology, aided by the Special Non-invasive Advances in Fetal and Neonatal Evaluation Network [55]. In Denmark, NIPD testing is now implemented on a national basis to restrict anti-D immunoglobulin prophylaxis to those carrying a Rhesus positive fetus. NIPD at 25 weeks of gestation can detect 99.9% of Rhesus positive fetuses and reduce unnecessary prenatal RhD prophylaxis in 97.3% of women carrying an RhD-negative fetus [56].

NIPD for other single gene disorders has received relatively less attention than Rhesus typing due to the need for disease-specific or patient-specific assay development. However, a number of disorders have been detected using cell-free fetal DNA in proof-of-principle studies, including hemoglobinopathies [57] and fetal/neonatal alloimmune thrombocytopenia [58]. The use of digital PCR may improve detection of paternally inherited mutations and facilitate further clinical applications [59, 60].

However, it is the enormous capabilities of next generation sequencing that may rapidly advance NIPD for single gene disorders. A recent proof of principle study of the noninvasive diagnosis of congenital adrenal hyperplasia before 9 weeks gestation using next generation DNA sequencing suggests that NIPD for a wider range of autosomal recessive disorders may become a clinical reality in the near future [61].

2.2.3 Aneuploidy Detection Using Cell-Free DNA

The diagnosis of fetal aneuploidy using cell-free DNA in maternal plasma poses a much greater technical challenge than the detection of paternally inherited fetal sequences. Detection of fetal aneuploidy from maternal plasma requires the determination of relative chromosome dosage in the fetus from a mixed population of maternal and placental cell-free DNA fragments. Furthermore, DNA fragments of fetal origin are not readily distinguishable from those of maternal origin. The recent application of next generation sequencing techniques to this task has led to revolutionary advances in noninvasive prenatal testing for aneuploidy.

Sequencing is the determination of the individual base order of nucleotide bases in a sample of DNA or RNA. "First generation," or Sanger sequencing, was the primary method of sequencing dating from the 1980s. This method is very accurate and can sequence very long stretches of DNA (500–600 bases per read), but is relatively slow and not conducive to high throughput. Next generation sequencing is based on similar approach of synthesizing DNA from single stranded genomic DNA template but it performs multiple short reads simultaneously, in a "massively parallel" fashion. In massively parallel sequencing (MPS), only a fraction of each DNA fragment is actually sequenced. A 36-base pair read is typically sufficient to map a DNA fragment to a unique location in the human genome and thus identify its chromosome of origin. Hence, sequencing for noninvasive prenatal testing for fetal aneuploidy (NIPT) does not aim to reconstruct the actual fetal or maternal genome, but simply determines the relative contribution of chromosomes to the cell-free population in maternal plasma. This approach is based on the assumption that the entire genome is represented in maternal plasma at a constant relative proportion. If there is more than expected cell-free DNA originating chromosome 21, this is evidence of a pregnancy affected by trisomy 21. However, the mean proportion of cell-free DNA of placental origin in maternal plasma is only 10% at 13 weeks gestation [62]. The high background level of maternal cell-free DNA means that high precision counting is required to detect an affected pregnancy.

Since 2011, multiple groups have demonstrated the clinical validity of a DNA-based sequencing approach for fetal aneuploidy in high risk women. The various terms noninvasive prenatal testing (NIPT), noninvasive prenatal screening (NIPS), and noninvasive DNA-based testing (NIDT) have been coined to distinguish this test from NIPD, as it is not considered a diagnostic test.

Various methods exist, including MPS of the whole genome (random sequencing) [63–68], chromosome selective approaches using targeted assays [69–72], or single nucleotide polymorphism-based assays [73, 74]. The MPS method has the potential to provide information across the entire genome, including detection of whole chromosome and subchromosomal abnormalities [64, 75, 76]. However, targeted approaches have much lower sequencing requirements as only DNA fragments unique to the chromosomes of interest are sequenced, and therefore have advantages in cost and throughput.

The extremely high sensitivity (98.58–100%) and specificity (97.95–100%) of NIPT outperform any screening method for aneuploidy to date [77]. It is also effective from 10 weeks gestation on, with no upper gestational age limit, greatly improving the flexibility of timing of testing. Professional societies have now endorsed its use in high risk women, but emphasize that it remains a screening, not a diagnostic test [78, 79]. Given the relatively low a priori risk of an affected fetus even in high risk groups, and the potentially serious consequences of a false positive result, confirmatory invasive testing is still required after an abnormal NIPT result [80]. As test performance is not affected by maternal age, NIPT in low risk populations appears to perform just as well as in high risk populations [81–83].

In a direct clinical comparison between standard prenatal screening and DNA sequencing-based methods, the anticipated advantages of NIPT were confirmed [84]. Specifically, there was a much lower false positive rate with cell-free DNA-based testing vs routine screening for trisomy 21 (0.3% vs. 3.6%), with a corresponding higher positive predictive value of 45.5% vs. 4.2%.

The major limitation of NIPT is the high cost compared with current screening techniques. In most countries, this cost has been directly born by the patient or their private insurer, creating substantial issues with equity of access. Reductions in invasive testing rates have been widely reported since the introduction of NIPT into clinical practice but the many ethical and public health challenges associated with its implementation remain to be solved [85, 86].

3 Future Directions

The past 40 years have seen prenatal screening and diagnosis for aneuploidy become an integral part of pregnancy care. All women, regardless of background risk, are now offered some form of noninvasive testing for trisomy 21 [87]. The field has grown to encompass the various disciplines of epidemiology, laboratory medicine, obstetric ultrasound, clinical genetics, bioinformatics, genomics, genetic counseling, bioethics, and health economics. The final result of these developments has been the steady reduction in the number of women undergoing invasive testing, and an increase in the prenatal detection rate of Down syndrome [5, 88, 89].

The knowledge accumulated over several decades of screening with maternal serum biochemistry and ultrasound is now being rapidly eclipsed by advances in molecular genetics and direct analysis of fetal DNA using noninvasive methods. Noninvasive prenatal testing is no longer just about trisomy 21, 18, and 13. Noninvasive DNA-based testing for fetal aneuploidy has already expanded beyond these three common autosomal trisomies to include fetal sex, sex chromosome aneuploidy [90], selected microdeletion syndromes [91, 92], and genome-wide abnormalities [75]. It is now possible to interrogate the fetal genome at the same resolution as a chromosomal array [93] and to even reconstruct the entire fetal genome from maternal blood [94–96].

This represents the final convergence of the major themes in noninvasive prenatal testing from the past decades (Fig. 2). This paradigm shift has enormous ethical, medical, and resource implications for the field. We stand at the crossroads where noninvasive

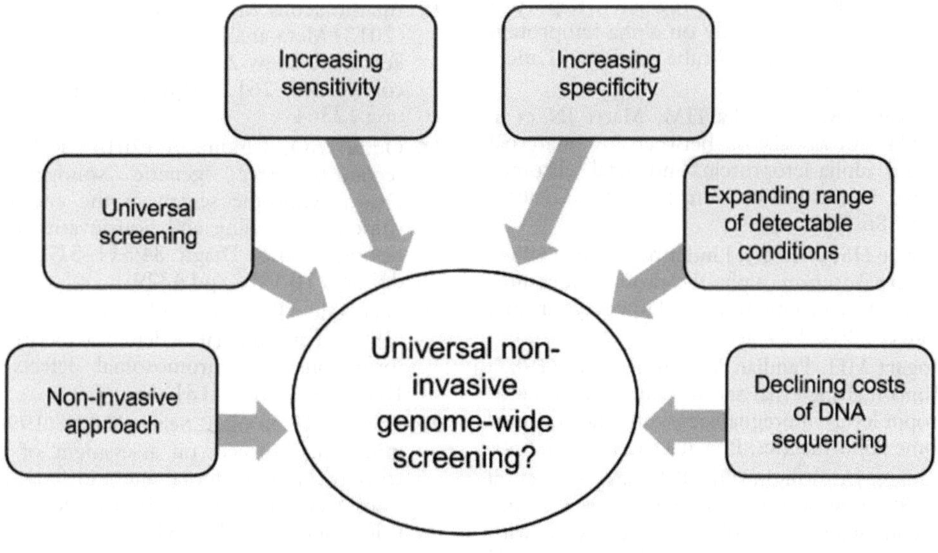

Fig. 2 Converging trends in screening for chromosomal abnormalities

prenatal testing is posed to move beyond the detection of common aneuploidies to encompass the whole range of human genetic variation. The major future challenges in the noninvasive detection of genetic abnormalities are therefore not simply technical, but ethical and social.

References

1. Valenti C, Schutta EJ, Kehaty T (1968) Prenatal diagnosis of Down's syndrome. Lancet 2:220
2. Tabor A, Alfirevic Z (2010) Update on procedure-related risks for prenatal diagnosis techniques. Fetal Diagn Ther 27:1–7. https://doi.org/10.1159/000271995
3. Nicolaides KH (2004) First trimester diagnosis of chromosomal defects. In: The 11–13+6 week scan. Fetal Medicine Foundation, London
4. de Graaf G, Haveman M, Hochstenbach R et al (2011) Changes in yearly birth prevalence rates of children with Down syndrome in the period 1986-2007 in The Netherlands. J Intellect Disabil Res 55:462–473. https://doi.org/10.1111/j.1365-2788.2011.01398.x
5. Cheffins T, Chan A, Haan EA et al (2000) The impact of maternal serum screening on the birth prevalence of Down's syndrome and the use of amniocentesis and chorionic villus sampling in South Australia. BJOG 107:1453–1459
6. Wald NJ, Cuckle H, Brock JH et al (1977) Maternal serum-alpha-fetoprotein measurement in antenatal screening for anencephaly and spina bifida in early pregnancy. Report of U.K. collaborative study on alpha-fetoprotein in relation to neural-tube defects. Lancet 1:1323–1332
7. Merkatz IR, Nitowsky HM, Macri JN et al (1984) An association between low maternal serum alpha-fetoprotein and fetal chromosomal abnormalities. Am J Obstet Gynecol 148:886–894
8. Cuckle HS, Wald NJ, Lindenbaum RH (1984) Maternal serum alpha-fetoprotein measurement: a screening test for Down syndrome. Lancet 1:926–929
9. Bogart MH, Pandian MR, Jones OW (1987) Abnormal maternal serum chorionic gonadotropin levels in pregnancies with fetal chromosome abnormalities. Prenat Diagn 7:623–630
10. Canick JA, Knight GJ, Palomaki GE et al (1988) Low second trimester maternal serum unconjugated oestriol in pregnancies with Down's syndrome. Br J Obstet Gynaecol 95:330–333
11. Wald NJ, Cuckle HS, Densem JW et al (1988) Maternal serum screening for Down's syndrome in early pregnancy. BMJ 297:883–887
12. Wald NJ, Rodeck C, Hackshaw AK et al (2003) First and second trimester antenatal screening for Down's syndrome: the results of the serum, urine and ultrasound screening study (SURUSS). J Med Screen 10:56–104
13. Malone FD, Canick JA, Ball RH et al (2005) First-trimester or second-trimester screening, or both, for Down's syndrome. N Engl J Med 353:2001–2011. https://doi.org/10.1056/NEJMoa043693
14. Bianchi DW, Crombleholme TM, D'Alton ME et al (2010) Fetology, 2nd edn. McGraw-Hill, New York, NY
15. Ewigman BG, Crane JP, Frigoletto FD et al (1993) Effect of prenatal ultrasound screening on perinatal outcome. RADIUS Study Group. N Engl J Med 329:821–827. https://doi.org/10.1056/NEJM199309163291201
16. Benacerraf BR (1996) Use of sonographic markers to determine the risk of Down syndrome in second-trimester fetuses. Radiology 201:619–620. https://doi.org/10.1148/radiology.201.3.8939206
17. Agathokleous M, Chaveeva P, Poon LC et al (2013) Meta-analysis of second-trimester markers for trisomy 21. Ultrasound Obstet Gynecol 41:247–261. https://doi.org/10.1002/uog.12364
18. Odibo AO, Ghidini A (2014) Role of the second-trimester 'genetic sonogram' for Down syndrome screen in the era of first-trimester screening and non-invasive prenatal testing. Prenat Diagn 34:511–517. https://doi.org/10.1002/pd.4329
19. Nicolaides KH, Azar G, Snijders RJ et al (1992) Fetal nuchal oedema: associated malformations and chromosomal defects. Fetal Diagn Ther 7:123–131
20. Snijders RJ, Noble P, Sebire N et al (1998) UK multicentre project on assessment of risk of trisomy 21 by maternal age and fetal nuchal-translucency thickness at 10-14 weeks of gestation. Lancet 352:343–346
21. Cicero S, Avgidou K, Rembouskos G et al (2006) Nasal bone in first-trimester screening for trisomy 21. Am J Obstet Gynecol

195:109–114. https://doi.org/10.1016/j.ajog.2005.12.057
22. Maiz N, Valencia C, Emmanuel EE et al (2008) Screening for adverse pregnancy outcome by ductus venosus doppler at 11-13+6 weeks of gestation. Obstet Gynecol 112:598–605. https://doi.org/10.1097/AOG.0b013e3181834608
23. Kagan KO, Valencia C, Livanos P et al (2009) Tricuspid regurgitation in screening for trisomies 21, 18 and 13 and turner syndrome at 11 +0 to 13+6 weeks of gestation. Ultrasound Obstet Gynecol 33:18–22. https://doi.org/10.1002/uog.6264
24. Nicolaides KH (2011) Screening for fetal aneuploidies at 11 to 13 weeks. Prenat Diagn 31:7–15. https://doi.org/10.1002/pd.2637
25. Malone FD (2005) Nuchal translucency-based Down syndrome screening: barriers to implementation. Semin Perinatol 29:272–276. https://doi.org/10.1053/j.semperi.2005.05.002
26. Cuckle H, Benn P, Wright D (2005) Down syndrome screening in the first and/or second trimester: model predicted performance using meta-analysis parameters. Semin Perinatol 29:252–257. https://doi.org/10.1053/j.semperi.2005.05.004
27. Schmorl CG (1893) Pathologisch-Anatomische Untersuchungen uber Puerperal Eklampsie [Pathological-anatomical explorations on puerperal eclampsia]. Verlag FCW Vogel, Leipzig
28. Walknowska J, Conte FA, Grumbach MM (1969) Practical and theoretical implications of fetal-maternal lymphocyte transfer. Lancet 1:1119–1122
29. Bianchi DW, Flint AF, Pizzimenti MF et al (1990) Isolation of fetal DNA from nucleated erythrocytes in maternal blood. Proc Natl Acad Sci U S A 87:3279–3283
30. Bianchi DW, Zickwolf GK, Weil GJ et al (1996) Male fetal progenitor cells persist in maternal blood for as long as 27 years postpartum. Proc Natl Acad Sci U S A 93:705–708
31. Busch J, Huber P, Pfluger E et al (1994) Enrichment of fetal cells from maternal blood by high gradient magnetic cell sorting (double MACS) for PCR-based genetic analysis. Prenat Diagn 14:1129–1140
32. Chen H, Griffin DK, Jestice K et al (1998) Evaluating the culture of fetal erythroblasts from maternal blood for non-invasive prenatal diagnosis. Prenat Diagn 18:883–892
33. Bianchi DW, Simpson JL, Jackson LG et al (2002) Fetal gender and aneuploidy detection using fetal cells in maternal blood: analysis of NIFTY I data. National Institute of Child Health and Development Fetal Cell Isolation Study. Prenat Diagn 22:609–615. https://doi.org/10.1002/pd.347
34. Huang Z, Fong CY, Gauthaman K et al (2011) Novel approaches to manipulating foetal cells in the maternal circulation for non-invasive prenatal diagnosis of the unborn child. J Cell Biochem 112:1475–1485. https://doi.org/10.1002/jcb.23084
35. Lo YM, Corbetta N, Chamberlain PF et al (1997) Presence of fetal DNA in maternal plasma and serum. Lancet 350:485–487. https://doi.org/10.1016/S0140-6736(97)02174-0
36. Alberry M, Maddocks D, Jones M et al (2007) Free fetal DNA in maternal plasma in anembryonic pregnancies: confirmation that the origin is the trophoblast. Prenat Diagn 27:415–418. https://doi.org/10.1002/pd.1700
37. Gupta AK, Holzgreve W, Huppertz B et al (2004) Detection of fetal DNA and RNA in placenta-derived syncytiotrophoblast microparticles generated in vitro. Clin Chem 50:2187–2190. https://doi.org/10.1373/clinchem.2004.040196
38. Masuzaki H, Miura K, Yoshiura KI et al (2004) Detection of cell free placental DNA in maternal plasma: direct evidence from three cases of confined placental mosaicism. J Med Genet 41:289–292
39. Guibert J, Benachi A, Grebille AG et al (2003) Kinetics of SRY gene appearance in maternal serum: detection by real time PCR in early pregnancy after assisted reproductive technique. Hum Reprod 18:1733–1736
40. Lo YM, Zhang J, Leung TN et al (1999) Rapid clearance of fetal DNA from maternal plasma. Am J Hum Genet 64:218–224. https://doi.org/10.1086/302205
41. Hui L, Vaughan JI, Nelson M (2008) Effect of labor on postpartum clearance of cell-free fetal DNA from the maternal circulation. Prenat Diagn 28:304–308. https://doi.org/10.1002/pd.1975
42. Rusterholz C, Messerli M, Hoesli I et al (2011) Placental microparticles, DNA, and RNA in preeclampsia. Hypertens Pregnancy 30:364–375. https://doi.org/10.3109/10641951003599571
43. Sifakis S, Zaravinos A, Maiz N et al (2009) First-trimester maternal plasma cell-free fetal DNA and preeclampsia. Am J Obstet Gynecol 201(472):e471–e477. https://doi.org/10.1016/j.ajog.2009.05.025
44. Caramelli E, Rizzo N, Concu M et al (2003) Cell-free fetal DNA concentration in plasma of

patients with abnormal uterine artery doppler waveform and intrauterine growth restriction—a pilot study. Prenat Diagn 23:367–371. https://doi.org/10.1002/pd.596

45. Hahn S, Rusterholz C, Hosli I et al (2011) Cell-free nucleic acids as potential markers for preeclampsia. Placenta 32(Suppl):S17–S20. https://doi.org/10.1016/j.placenta.2010.06.018
46. Chim SS, Tong YK, Chiu RW et al (2005) Detection of the placental epigenetic signature of the maspin gene in maternal plasma. Proc Natl Acad Sci U S A 102:14753–14758. https://doi.org/10.1073/pnas.0503335102
47. Chan KC, Ding C, Gerovassili A et al (2006) Hypermethylated RASSF1A in maternal plasma: a universal fetal DNA marker that improves the reliability of non-invasive prenatal diagnosis. Clin Chem 52:2211–2218. https://doi.org/10.1373/clinchem.2006.074997
48. Tsui NB, Lo YM (2008) A microarray approach for systematic identification of placental-derived RNA markers in maternal plasma. Methods Mol Biol 444:275–289. https://doi.org/10.1007/978-1-59745-066-9_22
49. Pang WW, Tsui MH, Sahota D et al (2009) A strategy for identifying circulating placental RNA markers for fetal growth assessment. Prenat Diagn 29:495–504. https://doi.org/10.1002/pd.2230
50. Whitehead CL, Tong S (2014) Measuring hypoxia-induced RNA in maternal blood: a new way to identify critically hypoxic fetuses in utero? Expert Rev Mol Diagn 14:509–511. https://doi.org/10.1586/14737159.2014.915749
51. Phillippe M (2014) Cell-free fetal DNA—a trigger for parturition. N Engl J Med 370:2534–2536. https://doi.org/10.1056/NEJMcibr1404324
52. Devaney SA, Palomaki GE, Scott JA et al (2011) Non-invasive fetal sex determination using cell-free fetal DNA: a systematic review and meta-analysis. JAMA 306:627–636. https://doi.org/10.1001/jama.2011.1114
53. Hill M, Finning K, Martin P et al (2011) Non-invasive prenatal determination of fetal sex: translating research into clinical practice. Clin Genet 80:68–75. https://doi.org/10.1111/j.1399-0004.2010.01533.x
54. Finning KM, Martin PG, Soothill PW et al (2002) Prediction of fetal D status from maternal plasma: introduction of a new non-invasive fetal RHD genotyping service. Transfusion 42:1079–1085
55. Chitty LS, van der Schoot CE, Hahn S et al (2008) SAFE—the special non-invasive advances in fetal and neonatal evaluation network: aims and achievements. Prenat Diagn 28:83–88. https://doi.org/10.1002/pd.1929
56. Clausen FB, Steffensen R, Christiansen M et al (2014) Routine non-invasive prenatal screening for fetal RHD in plasma of RhD-negative pregnant women-2 years of screening experience from Denmark. Prenat Diagn 34(10):1000–1005. https://doi.org/10.1002/pd.4419
57. Traeger-Synodinos J, Vrettou C, Kanavakis E (2011) Prenatal, non-invasive and preimplantation genetic diagnosis of inherited disorders: hemoglobinopathies. Expert Rev Mol Diagn 11:299–312. https://doi.org/10.1586/erm.11.7
58. Scheffer PG, Ait Soussan A, Verhagen OJ et al (2011) Non-invasive fetal genotyping of human platelet antigen-1a. BJOG 118:1392–1395. https://doi.org/10.1111/j.1471-0528.2011.03039.x
59. Barrett AN, Chitty LS (2014) Developing non-invasive diagnosis for single-gene disorders: the role of digital PCR. Methods Mol Biol 1160:215–228. https://doi.org/10.1007/978-1-4939-0733-5_17
60. Lo YM, Chiu RW (2010) Non-invasive approaches to prenatal diagnosis of hemoglobinopathies using fetal DNA in maternal plasma. Hematol Oncol Clin North Am 24:1179–1186. https://doi.org/10.1016/j.hoc.2010.08.007
61. New MI, Tong YK, Yuen T et al (2014) Non-invasive prenatal diagnosis of congenital adrenal hyperplasia using cell-free fetal DNA in maternal plasma. J Clin Endocrinol Metab 99:E1022–E1030. https://doi.org/10.1210/jc.2014-1118
62. Ashoor G, Syngelaki A, Poon LC et al (2013) Fetal fraction in maternal plasma cell-free DNA at 11-13 weeks' gestation: relation to maternal and fetal characteristics. Ultrasound Obstet Gynecol 41:26–32. https://doi.org/10.1002/uog.12331
63. Chiu RW, Akolekar R, Zheng YW et al (2011) Non-invasive prenatal assessment of trisomy 21 by multiplexed maternal plasma DNA sequencing: large scale validity study. BMJ 342:c7401. https://doi.org/10.1136/bmj.c7401
64. Bianchi DW, Platt LD, Goldberg JD et al (2012) Genome-wide fetal aneuploidy detection by maternal plasma DNA sequencing. Obstet Gynecol 119:890–901. https://doi.org/10.1097/AOG.0b013e31824fb482

65. Jiang F, Ren J, Chen F et al (2012) Non-invasive fetal trisomy (NIFTY) test: an advanced non-invasive prenatal diagnosis methodology for fetal autosomal and sex chromosomal aneuploidies. BMC Med Genet 5:57. https://doi.org/10.1186/1755-8794-5-57
66. Ehrich M, Deciu C, Zwiefelhofer T et al (2011) Non-invasive detection of fetal trisomy 21 by sequencing of DNA in maternal blood: a study in a clinical setting. Am J Obstet Gynecol 204 (205):e201–e211. https://doi.org/10.1016/j.ajog.2010.12.060
67. Palomaki GE, Kloza EM, Lambert-Messerlian GM et al (2011) DNA sequencing of maternal plasma to detect Down syndrome: an international clinical validation study. Genet Med 13:913–920. https://doi.org/10.1097/GIM.0b013e3182368a0e
68. Lau TK, Chen F, Pan X et al (2012) Non-invasive prenatal diagnosis of common fetal chromosomal aneuploidies by maternal plasma DNA sequencing. J Matern Fetal Neonatal Med 25:1370–1374. https://doi.org/10.3109/14767058.2011.635730
69. Ashoor G, Syngelaki A, Wagner M et al (2012) Chromosome-selective sequencing of maternal plasma cell-free DNA for first-trimester detection of trisomy 21 and trisomy 18. Am J Obstet Gynecol 206(322):e321–e325. https://doi.org/10.1016/j.ajog.2012.01.029
70. Sparks AB, Wang ET, Struble CA et al (2012) Selective analysis of cell-free DNA in maternal blood for evaluation of fetal trisomy. Prenat Diagn 32:3–9. https://doi.org/10.1002/pd.2922
71. Sparks AB, Struble CA, Wang ET et al (2012) Non-invasive prenatal detection and selective analysis of cell-free DNA obtained from maternal blood: evaluation for trisomy 21 and trisomy 18. Am J Obstet Gynecol 206:319e311–319e319. https://doi.org/10.1016/j.ajog.2012.01.030
72. Norton ME, Brar H, Weiss J et al (2012) Non-invasive chromosomal evaluation (NICE) study: results of a multicenter prospective cohort study for detection of fetal trisomy 21 and trisomy 18. Am J Obstet Gynecol 207 (137):e131–e138. https://doi.org/10.1016/j.ajog.2012.05.021
73. Zimmermann B, Hill M, Gemelos G et al (2012) Non-invasive prenatal aneuploidy testing of chromosomes 13, 18, 21, X, and Y, using targeted sequencing of polymorphic loci. Prenat Diagn 32:1233–1241. https://doi.org/10.1002/pd.3993
74. Nicolaides KH, Syngelaki A, Gil M et al (2013) Validation of targeted sequencing of single-nucleotide polymorphisms for non-invasive prenatal detection of aneuploidy of chromosomes 13, 18, 21, X, and Y. Prenat Diagn 33:575–579. https://doi.org/10.1002/pd.4103
75. Lau TK, Cheung SW, Lo PS et al (2014) Non-invasive prenatal testing for fetal chromosomal abnormalities by low-coverage whole-genome sequencing of maternal plasma DNA: review of 1982 consecutive cases in a single center. Ultrasound Obstet Gynecol 43:254–264. https://doi.org/10.1002/uog.13277
76. Srinivasan A, Bianchi DW, Huang H et al (2013) Non-invasive detection of fetal sub-chromosome abnormalities via deep sequencing of maternal plasma. Am J Hum Genet 92:167–176. https://doi.org/10.1016/j.ajhg.2012.12.006
77. Mersy E, Smits LJ, van Winden LA et al (2013) Non-invasive detection of fetal trisomy 21: systematic review and report of quality and outcomes of diagnostic accuracy studies performed between 1997 and 2012. Hum Reprod Update 19:318–329. https://doi.org/10.1093/humupd/dmt001
78. Benn P, Borell A, Chiu R et al (2013) Position statement from the Aneuploidy Screening Committee on behalf of the Board of the International Society for Prenatal Diagnosis. Prenat Diagn 33:622–629. https://doi.org/10.1002/pd.4139
79. American College of O, Gynecologists Committee on G (2012) Committee Opinion No. 545: Non-invasive prenatal testing for fetal aneuploidy. Obstet Gynecol 120:1532–1534. https://doi.org/10.1097/01.AOG.0000423819.85283.f4
80. Ohno M, Caughey A (2013) The role of non-invasive prenatal testing as a diagnostic versus a screening tool—a cost-effectiveness analysis. Prenat Diagn 33:630–635. https://doi.org/10.1002/pd.4156
81. Nicolaides KH, Syngelaki A, Ashoor G et al (2012) Non-invasive prenatal testing for fetal trisomies in a routinely screened first-trimester population. Am J Obstet Gynecol 207(374): e371–e376. https://doi.org/10.1016/j.ajog.2012.08.033
82. Dan S, Wang W, Ren J et al (2012) Clinical application of massively parallel sequencing-based prenatal non-invasive fetal trisomy test for trisomies 21 and 18 in 11,105 pregnancies with mixed risk factors. Prenat Diagn 32:1225–1232. https://doi.org/10.1002/pd.4002
83. Gil MM, Quezada MS, Bregant B et al (2013) Implementation of maternal blood cell-free DNA testing in early screening for aneuploidies. Ultrasound Obstet Gynecol 42:34–40. https://doi.org/10.1002/uog.12504

84. Bianchi DW, Parker RL, Wentworth J et al (2014) DNA sequencing versus standard prenatal aneuploidy screening. N Engl J Med 370:799–808. https://doi.org/10.1056/NEJMoa1311037
85. Bianchi DW, Wilkins-Haug L (2014) Integration of non-invasive DNA testing for aneuploidy into prenatal care: what has happened since the rubber met the road? Clin Chem 60:78–87. https://doi.org/10.1373/clinchem.2013.202663
86. Hui L, Hyett J (2013) Non-invasive prenatal testing for trisomy 21: challenges for implementation in Australia. Aust N Z J Obstet Gynaecol 53:416–424. https://doi.org/10.1111/ajo.12117
87. Bulletins ACoP (2007) ACOG Practice Bulletin No. 77: screening for fetal chromosomal abnormalities. Obstet Gynecol 109:217–227
88. Huang T, Watt H, Wald N et al (1998) Birth prevalence of Down's syndrome in England and Wales 1990 to 1997. J Med Screen 5:213–214
89. Lai FM, Woo BH, Tan KH et al (2002) Birth prevalence of Down syndrome in Singapore from 1993 to 1998. Singap Med J 43:070–076
90. Samango-Sprouse C, Banjevic M, Ryan A et al (2013) SNP-based non-invasive prenatal testing detects sex chromosome aneuploidies with high accuracy. Prenat Diagn 33:643–649. https://doi.org/10.1002/pd.4159
91. Peters D, Chu T, Yatsenko SA et al (2011) Non-invasive prenatal diagnosis of a fetal microdeletion syndrome. N Engl J Med 365:1847–1848. https://doi.org/10.1056/NEJMc1106975
92. Jensen TJ, Dzakula Z, Deciu C et al (2012) Detection of microdeletion 22q11.2 in a fetus by next-generation sequencing of maternal plasma. Clin Chem 58:1148–1151. https://doi.org/10.1373/clinchem.2011.180794
93. Yu SC, Jiang P, Choy KW et al (2013) Non-invasive prenatal molecular karyotyping from maternal plasma. PLoS One 8:e60968. https://doi.org/10.1371/journal.pone.0060968
94. Fan HC, Gu W, Wang J et al (2012) Non-invasive prenatal measurement of the fetal genome. Nature 487:320–324. https://doi.org/10.1038/nature11251
95. Kitzman JO, Snyder MW, Ventura M et al (2012) Non-invasive whole-genome sequencing of a human fetus. Sci Transl Med 4:137ra176. https://doi.org/10.1126/scitranslmed.3004323
96. Lo YM, Chan KC, Sun H et al (2010) Maternal plasma DNA sequencing reveals the genome-wide genetic and mutational profile of the fetus. Sci Transl Med 2:61ra91. https://doi.org/10.1126/scitranslmed.3001720

Part II

Preimplantation Genetic Testing

Chapter 4

Molecular Testing for Preimplantation Genetic Diagnosis of Single Gene Disorders

Rebekah S. Zimmerman, Jennifer Eccles, Chaim Jalas, Nathan R. Treff, and Richard T. Scott Jr.

Abstract

Preimplantation genetic testing has evolved tremendously from the early days of FISH detection for a select few chromosome aneuploidies to now combining the detection of all whole chromosome imbalances in conjunction with single gene disorder testing for inherited diseases. As universal carrier screening and exome or genome studies become more commonplace, more and more families are becoming interested in reducing the risk of having a child with a severe disease using preimplantation genetic testing. We describe here the use of quantitative PCR (qPCR) for the custom construction of single gene disorder testing plans for families, the validation of the probes designed, and the protocol for diagnosing an embryo biopsy. qPCR has been shown to have the lowest risk of failed amplification and allele dropout and thus the lowest risk of a misdiagnosis, while also currently providing the fastest protocol to allow for rapid turnaround of results.

Key words Single gene disorder, PGD, IVF, Preimplantation genetic diagnosis, qPCR

1 Introduction

During the earliest stage of preimplantation genetic diagnosis (PGD), the first patients to benefit were those at risk to have offspring with single gene disorders (SGD) and first attempts were aimed at ruling out X-linked disorders by targeting Y-specific probes [1]. Following those efforts, a successful outcome using PGD to address an increased risk of cystic fibrosis was reported [2]. Over 20 years later, the scope of PGD has expanded to include over 200 single disorders including adult-onset conditions, cancer predisposition syndromes, and HLA genotyping to identify sibling matches for bone marrow transplants [3, 4]. The advent of preimplantation genetic screening (PGS) for aneuploidy further broadened the applications of these technologies [5].

Unlike PGS for aneuploidy, which employs the same testing paradigm for use in multiple populations, PGD for SGD requires a case-specific workup that is designed to address the testing variables

Brynn Levy (ed.), *Prenatal Diagnosis*, Methods in Molecular Biology, vol. 1885, https://doi.org/10.1007/978-1-4939-8889-1_4,

associated with each unique gene, mutation(s), inheritance pattern, and family history. Of particular importance, is whether or not the laboratory is able to obtain additional samples from informative family members that are needed to build supporting linkage probes. This extensive and complex workup is required to address the diagnostic challenges that are inherent in testing small numbers of cells. Such challenges include amplification failure, allele drop out (ADO), and contamination [6, 7]. As a result, the testing approach for two couples seeking PGD for the same single gene disorder may be quite different.

Currently, the most rapidly advancing standard for PGD for SGD involves DNA amplification via quantitative polymerase chain reaction technology (qPCR) to detect mutations directly (when applicable) along with amplification of one or more closely linked polymorphic markers [8]. This strategy is designed to provide both a direct and indirect means of assessing genotype with the goal of increasing accuracy by reducing the risk of a false result related to ADO and increasing the tests ability to detect contamination. Validation studies have demonstrated the validity and diagnostic value of this approach and accuracy using this methodology is greater than 98% [8, 9].

The first step of the process involves creating a custom validation for a family (Fig. 1) which includes: (1) extraction of DNA from blood collected from both members of a couple who are going to be the biological parents of the embryo, (2) possible extraction of DNA from buccal swab samples collected from pertinent family members, (3) SNP microarray to screen multiple SNP probe candidates simultaneously for SNPs that are linked to the mutation/gene of interest, (4) selection of SNPs from the microarray and ordering of TaqMan PCR primers, (5) testing of the TaqMan PCR probes on the couple and possible family members to both determine the accuracy of the probe as well as determining the configuration of alleles, or phase, for the linkage probes to ensure correct interpretation of results in the future embryo biopsies. When possible the specific mutation(s) are targeted and then at least one linkage probe is selected upstream and downstream from the mutation site, usually within 1 Mb. For repeat expansion disorders, or when the mutation probe is not performing up to standards, a "linkage only" approach is used where at least four linkage markers are selected (two upstream and two downstream). In the case of microdeletions, two markers are selected within the deletion and at least one marker is selected upstream and downstream of the deletion of interest.

Once the laboratory has completed the validation process, genetic material from the embryo can then be analyzed. While it is possible to perform embryo biopsies during different stages of embryonic development, there is currently a shift away from cleavage stage (blastomere, day 3) biopsy, toward trophectoderm

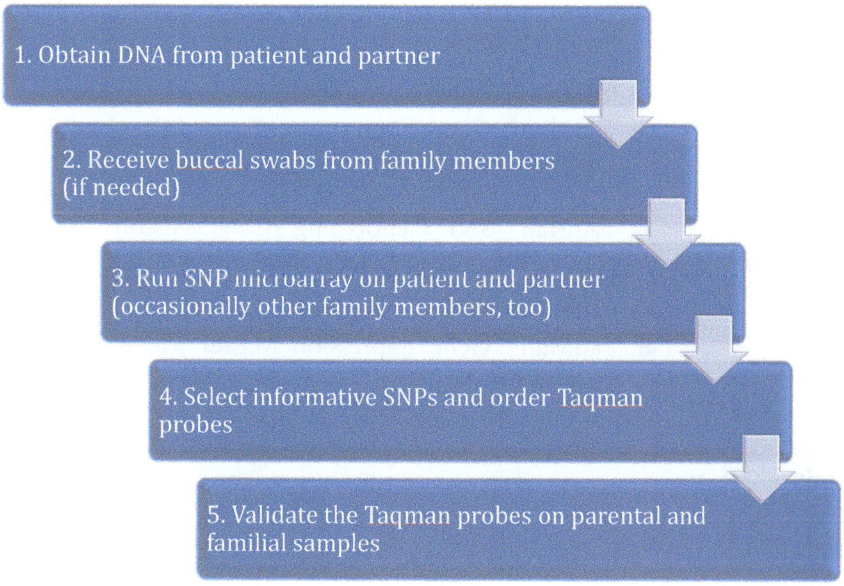

Fig. 1 Single gene disorders validation workflow

(blastocyst, days 5–6) biopsy, which has been shown to provide improved performance with regards to ADO and implantation rates [9, 10]. Current technology also allows for analysis of single gene disorders to be performed concurrently with PGS for aneuploidy, which provides further information regarding whether an embryo is suitable for transfer [8, 11].

The following report presents the protocol for the workup and embryo PGD for single gene disorders in a clinical diagnostic laboratory using real-time quantitative PCR.

2 Materials

2.1 Genomic DNA Extraction from Peripheral Blood

1. QIAamp DNA blood maxi kit (Qiagen, Germantown, MD, USA).
2. QIAGEN Protease (Qiagen, Germantown, MD, USA).
3. Prepare the protease by pipetting 5.5 mL distilled water into a vial of lyophilized QIAGEN Protease. Label the cap with date it was constituted (*see* **Notes 1** and **2**).
4. 100% ethyl alcohol (ethanol).

2.2 Genomic DNA Extraction from Buccal Swabs

1. Gentra Puregene Buccal Cell Kit for buffers (Qiagen, Germantown, MD, USA).
2. DNeasy Blood and Tissue Kit for collection tubes and spin columns (Qiagen, Germantown, MD, USA).
3. 100% ethyl alcohol (ethanol).

2.3 TaqMan Genotyping PCR for Probe Validation

1. TaqMan® SNP Genotyping Assays, custom ordered for each family (Life Technologies, Carlsbad, CA, USA).
2. Molecular Biology Grade water.
3. TaqMan® Gene Expression Master Mix (Life Technologies, Carlsbad, CA, USA).

2.4 TaqMan Genotyping PCR for Embryo Testing

1. TaqMan® SNP Genotyping Assays, custom ordered for each family (Life Technologies, Carlsbad, CA, USA).
2. Molecular Biology Grade water.
3. TaqMan® Gene Expression Master Mix (Life Technologies, Carlsbad, CA, USA).

3 Methods

3.1 Genomic DNA Extraction from Peripheral Blood

Peripheral blood is strongly recommended for patients for which SNP arrays will be performed.

1. Mix Buffer AL from the QIAamp DNA blood maxi kit thoroughly by shaking before use.
2. Make sure ethanol was added to buffers AW1 and AW2.
3. Preheat the water bath to 70 °C.
4. Pipet 500 μL QIAGEN Protease into the bottom of 50 mL centrifuge tubes.
5. Add 10 mL blood and mix briefly.
6. Bring the volume of the samples up to 10 mL with PBS (if necessary) before adding to the centrifuge tube.
7. Add 12 mL Buffer AL, and mix by inverting the tubes 15 times, followed by additional vigorous shaking for at least 1 min.
8. Incubate at 70 °C for 10 min.
9. Add 10 mL ethanol (96–100%) to the samples, and mix by inverting the tubes 10 times, followed by additional vigorous shaking.
10. Insert a VacConnector into each VacValve on the QIAvac manifold that is to be used. Insert the QIAamp Maxi column into the VacConnector. Open the corresponding VacValve. Close the main vacuum valve and switch on the vacuum pump.
11. Carefully transfer one half of the solution from the previous step onto the QIAamp Maxi column, taking care not to moisten the rim. Open the vacuum valve. If sample flow rates differ, close the VacValves where the lysate has already passed through. After all lysates have been drawn through the columns, close the main vacuum valve. Repeat this step.

12. Open the VacValve, and add 15 mL Buffer AW1 to the QIAamp Maxi columns, taking care not to moisten the rim. Open the main vacuum valve. After all of the Buffer AW1 has been drawn through the columns, close the main vacuum valve.
13. Open the VacValve, and add 15 mL Buffer AW2 to the QIAamp Maxi columns, take care not to moisten the rim. Open the main vacuum valve. After all of the Buffer AW1 has been drawn through the columns, close the main vacuum valve.
14. To dry the membranes, place the QIAamp Maxi column into the 50 mL centrifuge tube. Close the cap and centrifuge at 4500 × *g* for 15 min.
15. Place the QIAamp Maxi column in a new 50 mL centrifuge tube. Pipet 1.3 mL Buffer AE directly onto the membrane of the QIAamp Maxi column and close the cap. Incubate at room temperature for 5 min, and centrifuge at 4500 × *g* for 2 min.
16. Pipet 1.3 mL Buffer AE directly onto the membrane of the QIAamp Maxi column and close the cap. Incubate at room temperature for 5 min, and centrifuge at 4500 × *g* for 2 min.
17. Measure the concentration using NanoDrop ND-1000 and calculate the yield.
18. Aliquot 200 μL into 1.5 mL microtubes labeled with the sample ID. Quantify the DNA by Nanodrop and store at −20 °C.

3.2 Genomic DNA Extraction from Buccal Swabs

Extraction of DNA from buccal swabs is a modified protocol that combines the use of the Gentra Puregene Buccal Cell Kit with the Qiagen DNeasy Blood and Tissue kit.

1. Preheat water bath to 55°.
2. For each buccal swab, dispense 300 μL Cell Lysis Solution into a 1.5 mL microcentrifuge tube. Remove the collection brush from its handle using sterile scissors or a razor blade, and place the detached head in the tube containing the lysis solution.
3. Add 1.5 μL Puregene Proteinase K, mix by inverting 25 times, and incubate at 55 °C for at least 1 h (up to overnight for maximum yield).
4. Remove the collection brush head from the Cell Lysis Solution, scraping it on the sides of the tube to recover as much liquid as possible.
5. Add 300 μL 100% ethanol to the sample. Vortex mix for 15 s.

6. Carefully apply the entire sample (including any precipitate) to the DNeasy Mini Spin column placed in a 2 mL collection tube. Centrifuge at ≥6000 × *g* for 1 min. Discard the filtrate and the collection tube.
7. Place the DNeasy Mini Spin Column into a clean 2 mL collection tube. Add 500 μL Buffer AW1 without wetting the rim. Close the cap and centrifuge at ≥6000 × *g* for 1 min. Discard the filtrate and collection tube.
8. Place the DNeasy Mini Spin Column into another clean 2 mL collection tube. Carefully open the DNeasy Mini Spin Column and add 500 μL of Buffer AW2 without wetting the rim. Close the cap and centrifuge at full speed 20,000 × *g* for 1 min. Discard the filtrate, put the column back to the collection tube, close the cap, and centrifuge at full speed 20,000 × *g* for 2 min.
9. Discard the filtrate and collection tube. Place the DNeasy Mini Spin Column into a clean, sterile, 1.5 mL microfuge tube labeled with the sample ID. Carefully open the column and add 50 μL AE buffer. Incubate at room temperature (15–25 °C) for 2 min. Centrifuge at ≥6000 × *g* for 1 min.
10. Discard the filter column, close the 1.5 mL microcentrifuge tube, and store the DNA at 4 °C until needed for testing.

3.3 Informative Marker Selection

Any SNP array is suitable for this step. The greater the number of genome-wide SNPs, the better the likelihood of capturing informative SNPs.

1. Obtain the genotyping calls from the SNP array. Confirm that the coordinates of the SNPs on the array are from reference set hg19.
2. Find the closest informative marker that is upstream of the mutation/gene of interest (*see* Fig. 2 for examples of an informative marker). Be sure to select markers with the most significant *p* values (or confidence scores), as the DNA obtained from buccal swabs may have lower quality calls. Try to select markers within 1 Mb of the mutation/gene of interest to comply with ESHRE guidelines [9] and reduce the risk of recombination between markers.
3. Similarly, find the closest informative marker that is downstream of the mutation/gene of interest.
4. If the mutation will not be detected directly then select additional markers upstream and downstream.
5. Order all probes for the selected markers from the vendor, including the mutation specific assays.

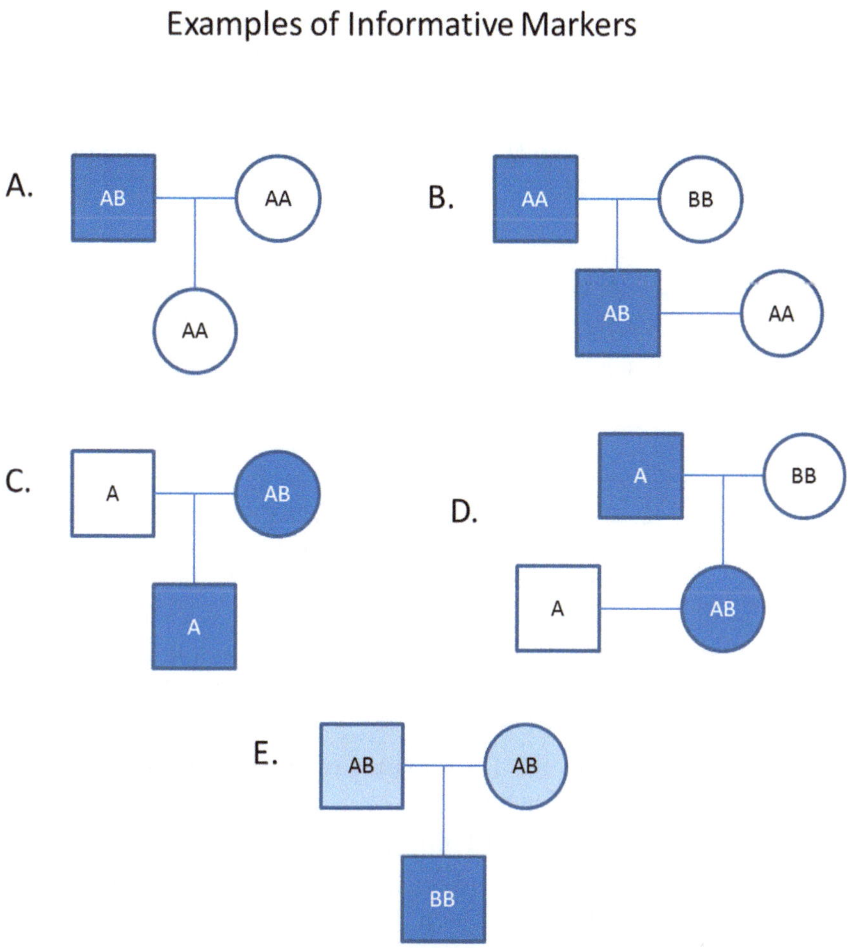

Fig. 2 Examples of informative markers. (**a**) Autosomal dominant condition with child with known genotype. (**b**) Autosomal dominant condition with no child, but affected parent one generation up. (**c**) X-linked condition (e.g., Fragile X) with child with known genotype (e.g., affected male). (**d**) X-linked condition with no children, but positive parent one generation up. (**e**) Autosomal recessive condition where both parents are carriers of the same mutation, with a child with a normal (non-carrier) or affected genotype

3.4 Taqman Genotyping PCR for Probe Validation

For each probe being used the following steps are required: Table 1 shows the volumes required and includes a 20% volume excess for each reagent to allow for pipetting variation.

3.4.1 Preparation of 20× Probes/Assays

1. Add TaqMan Gene Expression Mastermix to a labeled 1.5 mL tube.
2. Add Molecular Biology Grade water to the 1.5 mL tube.
3. Add the specific TaqMan assay to the 1.5 mL tube.
4. Vortex the tube for 10 s and spin down on short spin setting for 5 s.

Table 1
Example of volumes required for preparation of Taqman 20× probes/assays

	Amount for one reaction (μL)	Amount for 38 samples/ reactions	20% excess	Total volume
TaqMan gene expression master mix	2.5	95	19	114
Probe assay (20×)	0.125	4.75	0.95	5.7
MGB water	0.375	14.25	2.85	17.1
Total volume	3	114	22.8	136.8

3.4.2 Normalize gDNA

1. Thaw genomic DNA.
2. Calculate the amount of DNA required to normalize the sample to 5 ng/μL (if extracted from blood) or 10 ng/μL (if extracted from a buccal swab—*see* **Note 3**) in a total volume of 50 μL.
3. Calculate the amount of water required to normalize the sample by subtracting the amount in **step 2** from the total volume of 50 μL.
4. After the DNA master tube has thawed vortex the tube and spin down for 5 s.
5. Label one 1.5 mL tube for each sample with the sample ID.
6. Add water to each labeled tube according to the amount calculated in **step 3**.
7. Add DNA to each labeled tube according to the amount calculated in **step 2**.
8. Close each tube, vortex for 10 s and spin down.

3.4.3 PCR Setup for Probe Validation

1. Label a 384-well plate with the date the PCR is being performed.
2. Using a multi-pipettor, add 3 μL of the assay mixture into each designated well.
3. Using a multi-pipettor, add 2 μL of normalized DNA to each assigned well.
4. Include two "wild-type" controls and at least one "no template control" (NTC) for each assay being run.
5. Seal the plate with optical adhesive film.
6. Vortex the plate for 10 s and spin down in a microfuge for 1 min at 2000 rpm.
7. Place the plate inside a thermal cycler (*see* **Note 4**) previously programmed with the following program:

- Hold: 50 °C for 2 min, 95 °C for 10 min.
- Forty cycles: 95 °C for 15 s, 60 °C for 1 min.
- 4 °C Hold.

8. After the PCR program is complete remove the plate from the thermal cycler and transfer it to the 7900HT Fast Real-Time PCR System.
9. Perform allelic discrimination post-read per the manufacturer's instructions.
10. Analyze the genotyping calls using either SDS or TaqMan Genotyper.

3.4.4 TaqMan Genotyping PCR for Embryo Testing

This section of the protocol is intended to start on samples that have already been biopsied from an embryo on day 5 or 6 of development and lysed using standard lysing protocols.

1. Prepare Primer Pool: Mix 2.5 μL of each mutation assays and linkage assays for a specific SGD patient so that the final concentration for each assay will be 0.2×.
2. Prepare precoated plates containing the probes designed and validated previously.
3. Dilute all of the probe assays from 40× to 20× first with MBG water (50 μL of assay and 50 μL of water).
4. Then dilute the assays to 1× in a 96-well plate (7 μL of 20× assay and 133 μL of MBG water).
5. The 1× assay plate is aliquot into 6384-well plates by EP motion and dried by Genevac machine for 40 min.
6. Prepare the preamplification (PreAmp) reaction by combining the following for each reaction: 25 μL TaqMan PreAmp Master Mix, 12.5 μL PreAmp Primer Pool, 2.5 μL MBG Water.
7. Vortex and spin the combined reagents before use.
8. Add 40 μL of the mix to the side of the tube containing 10 μL of lysed embryo biopsy sample.
9. Cap the tube, spin down, vortex the tube, and spin down again.
10. Add the tubes to the thermal cycler (*see* **Note 4**) and run the following program:
    - Hold: 95 °C for 10 min.
    - Eighteen cycles: 95 °C for 15 s, 60 °C for 4 min.
    - 4 °C Hold.
11. Remove the tubes from the thermal cycler and spin down.
12. Using a 12-channel repeat pipette, aliquot 5 μL of each sample into precoated 384-well SGD plate.
13. Tap plate after adding samples to bring complete volume to bottom of well.

14. Seal the plate with optical film and spin down. After the spin seal edges tightly.
15. Run amplification in the thermal cycler (*see* **Note 4**) using the following program:
    - Hold: 50 °C for 2 min, 95 °C for 10 min.
    - Forty cycles: 95 °C for 15 s, 60 °C for 1 min.
    - 4 °C Hold.
16. After the PCR program is complete remove the plate from the thermal cycler and transfer it to the 7900HT Fast Real-Time PCR System.
17. Perform allelic discrimination post-read per the manufacturer's instructions.
18. Analyze the genotyping calls using either SDS or TaqMan Genotyper.

4 Notes

1. Dissolved QIAGEN Protease is stable for 2 months when stored at 2–8 °C.
2. For storage at −20 °C, prepare and freeze QIAGEN Protease stock solution in aliquots.
3. DNA from buccal swabs can often be contaminated with DNA from bacterial sources, so to account for those contaminants a higher concentration of DNA is used if the DNA was isolated from buccal swabs.
4. The GeneAmp PCR System 9700 is the preferred PCR thermal cycler.

Acknowledgments

Thank you to David Gabrielle, Anastasia Fedick, Xin Tao, Heather Garnsey, and Andrew Behrens for the assistance in the development and implementation of these protocols.

References

1. Handyside AH, Kontogianni EH, Hardy K et al (1990) Pregnancies from biopsied human preimplantation embryos sexed by Y-specific DNA amplification. Nature 344 (6268):768–770. https://doi.org/10.1038/344768a0
2. Handyside AH, Lesko JG, Tarin JJ et al (1992) Birth of a normal girl after in vitro fertilization and preimplantation diagnostic testing for cystic fibrosis. N Engl J Med 327(13):905–909
3. Findlay I, Ray P, Quirke P et al (1995) Allelic drop-out and preferential amplification in single cells and human blastomeres: implications for preimplantation diagnosis of sex and cystic fibrosis. Hum Reprod 10(6):1609–1618

4. Gianaroli L, Magli MC, Ferraretti AP et al (1999) Preimplantation diagnosis for aneuploidies in patients undergoing in vitro fertilization with a poor prognosis: identification of the categories for which it should be proposed. Fertil Steril 72(5):837–844
5. Zimmerman RS, Jalas C, Tao X et al (2016) Development and validation of concurrent preimplantation genetic diagnosis for single gene disorders and comprehensive chromosomal aneuploidy screening without whole genome amplification. Fertil Steril 105(2):286–294. https://doi.org/10.1016/j.fertnstert.2015.10.003
6. Verlinsky Y, Rechitsky S, Schoolcraft W et al (2001) Preimplantation diagnosis for Fanconi anemia combined with HLA matching. JAMA 285(24):3130–3133
7. Thornhill AR, Snow K (2002) Molecular diagnostics in preimplantation genetic diagnosis. J Mol Diagn 4(1):11–29. https://doi.org/10.1016/S1525-1578(10)60676-9
8. Scott RT Jr, Upham KM, Forman EJ et al (2013) Cleavage-stage biopsy significantly impairs human embryonic implantation potential while blastocyst biopsy does not: a randomized and paired clinical trial. Fertil Steril 100 (3):624–630. https://doi.org/10.1016/j.fertnstert.2013.04.039
9. Harton GL, De Rycke M, Fiorentino F et al (2011) ESHRE PGD consortium best practice guidelines for amplification-based PGD. Hum Reprod 26(1):33–40. https://doi.org/10.1093/humrep/deq231
10. Simpson JL (2010) Preimplantation genetic diagnosis at 20 years. Prenat Diagn 30 (7):682–695. https://doi.org/10.1002/pd.2552
11. Tao X, Su J, Pepe R, Northrop LE, Ferry KM, Treff NR (2011) PGD for monogenic disease by direct mutation analysis alone in 2 or more cells is more reliable than multiple marker analysis in single cells. Fertil Steril 96(3):S21

Chapter 5

Detection of Aneuploidy and Unbalanced Rearrangements Using Comparative Genomic Hybridization Microarrays

Lorena Rodrigo Vivó and Carmen Rubio Lluesa

Abstract

Comparative genomic hybridization arrays (aCGH) allow the analysis of all 24 chromosome aneuploidies and chromosome rearrangements in the same single (or few) biopsied cells in a short period (less than 24 h). When applied to preimplantation genetic diagnosis (PGD) and screening (PGS) this technique can improve the selection of embryos for transfer and therefore also the reproductive outcomes. In this chapter, we describe the CGH microarray protocol for PGS and PGD used in our laboratory.

Key words Preimplantation genetic screening (PGS), Preimplantation genetic diagnosis (PGD), Aneuploidy, Chromosomal rearrangement, Array CGH, Whole genome amplification

1 Introduction

Aneuploidy may be a contributing factor to the reproductive problems in normal-karyotype infertile couples with advanced maternal age, recurrent pregnancy loss, repetitive implantation failure, or even male infertility [1]. For this reason preimplantation genetic screening (PGS) is often used to select euploid embryos before their placement into the uterus in in vitro fertilization (IVF) treatments. Over the last 20 years the technology used for chromosome screening has dramatically changed; whereas in 1995 the fluorescence in situ hybridization (FISH) technique could only be applied in single cells for the analysis of a limited number of chromosomes, from 2008 comparative genomic hybridization arrays (aCGH) have allowed all 24 chromosomes to be analyzed, not only in single cells but also in trophectoderm biopsies. Additional microarray platforms using different techniques such as single nucleotide polymorphisms (SNPs, in 2010) or quantitative polymerase chain reaction (qPCR, in 2013) have also been successfully applied in PGS [2]. Consequently, embryologists can now use PGS in several groups of infertile couples as a tool to be used in addition to

Brynn Levy (ed.), *Prenatal Diagnosis*, Methods in Molecular Biology, vol. 1885, https://doi.org/10.1007/978-1-4939-8889-1_5,

morphological criteria to help select embryos with the best chance of giving rise to a successful pregnancy.

Patients who carry chromosomal rearrangements have a high risk of having unbalanced pregnancies resulting in miscarriages or abnormal offspring. Preimplantation genetic diagnosis (PGD) is a potent tool which helps to avoid the transfer of embryos carrying unbalanced rearrangements into the uterus. Selecting a normal or balanced embryo for transfer increases the chances of having a healthy, live, newborn child, and decreases the potential for stress and difficult decisions that these couples usually have to make in the case of an unbalanced pregnancy. For many years the FISH technique has been used to analyze embryos in chromosomal rearrangement carriers. Specific strategies using different fluorescent DNA probes must be tested and applied in each particular couple, and no chromosomes other than those implicated in the rearrangement can usually be analyzed. In contrast, the aCGH approach offers the advantage of detecting rearrangement and aneuploidy unbalances for every chromosome at the same time and in the same single cell or trophectoderm biopsy [3]. However, unfortunately, only chromosome rearrangements with translocated fragment sizes larger than the resolution of the microarray platform can be addressed with this technique, meaning that the remaining cases must still be analyzed using the FISH technique.

The aim of this chapter is to describe, in detail, the Illumina® aCGH microarray 24sure and 24sure + protocols (for PGS and PGD respectively) used in our laboratory. These microarray platforms are based on BACs (bacterial artificial chromosomes), and contain spots with normal DNA fragments representing the whole genome. The technology uses a microarray-based genomic hybridization approach to investigate whole chromosome copy number and sub-chromosomal structural imbalances in a 12-h protocol. Regardless of whether a single cell or trophectoderm biopsy is used, the genome must be amplified to obtain sufficient DNA for the analysis. This amplified DNA is labeled with Cyanine 3 (Cy3) or Cyanine 5 (Cy5) fluorophores and is hybridized to the array platform. Female and male euploid DNA are also labeled and hybridized and used as references. After hybridization, the arrays are washed and scanned using a dual-channel scanner: the green channel (532 nm) for excitation and reading the Cy3 signal, and the red channel (635 nm) for excitation and reading of the Cy5 signal. The images generated are analyzed by the software provided by the array manufacturer, which generates a plot representing the sample DNA quantity compared to the reference DNA. Interpretation of the plots allows DNA gains or losses in the sample to be determined by comparing them to the hybridized references.

2 Materials

1. 100–130 μm diameter micro glass capillaries.
2. Mouth aspiration system/striper.
3. Stereomicroscope for cell manipulation.
4. Hybridization chamber.

2.1 Cell Loading Consumables

1. 20× PBS.
2. Double-distilled autoclaved water.
3. Mineral oil.

2.2 aCGH Consumables

1. SurePlex Single Cell Whole Genome Amplification Kit (Illumina, San Diego, CA, USA): Contains cell extraction buffer; extraction enzyme dilution buffer; extraction enzyme; pre-amplification buffer; pre-amplification enzyme; amplification buffer; amplification enzyme; nuclease-free water.
2. Fluorescent dCTP Labelling System (Illumina, San Diego, CA, USA): Contains reaction buffer; dCTP-labeling mix; Cy3 dCTP; Cy5 dCTP; Klenow enzyme; dextran sulfate Hybridization Buffer.
3. SureRef DNA (Illumina, San Diego, CA, USA): Contains male and female amplified genomic DNA ready for use as hybridization references.
4. COT Human DNA (Illumina, San Diego, CA, USA).
5. 20× SSC Buffer, pH 7.0.
6. 15 pg genomic DNA for positive amplification control (produced in house).
7. 24sure and 24sure + BAC array slides (Illumina, San Diego, CA, USA).

2.3 Solutions (See Notes 1 and 2)

2.3.1 Solutions for Cell Loading

1. 1× PBS: Autoclave the 20× PBS. Prepare 1 mL of 1× PBS in a sterile, autoclaved 1.5 mL tube by mixing 50 μL of the autoclaved 20× PBS in 950 μL of the double-distilled autoclaved water; vortex and briefly centrifuge it. Dispense 2.5 μL of 1× PBS into autoclaved 0.2 mL PCR tubes. Prepare as many tubes as the number of embryo biopsies. Prepare two additional tubes to be used as positive and negative PCR controls.
2. 1% Polyvinylpyrrolidone (PVP) Solution: In an autoclaved, sterile 1.5 mL tube, dilute 0.01 g of polyvinylpyrrolidone in 1 mL of 1× PBS. Vortex and briefly centrifuge.

2.3.2 Hybridization

1. 50% Formamide/2× SSC Solution: 3 mL formamide +3 mL 2× SSC solution.

2.3.3 Slide Washing Buffers (See **Notes 3** and **4**)

1. 20× SSC, adjusted to pH 7.0. Store all of the buffers at room temperature.
2. 2× SSC/0.05%Tween 20: 100 mL 20× SSC + 899.5 mL double-distilled water +0.5 mL Tween 20.
3. 1× SSC: 25 mL 20× SSC + 475 mL double-distilled water.
4. 0.1× SSC: 5 mL 20× SSC + 995 mL double-distilled water.

3 Methods

The protocols described in this chapter are based on the protocols recommended by the array manufacturer, Illumina [4, 5] (*see* **Note 5**).

3.1 Cell Loading (See Notes 6–8)

The single cell, or the few biopsied trophectoderm cells, should be washed before amplification to minimize non-cellular DNA contamination. After this, the samples are loaded into 0.2 mL PCR tubes in order to start the amplification.

1. Use one capillary for each individual cell or trophectoderm biopsy.
2. Briefly centrifuge the 0.2 mL PCR sterile tubes containing 2.5 μL 1× PBS to avoid the formation of bubbles inside them.
3. Prepare a petri dish (for each biopsied embryo) containing a row with three droplets of 5 μL 1% PVP solution and cover with mineral oil. Capture the cell or trophectoderm biopsy with the capillary and rinse it by passing it through each of these droplets (release it in the first droplet, recapture it and transfer it into the second droplet; repeat for the third droplet).
4. Deposit each biopsied cell, or trophectoderm cell sample, into a 0.2 mL PCR sterile tube under the stereoscope. The cell (s) release should be observed by the embryologist and done with a minimal volume of washing media (maximum 0.5 μL). Cap the PCR tube and place inside a cold rack.
5. Store at −20 °C until amplification, or maintain at 4 °C if the amplification procedure is immediate.

3.2 Sample Amplification

3.2.1 Cell Lysis and DNA Extraction in the Pre-PCR Lab (See Notes 7–10)

1. Defrost the positive control genomic DNA; vortex and briefly centrifuge it. Store it in a rack.
2. Organize the batch of samples to be amplified and calculate the buffer quantities for the different master mixes (*see* quantities indicated in the protocol).
3. Defrost a vial of Cell Extraction Buffer and Extraction Enzyme Dilution Buffer, vortex and briefly centrifuge it.

4. Transfer the 0.2 PCR tubes containing the samples from the batch into a cold rack. Prepare two additional tubes containing 2.5 μL 1× PBS for positive and negative PCR controls.
5. Briefly centrifuge all the tubes before starting the amplification.
6. Prepare a master mix in a 1.5 mL Eppendorf tube as follows: For each sample, use 3 μL cell extraction buffer, 4.8 μL extraction enzyme dilution buffer, and 0.2 μL extraction enzyme. Scale the amounts according to the number of samples being processed. Add the Extraction Enzyme at the last minute and mix by inversion (or a very short vortex burst). Briefly centrifuge and keep the master mix in a cold rack.
7. Add 8 μL of freshly prepared master mix to each sample and the controls. Briefly centrifuge.
8. Take the samples in the cold rack to the post-PCR lab and add 1 μL of control DNA to the positive control tube. Incubate the samples in a PCR thermo-cycler with the lid preheated to 95 °C (for approximately 15 min) prior to starting the reaction, and use the following program settings: 75 °C for 10 min, 95 °C for 4 min and hold at room temperature.

3.2.2 Pre-Amplification in the Pre-PCR Lab (See Notes 7–10)

1. In pre-PCR lab, defrost a vial of Pre-amplification Buffer, vortex and briefly centrifuge it.
2. Prepare a master mix in a 1.5 mL Eppendorf tube as follows: For each sample, use 4.8 μL pre-amplification buffer and 0.2 μL pre-amplification enzyme. Scale the amounts according to the number of samples being processed. Add the pre-amplification Enzyme at the last minute and mix by inversion (or a very short vortex burst). Briefly centrifuge and keep the master mix in a cold rack.
3. Collect the PCR tubes from thermo-cycler in the post-PCR lab into a cold rack.
4. In pre-PCR lab, add 5 μL of freshly prepared master mix to each sample and the controls. Briefly centrifuge.
5. Take the samples to the post-PCR lab in cold rack and incubate them in a PCR thermal cycler with the lid preheated to 99 °C (for 1 h 10 min) and use the following program settings:
   - One cycle: 95 °C for 2 min.
   - Twelve cycles: 95 °C for 15 s, 15 °C for 50 s, 25 °C for 40 s, 35 °C for 30 s, 65 °C for 40 s, 75 °C for 40 s.
   - 4 °C Hold.

3.2.3 Amplification (See Notes 7–10)

1. In pre-PCR lab, defrost a vial of Amplification Buffer and a vial of Nuclease-free water, vortex and briefly centrifuge it.

2. Prepare a master mix in a 1.5 mL Eppendorf tube as follows: For each sample, use 34.2 μL nuclease-free water, 25 μL amplification buffer, and 0.8 μL amplification enzyme. Scale the amounts according to the number of samples being processed. Add the amplification enzyme at the last minute and mix by inversion (or a very short vortex burst). Briefly centrifuge and keep the master mix in a cold rack.
3. Collect the PCR tubes from the thermo-cycler in the post-PCR lab into a cold rack.
4. In pre-PCR lab, add 60 μL of freshly prepared master mix to each sample and the controls. Briefly centrifuge.
5. Take the samples in a cold rack to the post-PCR lab and incubate the samples in a PCR thermal cycler with the lid preheated to 99 °C (for approximately 40 min) and then apply the following program settings:
   - One cycle: 95 °C for 2 min.
   - Fifteen cycles: 95 °C for 15 s, 65 °C for 1 min, 75 °C for 1 min.
   - 4 °C Hold.
6. Place the PCR tubes into a cold rack (in the fridge at 4 °C) and check for sample amplification by agarose gel electrophoresis (*see* **Note 11**).

3.3 Sample Labeling

After amplification, samples and reference DNAs are labeled with Cy3 and Cy5 fluorophores using random primers. The 24sure® microarray used for PGS is a single channel platform in which the test samples are labeled and hybridized against each other and are compared to male and female DNA references which are hybridized in a different sub-array. In contrast, the 24sure + ® microarray used for PGD is a dual channel platform in which the test and reference samples are hybridized onto the same sub-array. The manufacturer provides an excel workbook template for planning the sample labeling and distribution in the 96-well plate, and automatically calculates the proportion of labeling reagents to prepare for the mix. Moreover, by introducing the microarray slide barcodes into the planning software it specifies the slide position for hybridization of each sample.

1. Defrost the Reaction Buffer, Primer Solution, dCTP labeling mix, Cy3, Cy5, and SureRef Male® and SureRef Female®, vortex and briefly centrifuge them, and keep them in a cold rack.
2. Introduce the sample batch and microarray barcodes into the planning software, and distribute the 0.2 mL tubes with the amplified samples into the rack according to the planning software specifications.

3. Add 5 μL of Primer solution to the 96-well plate.
4. Add 8 μL of male and female DNA reference samples according to the order specified by the planner.
5. Using a multichannel pipette add 8 μL of amplified DNA product following the order specified by the planner.
6. Seal the plate with adhesive film and briefly centrifuge (20 s).
7. Denature the DNA at 94 ° C for 5 min in the thermo-cycler and then keep it at 4 °C (in a cooled rack) for 5 min.
8. Prepare the Cy3 master mix in a 1.5 mL Eppendorf tube as follows: For each sample use 5 μL reaction buffer, 5 μL dCTP mix, 1 μL Cy3, 1 μL Klenow. Scale the amounts according to the number of samples being processed. Remove the Klenow enzyme from the freezer and add it to the master mix at the last minute. Mix by inversion (or a very short vortex burst). Briefly centrifuge and keep the master mix in a cold rack.
9. Prepare the Cy5 master mix in a 1.5 mL Eppendorf tube as follows: For each sample use 5 μL reaction buffer, 5 μL dCTP mix, 1 μL Cy5, 1 μL Klenow. Scale the amounts according to the number of samples being processed. Remove the Klenow enzyme from the freezer and add it to the master mix at the last minute. Mix by inversion (or a very short vortex burst). Briefly centrifuge and keep the master mix in a cold rack.
10. Dispense 12 μL of the Cy3 or Cy5 mix into each well according to the planning software specifications, and always work with the plate in a cooled rack.
11. Seal the plate with adhesive film and briefly centrifuge (20 s).
12. Incubate at 37 °C for 2 h in the thermal cycler to allow labeling to take place, and then store the plate in a cold rack.

3.4 Combination, Volume Reduction, and Hybridization

1. Defrost the COT Human DNA; vortex and briefly centrifuge it and keep it in a cold rack.
2. Warm the dextran sulfate Hybridization Buffer to 75 °C.
3. In a fume cabinet, prepare the hybridization chambers by lining the bottom of the chamber with a paper towel soaked in the 50% Formamide/2× SSC solution.
4. Pulse spin the 96-well plate from the labeling step to collect the content at the bottom of the wells, and transfer the plate to a cold rack.
5. Add 25 μL COT Human DNA to each well of the 96-well plate containing Cy5 labeling products.
6. Using a multichannel pipette, combine Cy3 with the corresponding Cy5-labeled DNA as set out in the schema.

7. Transfer the plate to a pre-warmed centrifugal evaporator with the wells uncovered. Evaporate under centrifuge at 75 °C until around 3 μL remains in each tube/well (approximately 1 h).
8. Transfer the plate to a pre-warmed thermo-block (75 °C) and add 21 μL of DS Hybridization Buffer to each well. Resuspend the pellet, ensuring that it is completely dissolved. Pulse centrifuge to collect the contents into the bottom of the wells.
9. Seal the plate and denature it at 75 °C for a further 10 min, centrifuge it for 20 s, and allow it to cool to room temperature.
10. Apply 18 μL of labeled DNA solution to each cover slip (22 × 22) and lower the slide (barcode-down) onto the cover slip for each hybridization area in a fume cabinet.
11. Use the hybridization template to position the cover slips and to confirm which labeled DNAs are loaded onto each hybridization area.
12. Place the arrays into the hybridization chamber. Seal them and incubate in a water bath set at 48 °C for 3–16 h.

3.5 Slide Washing

To remove the unhybridized DNA from the array, the slides must be washed under stringent salt concentration and temperature conditions.

1. Warm the 0.1× SSC solution to 60 °C in a Clear Hybex® Hybridization System.
2. Remove the cover slips from each slide by manually agitating them in 2× SSC/0.05%Tween20 at room temperature in a fume cabinet. Immediately transfer them to a stainless steel rack sitting in a staining jar containing 2× SSC/0.05% Tween20 solution. Repeat this process for all the slides.
3. Once the rack is fully loaded replace lid, turn on the stirrer, and clean the slides for 10 min at room temperature. Transfer the stainless steel rack to a staining jar containing 1× SSC solution, turn on the stirrer, and clean them for 10 min at room temperature.
4. Transfer the stainless steel rack to the Clear Hybex® Hybridization System containing 0.1× SSC solution at 60 °C and wash them for 5 min without agitation.
5. Transfer the stainless steel rack to a staining jar containing 0.1× SSC solution, turn on the stirrer, and clean them for 1 min at room temperature.
6. Immediately dry the slides by centrifugation at 180 × *g* for 3 min and store them in an opaque box. To enable more efficient drying, the slide codes should face toward the centrifuge rotor.

3.6 Scan the Slides

Use a dual-channel scanner to excite the Cy3 and Cy5 hybridized fluorophores and to record the emission signals as TIFF image files. Use the green laser (532 nm wavelength) to excite and read the Cy3 signal, and the red laser (635 nm wavelength) to excite and read the Cy5 signal. 24sure® and 24sure + ® slides should be scanned at a 10 μm resolution. To simplify the workflow and minimize errors, we recommended that the slide barcode appears in the image file name, with a TOP or BOTTOM suffix to identify which hybridization area is included in the image file.

3.7 Data Analysis and Interpretation

Use the specific array software to turn the scanned images into clear profiles from which whole chromosome aneuploidy and sub-chromosomal structural imbalances can be analyzed. The software processes the TIFF image files and normalizes the fluorescent intensities emitted by the Cy3 and Cy5 channels. The data are processed and represented in a log2 ratio scale plot. The data from each chromosome are plotted as green dots on a fused chart display, representing the data from the sample tested versus the reference DNA. For 24sure® microarrays the software compares each sample with both male and female references whereas for 24sure + ® microarrays, comparisons are made only with male reference DNA. The X chromosome log2 ratio (termed X-separation) is compared with the log2 ratios of each chromosome to highlight aneuploidy calls as gains [+] or losses [−] [6]. According to these comparisons, we call a normal sample when there are not any spot deviations from the reference DNA for any of the chromosomes shown on the plot (Fig. 1). A sample is considered as abnormal with specific chromosome aneuploidies (full chromosome gains or losses) when the plot shows all the dots for these chromosomes within the upper or lower normal confidence lines defined by the reference DNA. The presence of aneuploidies for most of the chromosomes in the same specimen is interpreted as an abnormal chaotic pattern. Partial gains or losses for specific segments of a chromosome are considered as segmental aneuploidies when the size is higher than the resolution of the platform. Segmental aneuploidies for the chromosomes involving the rearrangement are the most commonly expected unbalances found in chromosomal rearrangement carriers. In these cases, platforms with a higher resolution are recommended (e.g., 24sure + ®, with a higher number of BACs representing pericentromeric and subtelomeric regions, *see* Fig. 2). The samples resulting in amplification failure show a typical pattern of XXY for sex chromosomes with a chromosome 19 gain.

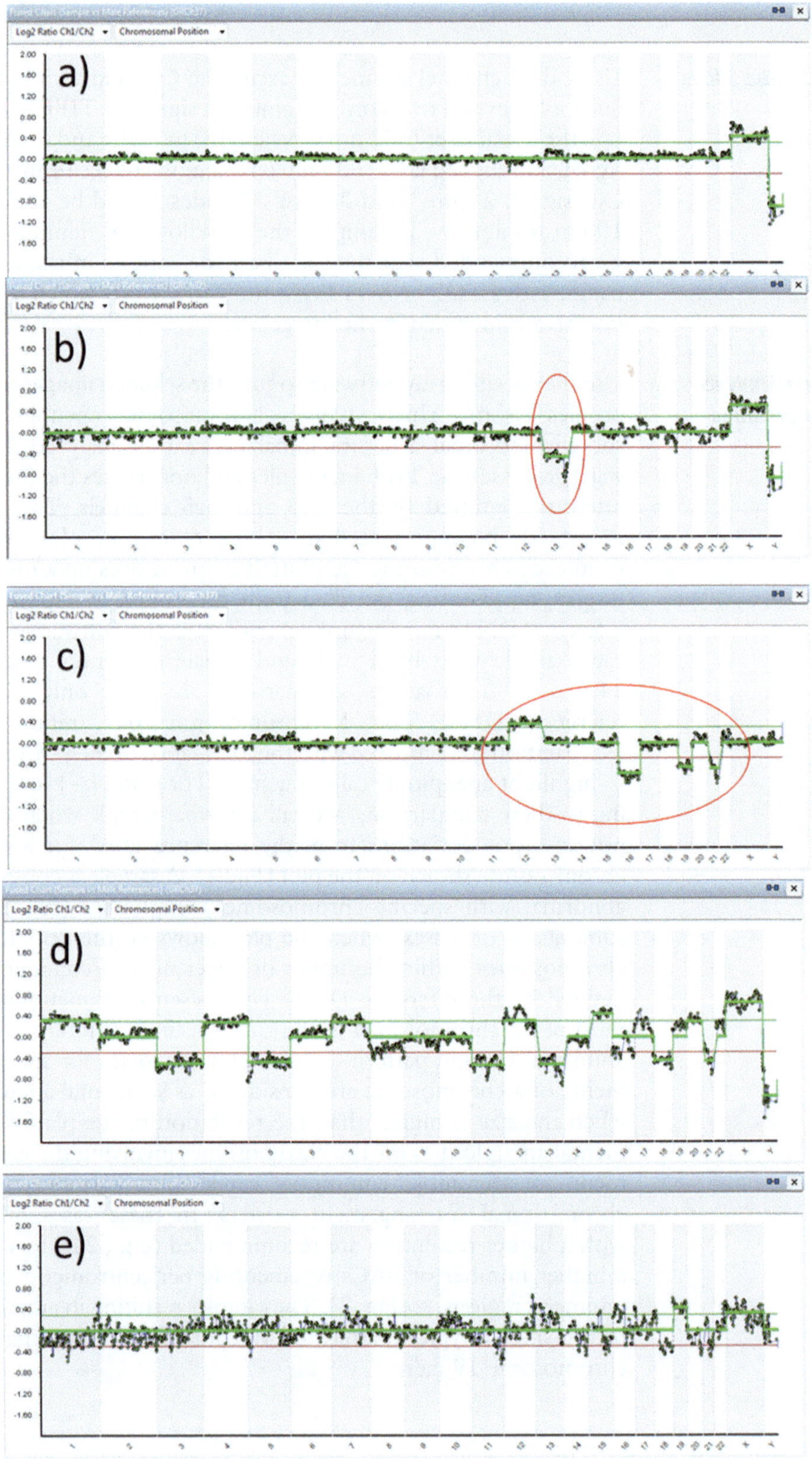

Fig. 1 PGS on a single cell using the 24sure array (20 Mb optimal resolution, but can achieve 10 Mb). (**a**) Normal XX embryo vs male reference. (**b**) Abnormal embryo with single aneuploidy, monosomy 13. (**c**) Complex abnormal embryo (between 2–5 aneuploid chromosomes). (**d**) Chaotic abnormal embryo (most of the chromosomes are abnormal). (**e**) Profile for a sample with amplification failure

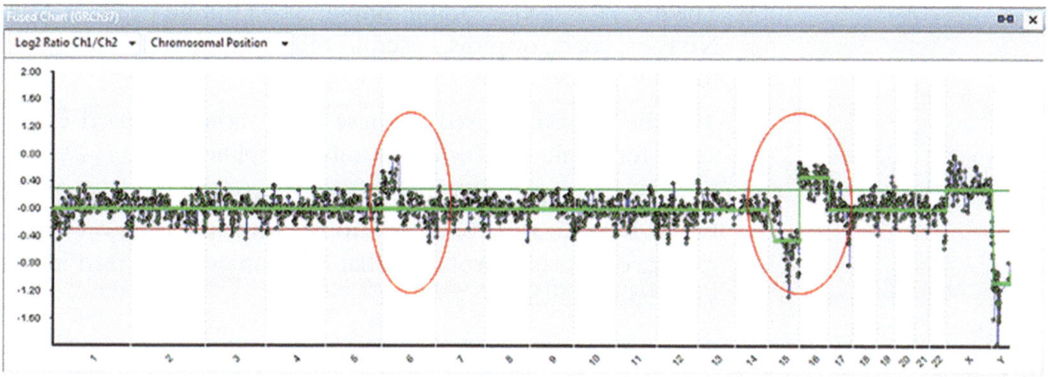

Fig. 2 PGS on a trophectoderm biopsy using the 24sure + array (10 Mb optimal resolution but can achieve 2 Mb) from a patient carrying a balanced reciprocal translocation, 46,XX,t(6;15)(p12;q14). The result shows an embryo with an unbalanced translocation (partial gain of 6p, a partial loss of 15q) as well as a complete gain of chromosome 16

4 Notes

1. Due to the low quantity of DNA we are working with for these PGS and PGD experiments it is very important to work in conditions of maximum sterility: i.e., a cap, lab coat, and gloves should be worn; gloves should be alcohol sterilized before starting any work. It is also important not to touch any surface without gloves.
2. Work should be undertaken in a vertical flow cabinet. Treat the cabinet with ultraviolet light for 10 min before starting the process. Clean the hood, materials, and instruments with alcohol.
3. Work in a clean area using a lab coat and gloves.
4. Store all of the buffers at room temperature.
5. We recommend that each step of the protocol in which the samples are transferred to new tubes, plates, or slides is verified by a second researcher.
6. We recommend working in a room separate from the IVF laboratory; avoid manipulating DNA in this room, or storing manipulated DNA samples in the freezer and fridge where the reaction solutions are stored.
7. Before starting, wear a cap, lab coat, and gloves. Alcohol sterilize gloves before starting any work. Do not touch any surface without gloves.
8. Work in a laminar flow cabinet and under the stereomicroscope. Treat the cabinet with ultraviolet light for 10 min before starting the process. Clean the hood, materials, and instruments with alcohol.

9. The pre-PCR lab for sample amplification should be DNA-free. No caps, coats, or gloves used in other labs should be allowed to enter this lab.
10. The thermo-cycler used in these steps should be used exclusively for single- or low-cell number amplification.
11. It is important to check the sample amplification products before hybridization because samples with amplification failure can have the same profile as that of samples hybridized in the same sub-array area.

References

1. Rodrigo L, Mateu E, Mercader A et al (2014) New tools for embryo selection: comprehensive chromosome screening by array comparative genomic hybridization. Biomed Res Int 2014:517125. https://doi.org/10.1155/2014/517125
2. Handyside AH (2013) 24-chromosome copy number analysis: a comparison of available technologies. Fertil Steril 100(3):595–602. https://doi.org/10.1016/j.fertnstert.2013.07.1965
3. Alfarawati S, Fragouli E, Colls P et al (2011) First births after preimplantation genetic diagnosis of structural chromosome abnormalities using comparative genomic hybridization and microarray analysis. Hum Reprod 26(6):1560–1574. https://doi.org/10.1093/humrep/der068
4. Illumina (2015) 24sure microarray single channel reference guide. https://support.illumina.com/content/dam/illumina-support/documents/documentation/chemistry_documentation/arraykits/24sure/24sure-microarray-single-channel-reference-guide-15056064-c.pdf
5. Illumina (2015) 24sure microarray dual channel reference guide. https://support.illumina.com/content/dam/illumina-support/documents/documentation/chemistry_documentation/arraykits/24sure/24sure-microarray-dual-channel-reference-guide-15056062-c.pdf
6. Illumina (2014) A technical guide to aneuploidy calling with 24sure single channel. https://support.illumina.com/content/dam/illumina-support/documents/documentation/chemistry_documentation/arraykits/24sure/A-Technical-Guide-to-Aneuploidy-Calling-24sure-15056973-A.pdf

Chapter 6

Aneuploidy Screening using Next Generation Sequencing

Cengiz Cinnioglu, Refik Kayali, Tristan Darvin, Adedoyin Akinwole, Milena Jakubowska, and Gary Harton

Abstract

Chromosomal aneuploidy is recognized to be a significant contributing factor in implantation failure and spontaneous miscarriage Hellani et al. (Reprod Biomed Online 17:841–847, 2008), Vanneste et al. (Nat Med 15:577–583, 2009) and is likely to be responsible for the majority of IVF failure [Baltaci et al. (Reprod Biomed Online 12:77–82, 2006), Munne (Placenta 24:S70–76, 2003)]. Preimplantation genetic testing for aneuploidy (PGT-A) screening, formerly termed preimplantation genetic screening (PGS), enables the assessment of the numeric chromosomal constitution in blastomere and/or trophectoderm biopsy before embryo transfer.

Preimplantation genetic testing for aneuploidy (PGT-A) has been proven to improve the selection of embryos for transfer and therefore also assisted reproductive technology (ART) cycles. In this chapter we describe the current gold standard platform for PGT-A, next generation sequencing (NGS) protocol used in our laboratory.

Key words Preimplantation genetic testing for aneuploidy (PGT-A), Aneuploidy, Next generation sequencing (NGS), Whole genome amplification (WGA)

1 Introduction

One of the most common genetic abnormalities in human embryos is aneuploidy [1–3] which contributes to increased reproductive issues of infertile couples including lack of implantation, recurrent implantation failure, miscarriage, and birth of children affected with various abnormalities associated with poor reproductive outcomes [4–6]. To increase both the implantation and pregnancy rates for these couples, performing PGT-A as a part of the fertility treatment is recommended. There are several indications for PGT-A, the most common being advanced maternal age (AMA-typically female patients older than 35 years at the time of IVF treatment). A study on polar body biopsies indicates that the aneuploidy of chromosomes 13, 16, and 18 increases from 20% to 60% for women in age group 35–43 [7]. Among other frequent

Brynn Levy (ed.), *Prenatal Diagnosis*, Methods in Molecular Biology, vol. 1885, https://doi.org/10.1007/978-1-4939-8889-1_6,

indications for PGT-A are recurrent miscarriage, repetitive implantation failure (RIF), male factor, and previous aneuploidy conception [8].

Techniques used in PGT-A have changed significantly in the last 20 years. Up until 2010, the most common way to diagnose embryos with aneuploidy was through fluorescence in situ hybridization (FISH). The major limiting factor to this procedure is an inability to test for the full chromosome complement (24 chromosomes in one test). In practice, only selected chromosomes are tested using FISH: most commonly, chromosomes 15, 16, 17, 18, 21, 22, X and Y [9]. To increase the number of chromosomes that can be analyzed simultaneously, new techniques were introduced including quantitative polymerase chain reaction (qPCR), single nucleotide polymorphism arrays (SNP arrays), and array comparative genomic hybridization (aCGH) [10]. All 24 chromosomes can be tested at the same time using these methods. The latest development in the aneuploidy screening field is the development of next generation sequencing (NGS) platforms for the analysis of the chromosome complement in early human embryos. Early stages of NGS involved a number of manual pipetting steps including whole genome amplification (WGA), library preparation, and sequencing chip loading ahead of sequencing which can be done using a number of NGS platforms commercially available. In our laboratories, we began NGS using the personal genome machine (PGM) from Thermo Fisher (San Francisco, CA). Recently, our laboratories have begun using new technology including robotics and machines such as Ion GeneStudio™ S5 with the Ion Chef™ system which allows for an automated chip loading and ability to analyze up to 96 samples simultaneously in less than 24 h. This makes this system the most costs effective, high throughput NGS system currently available commercially [11].

The objective of this chapter is to describe our use of the NGS platform from Thermo Fisher which utilizes semi-conductor sequencer sequencing and proprietary algorithms to allow for high throughput, high resolution NGS testing for PGT-A. All PGT-A protocols begin with a whole genome amplification step which allows for general amplification of the entire genome from one to a few cells from early human embryos. The aim of this step is twofold: to obtain sufficient amounts of deoxyribonucleic acid (DNA) for further processing and to incorporate specific, unique DNA barcodes to each embryo biopsy sample. By adding unique barcodes to each embryo biopsy sample, multiple samples from different embryos and/or different patients can be mixed together prior to sequencing allowing for high throughput NGS. Following WGA, 5 μL of each sample is taken and pooled or mixed with other samples, followed by a purification step which separates impurities from the double stranded DNA (dsDNA). The purified pool is quantified using Qubit (Thermo Fisher Scientific, USA) and the pool is diluted using nuclease-free water to obtain 18 pM concentration of DNA. The pooled DNA is then ready for the next step with is isothermal amplification (IA) (see Subheading 3.4). Following IA, the samples can be loaded on the semi-conductor chip. During the loading procedure, the DNA is fragmented, or cut, into smaller segments that can be attached to tiny beads used in sequencing. Each bead is the deposited into one well on the chip [12]. The chip, loaded with beads covered with DNA fragments, is then placed in the sequencer where a series of nucleotides are flowed across each bead, one nucleotide at a time. When the next nucleotide in the segment is incorporated, a hydrogen ion is released, which changes the pH in the solution in the chip's well. Changes of pH are measured and converted into voltage. By measuring the pH of each well during each nucleotide flow, incorporation of the next nucleotide is assessed and noted by the system. Once each nucleotide has been incorporated, the sequence of each unique DNA fragment can be cataloged and used later in the process [13]. Once completed, the sequence of each sample is aligned with a reference human genome. This is the followed by use of the Ion Reporter™ software which calculates the number of copies of each DNA fragment across the entire genome. This allows for analysis of chromosome copy number as well as measurement of small gains/losses [14]. Graphs are generated, and initial calls are determined by the Ion Reporter™ software. This step is then followed by analysis of the graphs by highly trained technologists in our laboratory based on training and use of control cell lines in each experiment with known chromosome abnormalities. These controls were purchased by Coriell cell repositories (https://www.coriell.org/) that were used initially for validation purposes and are now used in each experiment as positive controls.

2 Materials

1. Stereo Microscope for Cell Manipulation.
2. Stripper micropipette (Vitrolife, Colorado, USA).
3. 96-Well Thermal Cycler with heated lid (0.2 mL block for standard PCR amplification).
4. 96-Well Retainer for transferring tubes.
5. Microcentrifuge (capable of >15,500 × *g*, fits 1.5 mL and 0.2 mL microcentrifuge tubes).
6. DynaMag™ -2 magnet (Thermo Fisher Scientific, Waltham, MA).
7. Qubit™ 3.0 Fluorometer.
8. Heat block.

9. Ion OneTouch™ ES Instrument (Thermo Fisher Scientific, Waltham, MA).
10. 18-MΩ water purification system.
11. Multistage (dual-stage) gas regulator (0-50 PSI, 2-3 Bar output).
12. Ion Personal Genome Machine™ (PGM™) System (Thermo Fisher Scientific, Waltham, MA).
13. Ion Chip™ Minifuge (Thermo Fisher Scientific, Waltham, MA).
14. Vacuum filtration system.
15. 0.2 mL PCR tubes, Flat Cap (do not use polystyrene tubes).
16. 1.5 mL Eppendorf LoBind™ Tubes (DNA).
17. 2.0 mL Eppendorf LoBind™ Tubes (DNA).
18. Low TE (10 mM Tris pH 8.0, 0.1 mM EDTA).
19. Nuclease-free water.
20. NaOH (10 M), molecular biology grade.
21. 1 L Glass bottle.
22. 0.22 μm vacuum filter.

2.1 Cell Loading

1. 100–130 μm diameter micro glass capillaries.
2. 20× Phosphate Buffered Saline (PBS).
3. Double-distilled autoclaved water.
4. Mineral oil.
5. Polyvinylpyrrolidone (PVP).

2.2 Library Preparation, Purification, and Quantification

1. Ion SingleSeq™ Kit (Thermo Fisher Scientific, Waltham, MA): Contains: cell extraction buffer, extraction enzyme dilution buffer, extraction enzyme, pre-amplification buffer, pre-amplification enzyme, amplification buffer, amplification enzyme, nuclease-free water, Ion SingleSeq™ Barcode Set, Human CEPH Genomic DNA Control 100 μg/mL.
2. Agencourt™ AMPure™ XP Reagent (Beckman Coulter, Indianapolis, IN).
3. Qubit™ dsDNA High Sensitivity (HS) Assay Kit (Thermo Fisher Scientific, Waltham, MA): Contains: Qubit™ dsDNA HS Reagent (Component A), Qubit™ dsDNA HS Buffer (Component B), Qubit™ Standards (Component C and D).
4. Qubit™ Assay Tubes (Thermo Fisher Scientific, Waltham, MA).

2.3 Isothermal Amplification and Enrichment

1. Ion PGM™ Template IA Supplies (Thermo Fisher Scientific, Waltham, MA): Eppendorf™ LoRetention Dualfilter—300 μL PCR pipette tips, 8-well strips.
2. Ion PGM™ Template IA Reagents 500 (Thermo Fisher Scientific, Waltham, MA): Ion PGM™ Template IA Pellets 500, Ion PGM™ Template IA ISP Dilution Buffer, Ion PGM™ Template IA Start Solution.
3. Ion PGM™ Template IA Reactions 500 (Thermo Fisher Scientific, Waltham, MA): Ion PGM™ Template IA Ion Sphere Particles™, Ion PGM™ Template IA Primer Mix S, Ion PGM™ Template IA Rehydration Buffer.
4. Ion PGM™ Template IA Solutions 500 (Thermo Fisher Scientific, Waltham, MA): Ion PGM™ Template IA Stop Solution, Ion PGM™ Template IA Recovery Solution, Ion PGM™ Template IA Wash Solution, MyOne™ Beads Wash Solution, Neutralization Solution, Tween™ Solution.
5. Ion PGM™ Enrichment Beads (Thermo Fisher Scientific, Waltham, MA): Contains Dynabeads™ MyOne™ Streptavidin C1 Beads.

2.4 Sequencing, Initialization, and Cleaning

1. Ion PGM™ Sequencing Supplies (Thermo Fisher Scientific, Waltham, MA): Contains: Wash 1 Bottle with label (250 mL), Wash 3 Bottle with label (250 mL), Ion PGM™ Reagent Bottle Sipper Tubes, Ion PGM™ Wash Bottle Sipper Tubes, Reagent Bottles with labels (50 mL).
2. Ion PGM™ Hi-Q™ View Sequencing Reagents (Thermo Fisher Scientific, Waltham, MA): Contains: Ion PGM™ Hi-Q™ View Sequencing Polymerase, Sequencing Primer, Control Ion Sphere™ Particles.
3. Ion PGM™ Hi-Q™ View Sequencing Solutions (Thermo Fisher Scientific, Waltham, MA): Contains: Ion PGM™ Hi-Q™ View Sequencing W2 Solution, Ion PGM™ Cleaning Tablet, Annealing Buffer, Ion PGM™ Hi-Q™ View Sequencing W3 Solution.
4. Ion PGM™ Hi-Q™ View Sequencing dNTPs (Thermo Fisher Scientific, Waltham, MA): Contains: Ion PGM™ Hi-Q™ View Sequencing dGTP, Ion PGM™ Hi-Q™ View Sequencing dCTP, Ion PGM™ Hi-Q™ View Sequencing dATP, Ion PGM™ Hi-Q™ View Sequencing dTTP.
5. Ion PGM™ Wash 2 Bottle Kit (Thermo Fisher Scientific, Waltham, MA): Contains: Wash 2 Bottle with label (2 L), Wash 2 bottle condition solution.
6. Ion Chip Kits (Thermo Fisher Scientific, Waltham, MA): Contains: Ion 318™ Chip v2 BC.

2.5 Cell Loading

1. 1× PBS: Autoclave the 20× PBS. Prepare 1 mL of 1× PBS in a sterile, autoclaved 1.5 mL tube by mixing 50 μL of the autoclaved 20× PBS in 950 μL of the double-distilled autoclaved water; vortex and briefly centrifuge it. Dispense 2.5 μL of 1× PBS into autoclaved 0.2 mL PCR tubes. Prepare as many tubes as the number of embryo biopsies. Prepare two additional tubes to be used as positive and negative PCR controls.
2. 1% Polyvinylpyrrolidone (PVP) Solution: In an autoclaved, sterile 1.5 mL tube, dilute 0.01 g of polyvinylpyrrolidone in 1 mL of 1× PBS. Vortex and briefly centrifuge.

2.6 Purification and Quantification

1. 70% Ethanol: In a sterile 1.5 mL tube, dilute 210 μL of 100% ethanol in 90 mL of nuclease-free water. Vortex and briefly centrifuge.
2. Qubit™ Working Solution: In a sterile 1.5 mL tube, combine 1194 μL of Qubit™ dsDNA HS Buffer with 6 μL of Qubit™ dsDNA HS Reagent. Vortex, briefly centrifuge, and store in a dark area.

2.7 Isothermal Amplification and Enrichment

1. Melt-Off Solution: In a sterile 1.5 mL tube, combine 280 μL of Tween™ Solution and 40 μL of 1 M NaOH. Vortex and briefly centrifuge.
2. 1 M NaOH: In a sterile 1.5 mL tube, dilute 100 μL of 10 M NaOH in 900 μL of nuclease-free water. Vortex and briefly centrifuge.

2.8 Sequencing, Initialization, and Cleaning

1. 1 M NaOH: In a sterile 1.5 mL tube, dilute 100 μL of 10 M NaOH in 900 μL of nuclease-free water. Vortex and briefly centrifuge.
2. Chlrorite Cleaning Solution: In a 1 L glass bottle, combine 1 L of 18 MΩ water Ion Cleaning tablet (chlorite tablet). Allow the tablet to dissolve completely. After the tablet has dissolved, add 1 mL of 1 M NaOH and filter the solution using a 0.22 μm filter.
3. 100 nM NaOH: In a sterile 1.5 mL tube, dilute 50 μL of 1 M NaOH in 450 μL of nuclease-free water.
4. Wash 2 Solution: Rinse the Wash 2 Bottle (2 L) 3 times with 200 mL of 18 MΩ water. Fill with 2 L of 18 MΩ water, an entire bottle of Ion PGM™ Hi-Q™ View Sequencing W2 Solution, and 70 μL of 100 nM NaOH. Invert 5 times to mix thoroughly.

3 Methods

The protocols described in this chapter are based on the protocols recommended by the NGS manufacturer, Thermo Fisher Scientific.

3.1 Cell Loading

The single cell, or 3–5 cells biopsied from the trophectoderm of blastocyst stage embryos, should be washed before amplification to minimize non-cellular DNA contamination. After this, the samples are loaded into 0.2 mL PCR tubes to start the amplification process.

1. Use one capillary Stripper tip for each individual cell or trophectoderm biopsy.
2. Briefly centrifuge the 0.2 mL PCR sterile tubes containing 5 μL 1× PBS to avoid the formation of bubbles inside them.
3. Prepare a petri dish (one for each biopsied embryo) containing a row with three droplets of 5 μL PBS/1% PVP solution and cover with mineral oil. Capture the cell or trophectoderm biopsy with the capillary and rinse it by passing it through each of these droplets (release it in the first droplet, recapture it, and transfer it into the second droplet; repeat for the third droplet).
4. Deposit each biopsied cell, or trophectoderm cell sample, into a 0.2 mL PCR sterile tube under the stereoscope. The cell (s) release should be observed by the embryologist and done with a minimal volume of washing media (maximum 0.5 μL). Cap the PCR tube and place inside a cold rack.
5. Store at −20 °C until amplification or maintain at 4 °C if the amplification procedure is immediate.

3.2 Sample Amplification

Due to the low quantity of DNA we are working with for these PGT-A experiments it is very important to work in conditions of maximum sterility: i.e., a cap, lab coat, and gloves should be worn; gloves should be alcohol sterilized before starting any work. It is also important not to touch any surface without gloves. Work should be done in a vertical flow hood. Sterilize the hood with UV light for 10 min prior to starting the process. Clean the hood, materials, and equipment with alcohol. Store all reagents in their appropriate temperatures. We recommend that each step of the protocol in which the samples are transferred to new tubes, plates, or slides is verified by a second researcher. We recommend working in Pre-PCR room separate from the IVF laboratory. It is crucial to perform gel electrophoresis during the whole genome amplification process to determine if amplification has been successful or not.

3.2.1 Cell Lysis and DNA Extraction

1. Defrost the positive control genomic DNA; vortex and briefly centrifuge it. Store it in a rack.
2. Organize the batch of samples to be amplified and calculate the buffer quantities for the different master mixes.
3. Defrost a vial of cell extraction buffer and extraction enzyme dilution buffer, vortex and briefly centrifuge it.
4. Transfer the 0.2 mL PCR tubes containing the samples from the batch into a cold rack. Prepare one tube containing 2.0 μL CEPH DNA (10 pg DNA) and 5.0 μL washing buffer for the positive control and one tube containing only 5.0 μL washing buffer for the negative control. Briefly centrifuge all the tubes before starting the amplification.
5. Add 2.5 μL cell extraction buffer to each tube and briefly centrifuge to collect the contents.
6. Prepare a master mix in a 0.2 mL microcentrifuge tube as follows: For each sample, use 4.8 μL extraction enzyme dilution buffer and 0.2 μL extraction enzyme. Scale the amounts according to the number of samples being processed. Add the extraction enzyme at the last minute and mix by inversion (or a very short vortex burst). Briefly centrifuge and keep the master mix in a cold rack.
7. Add 5 μL of freshly prepared master mix to each sample and the controls. Briefly centrifuge.
8. Incubate the samples in a PCR thermal cycler with the lid preheated to 95 °C prior to starting the reaction and use the following program settings:
   - One Cycle: 75 °C for 10 min.
   - One Cycle: 95 °C for 4 min.
   - 22 °C Hold.

3.2.2 Pre-amplification

1. Defrost a vial of pre-amplification buffer, vortex and briefly centrifuge it.
2. Prepare a master mix in a 0.2 mL microcentrifuge tube as follows: For each sample, use 4.8 μL pre-amplification buffer and 0.2 μL pre-amplification enzyme. Scale the amounts according to the number of samples being processed. Add the pre-amplification enzyme at the last minute and mix by inversion (or a very short vortex burst). Briefly centrifuge and keep the master mix in a cold rack.
3. Under a pre-PCR hood, to add 5 μL of freshly prepared master mix to each sample and the controls. Briefly centrifuge.

4. Incubate them in a PCR thermal cycler with the lid preheated to 95 °C and use the following program settings:
   - One cycle: 95 °C for 2 min.
   - Twelve cycles: 95 °C for 15 s, 15 °C for 50 s, 25 °C for 40 s, 35 °C for 30 s, 65 °C for 40 s, 75 °C for 40 s.
   - 4 °C Hold.
5. Place the PCR tubes into a cold rack (or in the fridge at 4 °C) and check for sample pre-amplification by agarose gel electrophoresis.

3.2.3 Amplification

1. Defrost a vial of amplification buffer and a vial of nuclease-free water, vortex and briefly centrifuge it.
2. Prepare a master mix in a 1.5 mL Eppendorf tube as follows: For each sample, use 2.5 μL nuclease-free water, 27 μL amplification buffer, and 0.5 μL amplification enzyme. Scale the amounts according to the number of samples being processed. Add the amplification enzyme at the last minute and mix by inversion (or a very short vortex burst). Briefly centrifuge and keep the master mix in a cold rack.
3. Under a pre-PCR hood, add 30 μL of freshly prepared master mix to each sample and the controls. Briefly centrifuge.
4. Retrieve the Ion SingleSeq™ Barcode Set, sterilize the surface with 70% ethanol, and open carefully. Verify the position of the samples in accordance with run workflow. Add 5.0 μL of the respective barcode to their respective samples.
5. Mix the samples by inversion and incubate the samples in a PCR thermal cycler with the lid preheated to 95 °C and use following program settings:
   - One cycle: 95 °C for 2 min.
   - Four cycles: 95 °C for 20 s, 50 °C for 25 s, 752 °C for 40 s.
   - Twelve cycles: 95 °C for 20 sec, 72 °C for 55 sec.
   - 4 °C Hold (*see* **Note 1**).

3.3 Library Purification

1. Add 5 μL of each library to a new 200 μL microcentrifuge tube to create an equivolume pool. Vortex the tube to mix and pulse-spin to collect contents at the bottom of the tube (*see* **Note 2**).
2. Incubate the pool in thermal cycler with the lid preheated to 95 °C and use following program settings:
   - One cycle: 70 °C for 2 min.
   - 22 °C Hold.

3. Pulse-spin the tube to collect contents, then transfer the heated library pool to a fresh 1.5 mL Eppendorf DNA LoBind™ Tube.
4. Total the volumes of libraries added to the pool and add equal volume of AMPure™ XP beads. Vortex briefly, pulse-spin the tube to collect contents, then incubate for 5 min at room temperature.
5. Place the tube on the DynaMag™-2 magnet, then wait 5 min for beads to aggregate to the side of the tube.
6. At the end of the 5 min, aspirate the supernatant carefully and discard. Wash beads with 150 μL of freshly prepared 70% ethanol while the tube is still on the magnet and incubate for 30 s.
7. Aspirate and discard the wash solution. Repeat with a second wash, incubate for 30 s, and aspirate the wash solution.
8. Allow the beads to dry at room temperature for 3–4 min with the tube on the magnet. Then, remove the tube from the magnet and resuspend beads in 200 μL of Low TE, vortex thoroughly, and pulse-spin to collect the contents.
9. Incubate the tube at room temperature for 1 min.
10. Place the tube on the DynaMag™-2 magnet, then wait 2–3 min for beads to aggregate to the side of the tube.
11. Transfer 195 μL of the supernatant containing the purified library pool to a fresh 1.5 mL Eppendorf DNA LoBind™ tube avoiding the carryover of beads. Label the tube accordingly (*see* **Note 3**).

3.4 Library Quantification

1. Vortex the purified pool thoroughly, pulse-spin to collect contents, and transfer 30 μL to a new 0.2 μL microcentrifuge tube.
2. Incubate the sample in a thermal cycler with the lid preheated to 95 °C and use following program settings:
   - One cycle: 70 °C for 2 min.
   - 4 °C Hold.
3. Prepare the Qubit™ Working Solution by diluting the Qubit™ dsDNA HS Reagent (Component A) 1:200 in Qubit™ dsDNA HS Buffer (Component B) in a centrifuge tube enough for the purified pool(s) plus two standards and vortex well.
4. Prepare the two standards by adding 190 μL Qubit™ Working Solution to two labeled Qubit™ Assay Tubes. Add 10 μL of each Qubit™ Standard #1 (Component C) and Qubit™ Standard #2 (Component D) to the appropriate tubes.
5. Prepare the unknowns by adding 198 μL Qubit™ Working Solution to labeled Qubit™ Assay Tubes, 2 tubes per pool to

create an average. Add 2 μL of the heated library pool to the appropriate sample tube.

6. Vortex each of the tubes for 2–3 s, avoid creating bubbles. Incubate the tubes in the dark at room temperature for 2 min.
7. On a Qubit™ 3.0 Fluorometer, select "dsDNA Assay" and then select "dsDNA High Sensitivity." Choose "Read Standards" to measure standards that will generate a standard curve.
8. Set the roller wheel to 2 μL and the units to ng/μL. Read the standards and records the values. Calculate the average purified pool and immediately proceed to isothermal amplification reaction.

3.5 Isothermal Amplification (IA) Reaction

3.5.1 Preparation of Template-Positive Ion PGM™ Template IA Ion Sphere Particles (ISPs)

1. Turn on the heat block and set to 41 °C. Fill each of the wells with water.
2. Thaw the Ion PGM™ Template IA Primer Mix S and Ion PGM™ Template IA Rehydration Buffer on cold block. Place Ion PGM™ Template IA Pellet on cold block until needed.
3. Dilute the library pool to 2.0 nM based on the recorded average during the quantification step. Based on dilution calculation, use Low TE buffer to dilute.
4. Perform a 1:100 dilution using the freshly prepared 2.0 nM library pool and nuclease-free water to generate a 20 pM library pool.
5. Transfer 50 μL of 20 pM library pool to a new 0.2 mL PCR tube. Heat the pool in the thermal cycler with the lid preheated to 95 °C and use following program settings:
   - One cycle: 70 °C for 2 min.
   - 4 °C Hold.
6. Vortex the Ion PGM™ Template IA ISPs for 1 min.
7. In a new 2.0 mL Eppendorf DNA LoBind™ tube on a cold block, prepare the templating solution by combining the following: 130 μL Ion PGM™ Template IA ISP Dilution Buffer, 8.0 μL Ion PGM™ Template IA Primer Mix S, 21 μL Ion PGM™ Template IA ISPs, 10 μL of the preheated 20 pM purified library. Vortex the tube, pulse-spin to collect the contents, and place on cold block.
8. Invert the Ion PGM™ Template IA Rehydration Buffer 3 times to mix, the use 720 μL to rehydrate the Ion PGM™ Template IA Pellet. Vortex for 4 s at maximum setting, pulse-spin to collect the contents, and place on cold block.
9. Transfer the rehydrated IA pellet to the templating solution, vortex for 4 s, pulse-spin to collect contents, and store on cold block.

10. Invert the Ion PGM™ Template IA Start Solution 3 times to mix, then add 300 μL to the mixture using negative pipetting:
    - Set a 1 mL pipette to 300 μL. Press the pipette to the second stop and dip the tip into the Ion PGM™ Template IA Start Solution. Slowly release the pipette and allow 10 s for the contents to be fully drawn.
    - Dispense the contents to the mixture by pressing the pipette to the first stop and hold it. Allow 10 s for the contents to be dispensed. Some liquid will remain in the tip.
11. Vortex the tube ten times in 1 s pulses at maximum settings. Invert the tube and repeat the ten 1 s pulses. Pulse-spin to collect the contents and place the tube on ice block.
12. Start the reaction by gently placing the tube in the preheated heat block. Make certain the tube is immersed in water. Incubate the IA reaction for 25 min at 41 °C.

3.5.2 Recovery of Template-Positive Ion PGM™ Template IA Ion Sphere Particles (ISPs)

1. Stop the IA reaction by removing the tube from the heat block and adding 650 μL of the Ion PGM™ Template IA Stop Solution. Vortex the tube thoroughly.
2. Centrifuge the tube at 7500 × *g* for 6 min.
3. Aspirate and discard the supernatant, being careful not to disturb the pellet. Leave approximately 100 μL in the tube.
4. Resuspend the pellet in 1 mL of the Ion PGM™ Template IA Recovery Solution. Resuspend by pipetting up and down. Vortex the mixture well, avoiding to create bubbles.
5. Add an additional 700 μL of the Ion PGM™ Template IA Recovery Solution and vortex thoroughly. Incubate for 5 min with 5 s of vortexing every minute.
6. Centrifuge the tube at 17,000 × *g* for 6 min.
7. Immediately remove and discard all the supernatant without disturbing the ISP pellet. Remove any bubbles prior to removing the bulk of the liquid to avoid frothing in subsequent steps.
8. Add 100 μL of the Ion PGM™ Template IA Wash Solution to the ISP pellet. Resuspend the templated ISPs complete by vortexing for 4 s at maximum speed, then pipetting the ISP suspension up and down four times (*see* **Note 4**).

3.6 Enrichment

3.6.1 Preparing the Melt-Off Solution and the Dynabeads™ MyOne™ Streptavidin C1 Beads

1. Prepare a melt-off solution as follows: In a sterile 1.5 mL Eppendorf tube, combine 280 μL of the Tween™ Solution and 40 μL of 1 M NaOH. Vortex well and briefly centrifuge.
2. Vortex the tube of Dynabeads™ MyOne™ Streptavidin C1 Beads for 30 s to resuspend the beads thoroughly. Briefly centrifuge the tube to collect the supernatant without getting beads.

3. Transfer 13 μL of Dynabeads™ MyOne™ Streptavidin C1 Beads in a sterile 1.5 mL Eppendorf tube. Place the tube on the DynaMag™-2 magnet for 2 min, then carefully remove, and discard the supernatant without disturbing the pellet.
4. Add 130 μL of the MyOne™ Beads Wash Solution to the pellet. Remove the tube from the magnet, vortex the tube for 30 s, then briefly centrifuge to collect the contents.

3.6.2 Filling the 8-Well Strip

1. Vortex the template-positive ISPs (~100 μL) and transfer all contents in Well 1 in a sterile 8-well strip.
2. Fill the remaining wells with the following:
   - Well 2: 130 μL of Dynabeads™ MyOne™ Streptavidin C1 Beads resuspended in MyOne™ Beads Wash Solution.
   - Well 3: 300 μL of Ion PGM™ Template IA Wash Solution.
   - Well 4: 300 μL of Ion PGM™ Template IA Wash Solution.
   - Well 5: 300 μL of Ion PGM™ Template IA Wash Solution.
   - Well 6: Empty.
   - Well 7: 300 μL of freshly prepared Melt-Off Solution.
   - Well 8: Empty.

3.6.3 Preparing the Ion OneTouch™ ES for Enrichment

1. Place a new tip in the Tip Loader. Take the Tip Arm and push down onto the tip and ensure that it is tightly secured. Once secure, return the Tip Arm back to its cradle ensuring it is in the correct orientation.
2. In a sterile 0.2 mL PCR tube, add 10 μL of Neutralization Solution and place it into the place holder on the device.
3. Place the 8-well strip in the slot, flushed all the way right. Pres Start/Stop to begin the run (~36 min).
4. Immediately after the run, securely close and remove the PCR tube containing the enriched ISPs. Invert the tube five times to mix the contents.
5. Discard the used tip and 8-well strip (*see* **Note 5**).

3.7 Preparing the PGM for Initialization

3.7.1 Condition the Wash 2 Bottle for Use

1. Fill a brand-new Wash 2 Bottle to the mold line (~2 L) with 18 MΩ water. Pour the entire contents of the Wash 2 Bottle Condition Solution and invert the mix five times.
2. Allow the bottle to sit at room temperature for at least 8 h before use.

3.7.2 Cleaning the PGM

1. If performing an 18 MΩ water cleaning, do the following:
   - Empty and remaining solution from all bottle and rinse them twice with 18 MΩ water.

- Add 250 mL of 18 MΩ water into the cleaning bottle and securely attach this to the W1 position. Place the remaining empty bottles in their respective W2 and W3 positions without screwing the caps on.
- Remove any dNTP conical tubes and leave used sipper tips attached. Place drip trays below.
- Ensure that a used chip is securely placed in the PGM.
- Press Clean on the PGM touchscreen and selection 18-MOhm water cleaning. Follow the onscreen instructions and allow cleaning to begin.
- Empty all wastes once complete.

2. If performing a Chlorite cleaning, do the following:
   - Empty and remaining solution from all bottle and rinse them twice with 18 MΩ water.
   - Fill a glass bottle with 1 L 18 MΩ water, then add an Ion Cleaning tablet (chlorite tablet). Allow the tablet to dissolve completely. When the tablet has completely dissolved, add 1 mL of 1 M NaOH and filter the solution using a 0.22 μm filter.
   - Add 250 mL of the filtered chlorite solution into the cleaning bottle and securely attach this to the W1 position. Place the remaining empty bottles in their respective W2 and W3 positions without screwing the caps on.
   - Remove any dNTP conical tubes and leave used sipper tips attached. Place drip trays below.
   - Ensure that a used chip is securely placed in the PGM.
   - Press Clean on the PGM touchscreen and selection chlorite cleaning. Follow the onscreen instructions and allow cleaning to begin.
   - Empty all wastes once complete.

3.7.3 Initializing the PGM

1. Remove the dNTP stock solutions from the freezer and begin thawing. Check the tank pressure for the nitrogen gas.
2. Rinse the conditioned Wash 2 Bottle 3 times with 200 mL of 18 MΩ water. Fill to the mold line with 18 MΩ water. Add the entire bottle of Ion PGM™ Hi-Q™ View Sequencing W2 Solution to the Wash 2 bottle.
3. Prepare 500 μL of 100 mM NaOH by diluting 50 μL of 1 M NaOH in 450 μL of nuclease-free water.
4. Add 70 μL of 100 nM NaOH to the Wash 2 Bottle. Cap the bottle and invert it five times to mix contents thoroughly.
5. Rinse the Wash 1 and Wash 3 bottles with 18 MΩ water.
6. Add 350 μL of 100 nM NaOH to the Wash 1 Bottle.

7. Add Ion PGM™ Sequencing W3 Solution to the 50 mL line marked on the Wash 3 Bottle.
8. Replace the sippers for the Wash Bottles, place the prepared bottles in their respective positions, and securely fasten the caps on each.
9. On the PGM, press Initialize and follow the instruction. Select Ion PGM™ Hi-Q™ View Sequencing Kit when prompted, then press next. Allow the PGM to complete the first portion of the initialization process.
10. Using the thawed dNTP stocks, transfer 20 μL of each dNTP stock solution to a new respective reagent bottle. Cap each bottle until ready for use.
11. After the PGM completes the first portion of the initialization process, replace the sippers for the dNTP slots, and securely fasten each dNTP bottle into their respective positions. Press next to allow the PGM to complete the final portion of the initialization process.
12. If the initialization was successful, then a notification stating Passed will appear on the screening. This will indicate that the PGM is ready for sequencing.

3.8 Starting a Sequencing Run

3.8.1 Create a Planned Run

1. On the Ion Torrent Server, create a Planned Run using Ion ReproSeq™ Aneploidy.
2. Follow the on-screen instructions and confirm the plan run details.

3.8.2 Preparing the Enriched, Template-Positive ISPs

1. Thaw the Sequencing Primer on ice.
2. Vortex the Control Ion Sphere™ Particles (ISPs), then briefly centrifuge to collect the contents. Add 5 μL if the Control ISPs to the enriched, template-positive ISPs. Mix well.
3. Centrifuge at 17,000 × *g* for 3 min.
4. Aspirate the supernatant and avoid disturbing the pellet. Leave ~15 μL in the tube.
5. Vortex the thawed primer for 5 s and add 12 μL to the enriched, template-positive ISPs. Vortex the mixture and briefly centrifuge.
6. Incubate the samples in a PCR thermal cycler with the lid preheated to 95 ° C prior to starting the reaction and use the following program settings:
   - One cycle: 95 °C for 2 min.
   - One cycle: 37 °C for 2 min.

3.8.3 Performing a Chip Check

1. On the initialized PGM, press Run and follow the instructions to perform chip check.
2. When prompted, place a new Ion 318™ Chip v2 BC into the chip deck, securely fasten the chip, and allow the PGM to calibrate the chip.

3.8.4 Binding the Sequencing Polymerase, Loading the Chip, and Starting the Run

1. After annealing the Sequencing Primer in the thermal cycler, add 3 μL of Ion PGM™ Hi-Q™ View Sequencing Polymerase to the ISPs. Mix by pipetting up and down, then allow the mixture to incubate at room temperature for 5 min.
2. Following chip calibration, retrieve the new chip and aspirate all liquid in the chip through the loading port. Using an Ion Chip™ Minifuge, place the chip upside-down with the tab pointing in. Centrifuge the chip for 10 s to remove of any liquid.
3. Place the chip on a first surface. After the incubation is complete, transfer 30 μL of ISPs to the chip by loading through the loading port. Add the dial by dialing down ~1 μL per sec. Pay attention to the dispersal of the liquid in the chip to ensure a homogenous distribution is done.
4. Using an Ion Chip™ Minifuge, place the chip right-side up with the tab point in and centrifuge for 1 min. Repeat the 1 min centrifuge this time with the chip tab point out.
5. Remove the chip and hold it at a 45° angle. Without removing the tip, slowly pipet the sample out and then back into the chip one time. Pipet slowly to avoid creating bubbles. Then remove as much liquid as possible.
6. Using an Ion Chip™ Minifuge, briefly centrifuge the chip upside-down with the tab point in.
7. Load the chip onto the PGM and follow the onscreen instructions.
8. Once all planned run details have been confirmed, begin the run. Sequencing will take ~2 h.

3.9 Data Analysis

Run data obtained by the PGT-A sequencer is processed and sent to Ion Torrent Browser Suite™ version 5.6.0 for generation of data files utilized for base calling and profile generation. Run quality control (QC) parameters must be met to emit diagnosis. QC is broken down into two components for run validation. (1) Run performance (all samples are analyzed with identified control) and (2) the analysis of each sample independently meets QC run metrics. Optimal run performance metrics are as follows: Loading >70%. Life Ion Sphere™ Particles (ISPS) >98%. Usable Reads >30%. Polyclonality <50%. Optimal sample parameters are as follows: Duplicate Reads <30%. Median of the Absolute values of all Pairwise Differences (MAPD) <0.35. Reads per sample >70,000.

If all QC parameters are met, diagnosis can begin. Runs should be repeated if run parameter values are below the optimal QC values determined by the manufacturer and internal validation protocol. Sequencing data obtained by the PGT-A sequencer is processed and sent to Ion Reporter™ version 5.4 software for data analysis. This software uses the bioinformatic tool ReproSeq Low-pass whole-genome aneuploidy workflow v1.0 to detect 24 chromosomes aneuploidies from a single whole-genome sample with low coverage (minimum 0.01×). Normalization is done using the bioinformatics baseline ReproSeq Low-Coverage Whole-Genome Baseline generated from multiple normal samples. Ion Reporter™ software generates a graph representing the copy number variation (CNV) of the sample analyzed compared to the reference bioinformatics baseline. An embryo is considered normal when it has no deviations from the reference bioinformatics baseline for any of the 24 chromosomes. PGT-A test has different diagnostic results, depending on which, the transference of the embryo would be recommended or not. An embryo is considered normal when all its chromosomes have two copies. An embryo is defined as abnormal by the presence of aneuploidy (chromosome gains or losses) when there are bins that are diverted into the upper (gain +) or lower part (loss -) of the graph. The aneuploidies could be for a full chromosome, when all the bins covering a chromosome are gained or lost, or partial aneuploidies, when the bins gained or lost represent only part of the chromosome. These abnormalities are usually called deletions or duplications. The presence of aneuploidies for most of the chromosomes on the same specimen is interpreted as a chaotic abnormal embryo. With this technique, it is not possible to identify deletions and duplications smaller than 10 Mb (the limit of resolution of this platform), balanced structural abnormalities, low level mosaic aneuploidy, uni-parental disomy (UPD), haploidy, and most polyploidies.

4 Notes

1. This is a safe stopping point. The amplified samples may be stored at −20 °C for up to 2 years.
2. When pooling fewer than 8 libraries, the pool volume drops below 40 μL. Add nuclease-free water to bring the final volume to 40 μL prior to library pool purification.
3. This is a safe stopping point. The purified pool may be stored at −20 °C for up to 1 week.
4. This is a safe stopping point. The templated ISPs may be stored at −20 °C for up to 1 week.
5. This is a safe stopping point. The templated ISPs may be stored at 4 °C for up to 3 days.

References

1. Hellani A, Abu-Amero K, Azouri J et al (2008) Successful pregnancies after application of array-comparative genomic hybridization in PGS-aneuploidy screening. Reprod Biomed Online 17(6):841–847
2. Vanneste E, Voet T, Le Caignec C et al (2009) Chromosome instability is common in human cleavage-stage embryos. Nat Med 15 (5):577–583. https://doi.org/10.1038/nm.1924
3. Fragouli E, Alfarawati S, Spath K et al (2013) The origin and impact of embryonic aneuploidy. Hum Genet 132(9):1001–1013. https://doi.org/10.1007/s00439-013-1309-0
4. Baltaci V, Satiroglu H, Kabukçu C et al (2006) Relationship between embryo quality and aneuploidies. Reprod Biomed Online 12 (1):77–82
5. Munne S (2003) Preimplantation genetic diagnosis and human implantation--a review. Placenta 24(Suppl B):S70–S76
6. Rodrigo L, Mateu E, Mercader A et al (2014) New tools for embryo selection: comprehensive chromosome screening by array comparative genomic hybridization. Biomed Res Int 2014:517125. https://doi.org/10.1155/2014/517125
7. Kuliev A, Zlatopolsky Z, Kirillova I et al (2011) Meiosis errors in over 20,000 oocytes studied in the practice of preimplantation aneuploidy testing. Reprod Biomed Online 22(1):2–8. https://doi.org/10.1016/j.rbmo.2010.08.014
8. Rubio C, Vera M, Lopez P et al (2018) Preimplantation genetic testing for aneuploidy: all you need to know. In: Simon C, Rubio C (eds) Handbook of new genetic diagnostic technologies in reproductive medicine, 1st edn. CRC Press, Taylor and Francis Group, Boca Raton
9. Stephenson MD, Awartani KA, Robinson WP (2002) Cytogenetic analysis of miscarriages from couples with recurrent miscarriage: a case-control study. Hum Reprod 17 (2):446–451
10. Sermon K, Capalbo A, Cohen J et al (2016) The why, the how and the when of PGS 2.0: current practices and expert opinions of fertility specialists, molecular biologists, and embryologists. Mol Hum Reprod 22(8):845–857. https://doi.org/10.1093/molehr/gaw034
11. Yan L, Huang L, Xu L et al (2015) Live births after simultaneous avoidance of monogenic diseases and chromosome abnormality by next-generation sequencing with linkage analyses. Proc Natl Acad Sci U S A 112 (52):15964–15969. https://doi.org/10.1073/pnas.1523297113
12. Ion ReproSeq™ PGS Kits—Ion S5™ System USER GUIDE. (2017) Thermo Fisher Scientific, Inc. https://assets.thermofisher.com/TFS-Assets/LSG/manuals/MAN0016712_IonReproSeqPGS_S5_UG.pdf. Accessed 4 March 2018
13. Merriman B, Ion TR, Team D et al (2012) Progress in ion torrent semiconductor chip based sequencing. Electrophoresis 33 (23):3397–3417. https://doi.org/10.1002/elps.201200424
14. Kung A, Munne S, Bankowski B et al (2015) Validation of next-generation sequencing for comprehensive chromosome screening of embryos. Reprod Biomed Online 31 (6):760–769. https://doi.org/10.1016/j.rbmo.2015.09.002

Part III

Traditional Prenatal Diagnosis

Chapter 7

DNA Extraction from Various Types of Prenatal Specimens

Odelia Nahum, Amanda Thomas, and Brynn Levy

Abstract

A prenatal noninvasive genetic screening test that yields a positive result typically warrants further direct assessment of fetal DNA following an invasive procedure. The precious nature of these invasively acquired samples, combined with the time sensitive nature with which results should be reported, demands that the methodologies used for analysis be quick, efficient, and dependable.

Prenatal diagnosis has been performed using DNA extracted from amniotic fluid and chorionic villi for several decades, and more recently methodologies have been developed to extract cell free fetal DNA from amniotic fluid. DNA extraction methodologies in these matrices should reliably and reproducibly isolate a sufficient quality and quantity of DNA for the intended downstream application, and make it possible to purify and concentrate samples that may arrive with suboptimal quality or quantity.

Phenol-Chloroform extraction followed by DNA precipitation in ethanol has historically been used for prenatal samples, but this methodology is labor intensive, time consuming, and requires use of toxic chemicals. There are now commercially available, solid phase-based kits for rapid and reproducible DNA extraction and purification, enabling simultaneous extraction of a large number of samples. Commercial kits are available for a variety of sample matrices including all prenatal specimen types, although other methodologies including organic or inorganic liquid phase extraction may also be utilized.

Here, we describe extraction using both commercially available kits for direct amniocytes and chorionic villi and cell free fetal DNA derived from amniotic fluid, as well as inorganic liquid phase extraction for tissue culture of amniocytes, CVS, and products of conception.

Key words DNA extraction, Amniotic fluid, Chorionic villi, Cell free amniotic fluid, Cell culture, DNA prep, Precipitation, cffDNA, Inorganic liquid phase extraction, DNA extraction kit

1 Introduction

Prenatal genetic diagnosis traditionally requires invasive procedures to acquire fetal DNA for direct analysis. A critical feature of prenatal diagnosis is the ability to return accurate results quickly and efficiently, so that time may be afforded for decision-making or additional testing. In the laboratory, the first step of many diagnostic techniques is the extraction of high quality DNA with sufficient yield for the intended downstream methodology. DNA extraction techniques should be robust and focused on maximizing the quality and quantity of isolated DNA, as low yield or poor quality DNA

Brynn Levy (ed.), *Prenatal Diagnosis*, Methods in Molecular Biology, vol. 1885, https://doi.org/10.1007/978-1-4939-8889-1_7,

may require an additional invasive procedure. Extraction methodologies should be fast, efficient, reliable, and reproducibly isolate a sufficient quantity of DNA that is free from contaminating compounds. All DNA extraction protocols should be optimized to isolate DNA at both the quality and quantity sufficient for the intended downstream application.

Historically, DNA from amniocytes and chorionic villi has been isolated using phenol-chloroform extraction followed by ethanol precipitation [1, 2]. While similar methodologies may still be utilized for DNA extraction of prenatal samples, they are labor intensive, time consuming, and require the use of toxic chemicals. Today, a variety of commercial kits are available that quickly and efficiently isolate DNA without compromising quantity or quality. The volume of sample required for sufficient DNA quantity will depend on the sample matrix and the intended downstream application. Generally the quantity of DNA attainable from amniotic fluid is lower than that of CVS [3], and this is reflected in the amount of sample required for sufficient DNA yield.

Today, DNA extraction directly from chorionic villi and amniocytes can generally be achieved with the same commercially available column-based kit, however, the initial sample preparation steps vary depending on the sample type. Prior to DNA extraction, chorionic villi samples should be cleaned and microdissection employed to remove as much maternal tissue as possible. Further disaggregation of the villi is achieved by treating with trypsin to remove the trophoblastic layer, and collagenase to digest the intercellular matrix. By contrast, extraction from direct amniocytes requires only centrifugation to collect the cells, followed by washing and resuspension. Centrifugation of amniotic fluid allows for separation of the amniocytes and supernatant. The amniotic supernatant contains a high fraction of fetal cell free DNA and may also be utilized for prenatal analysis.

Once amniocyte and CVS samples are prepared for extraction, a broad spectrum protease such as Proteinase K, a ribonuclease, and buffer containing a chaotrophic agent are added to the sample to remove protein and RNA. DNA is bound to the column, washed, and excess contaminates are filtered using a series of buffers with varying stringencies to remove organic contaminants and salts. DNA can be eluted using water. These commercially available stationary phase kits typically produce high quality DNA free of contaminants, with yield proportional to the volume of starting material.

It is highly recommended that a backup culture be established for every prenatal specimen being processed. Having backup cultures provides multiple benefits including (1) having fetal material available when the DNA quality/quantity from the uncultured tissue (chorionic villi or amniocytes) is suboptimal, (2) the downstream assay fails and needs to be repeated and (3) additional confirmatory tests are required or ordered. In addition, establishment of cell cultures may reduce the probability of maternal cell contamination for amniotic fluid contaminated with peripheral blood [4], and decrease the probability of DNA extraction failure for suboptimal CVS samples [5]. DNA extraction from cultured chorionic villi, cultured amniocytes, or cultured tissue derived from products of conception can be attained with commercially available kits, or inorganic liquid phase extraction as described here. Briefly, when flasks are approximately 70–80% confluent, cells are trypsinized, washed, and pelleted via centrifugation. Cells are lysed in a detergent-based solution, typically 10% SDS, followed by a high salt protein precipitation with ammonium acetate. DNA is precipitated from the supernatant and resuspended in a Tris-EDTA buffer solution. Spectrophotometric analysis can be used to confirm DNA concentration and purity.

While prenatal diagnosis has been carried out in amniocytes and chorionic villi for many decades, more recently the existence of cell free fetal DNA (cffDNA) in amniotic fluid has been recognized as a robust matrix for analysis of genetic information [6]. The amount of cell free fetal DNA present in amniotic fluid seems to be a function of both gestational age and ploidy status of the fetus (for review see Hui [7]). Initial attempts at utilizing DNA extraction methods similar to that of serum/plasma or body fluid modified for large volumes met only partial success [6], and only 40% of the samples extracted produced a sufficient yield for microarray analysis [8]. Modification of protocols to resemble DNA extraction from urine produced more sufficient yield of DNA [9], and this is the basis for the current cffDNA methodologies. Further optimization of the cffDNA purification protocol has led to the standardization of this methodology, which is now commercially available in cell free DNA extraction kits. Extraction of cffDNA from amniotic fluid utilizes amniotic fluid remaining after the amniocytes have been removed. Since this is typically >5 mL, DNA extraction methods are adapted for a larger volume of starting material. Briefly, amniotic fluid samples are added to a binding optimization buffer containing Proteinase K. Carrier RNA is added to increase the DNA yield of low concentration samples [10]. DNA is concentrated by passing the sample through a vacuum-based column. Bound DNA is washed several times with a series of buffers with varying stringencies, followed by a final wash in 100% ethanol. Elution is performed with molecular biology grade water.

In our hands, the methodologies discussed in this chapter have reliably and reproducibly extracted DNA at sufficient quantities, with a 260/280 ratio between 1.8 and 2.0, and 260/230 ratio greater than 1.5. All procedures should be independently optimized to extract DNA of prenatal samples to a concentration sufficient for the specific application for which it is intended.

2 Materials

2.1 DNA Extraction from Amniotic Fluid

1. AccuGENE 1× PBS (Lonza, Basel, Switzerland).
2. QIAmp DNA Blood Mini Kit (QIAGEN, Germantown, MD, USA).
3. Proteinase K (QIAGEN, Germantown, MD, USA).
4. RNase A Solution (100 mg/mL) (QIAGEN, Germantown, MD, USA).
5. 100% Ethanol.
6. Molecular Biology Grade Water.

2.2 DNA Extraction from Chorionic Villi

1. QIAmp DNA Blood Mini Kit (QIAGEN, Germantown, MD, USA).
2. Proteinase K (QIAGEN, Germantown, MD, USA).
3. RNase A Solution (100 mg/mL) (QIAGEN, Germantown, MD, USA).
4. 100% Ethanol.
5. Molecular Biology Grade Water.

2.3 DNA Extraction from Cultured Cells

DNA can be extracted from cultured chorionic villi, cultured amniotic fluid cells (amniocytes), or cultured tissue derived from products of conception.

1. Trypsin (TrypLE Express) (Gibco, Gaithersburg, MD).
2. Cell Lysis Solution (QIAGEN, Germantown, MD, USA).
3. Protein Precipitation Solution (Ammonium acetate 7.5 M).
4. RNase A Solution (QIAGEN, Germantown, MD, USA).
5. 100% isopropanol.
6. 70% ethanol.
7. TE Buffer.

2.4 DNA Extraction from Cell Free Amniotic Fluid

1. QIAamp circulating nucleic acid kit (QIAGEN, Germantown, MD, USA).
2. AccuGENE 1x PBS (Lonza, Basel, Switzerland).
3. 100% Ethanol.
4. Molecular Biology Grade Water.
5. Carrier RNA: Add 1550 μL buffer AVE from the kit to the tube containing 310 μg lyophilized carrier RNA to obtain a solution of 0.2 μg/μL. Dissolve it thoroughly and aliquot in 200 μL tubes. Store at −20 °C.

3 Methods

3.1 DNA Extraction from Amniotic Fluid

1. Spin the amniotic fluid (AF) specimen in a 15 mL tube at 2500 × *g* for 15 min at room temperature (*see* **Note 1**).
2. Remove the supernatant with a sterile transfer pipet to a new tube (*see* **Note 2**).
3. Tap the tube to resuspend the pellet.
4. Add 900 μL of 1× PBS to the tube using the PBS to wash the sides of the tube.
5. Spin the tube at 2500 × *g* for 1 min at room temperature.
6. Remove the supernatant and add it to the original supernatant tube, leaving the cell pellet with about 50 μL of supernatant.
7. Tap the tube to resuspend the pellet.
8. Add 475 μL of 1× PBS; tap the tube to mix ensuring that the pellet is completely resuspended.
9. Add 50 μL of Qiagen proteinase K into the sample and mix well by tapping.
10. Add 10 μL of RNAse A solution (100 mg/mL), mix by tapping.
11. Add 600 μL of buffer AL (mix the buffer thoroughly before adding).
12. Vortex the tube for at least a minute.
13. Incubate in a 70 °C ± 2 °C water bath for 10 min. Mix by inverting it 20 times and incubate again at 70 °C ± 2 °C for another 10 min (*see* **Note 3**).
14. Add 500 μL of room temperature 100% Ethanol. Mix well by vortexing for at least 1 min.
15. Transfer 700 μL of solution to QIAmp mini column in a 2 mL collection tube, being careful not to wet the rim of the column.
16. Microcentrifuge at 6000 × *g* for 1 min.
17. Discard the filtrate and return the column to the tube.
18. Repeat **steps 15–17** as necessary to filter remaining solution.
19. Add 500 μL of buffer AW1 (add ethanol to the buffer when using for the first time according to the manufacturer's instructions), being careful not to wet the rim of the column.
20. Centrifuge for 1 min at 6000 × *g*.
21. Discard the filtrate and return the column to the tube.
22. Add 500 μL of buffer AW2 (add ethanol to the buffer when using for the first time according to the manufacturer's instruction), being careful not to wet the rim of the column.
23. Centrifuge for 3 min at maximum speed.

24. Transfer the column to a new 1.5 mL tube, and centrifuge for another minute at maximum speed.
25. Place the column in a clean 1.5 mL tube and add 15 μL of H_2O (*see* **Note 4**).
26. Incubate at room temperature for 5 min.
27. Centrifuge for 1 min at 6000 × *g*.
28. Remove and discard the column and measure the DNA using any type of UV spectrophotometer (*see* **Notes 5–8**).

3.2 DNA Extraction from Chorionic Villi (See Note 9)

1. Add 180 μL of Buffer ATL to the cleaned and prepared CVS sample (If a precipitate has formed in Buffer ATL, dissolve by incubating at 56 °C).
2. Add 20 μL proteinase K, mix by vortexing, and incubate at 56 °C until the tissue is completely lysed. Incubation time will vary depending on the size of the tissue sample, with larger samples requiring longer incubation. Vortex occasionally during incubation to assist in lysis.
3. Briefly centrifuge the tube to remove drops from the inside of the lid.
4. If necessary, transfer the solution to a 1.5 mL tube.
5. Add 4 μL RNase A (100 mg/mL), mix by pulse-vortexing for 15 s, and incubate for 2 min at room temperature. Briefly centrifuge the tube to remove drops from inside the lid, then add 200 μL Buffer AL to the sample. Mix again by pulse-vortexing for 15 s, and incubate at 70 °C for 10 min. Briefly centrifuge the tube to remove drops from inside the lid (It is essential that the sample and Buffer AL are mixed thoroughly to yield a homogeneous solution).
6. Add 200 μL ethanol (96–100%) to the sample, and mix by pulse-vortexing for 15 s. After mixing, briefly centrifuge to remove drops from inside the lid (It is essential that the sample, Buffer AL, and the ethanol are mixed thoroughly to yield a homogeneous solution).
7. Carefully apply the mixture (including the precipitate) to the QIAamp Mini spin column (in a 2 mL collection tube) without wetting the rim. Close the cap, and centrifuge at 6000 × *g* for 1 min. Place the QIAamp mini spin column in a clean 2 mL collection tube, and discard the tube containing the filtrate.
8. Repeat **step** 7 as necessary to filter remaining mixture.
9. Carefully open the QIAamp Mini spin column and add 500 μL Buffer AW1 (add ethanol to the buffer when using for the first time according to the manufacturer's instructions) without wetting the rim. Close the cap, and centrifuge at 6000 × *g* for 1 min. Place the QIAamp Mini spin column in a clean 2 mL

collection tube, and discard the collection tube containing the filtrate.

10. Carefully open the QIAamp Mini spin column and add 500 μL Buffer AW2 (add ethanol to the buffer when using for the first time according to the manufacturer's instructions) without wetting the rim. Close the cap and centrifuge at full speed for 3 min.
11. Place the QIAamp Mini spin column in a new 2 mL collection tube and discard the old collection tube with the filtrate. Centrifuge at full speed for 1 min.
12. Place the QIAamp Mini spin column in a clean 1.5 mL microcentrifuge tube, and discard the collection tube containing the filtrate. Carefully open the QIAamp Mini spin column and add 25 μL distilled water. Incubate at room temperature for 5 min, and then centrifuge at 6000 × *g* for 1 min.
13. Remove and discard the column and Measure the DNA using any type of UV spectrophotometer (*see* **Notes 5–8**). If the yield of DNA is insufficient, an additional 20 μL of distilled water can be added to the QIAmp Mini spin column, incubated, and centrifuged as in **step 12**.

3.3 DNA Extraction from Cultured Cells

1. Remove the supernatant from a confluent cell culture flask. Save the supernatant in a 15 mL falcon tube.
2. Add 3 mL of Trypsin to flask and incubate for 3 min in the incubator.
3. Tap flask to loosen cells, and check that cells are loose under the microscope.
4. Add 1 mL of the supernatant back to the flask to wash it and transfer the complete solution to the same 15 mL falcon tube (which contains the remaining supernatant).
5. Centrifuge for 10 min at 600 × *g*. Remove the supernatant leaving behind 200 μL residual fluid. Thoroughly suspend the pellet in the residual fluid by pipetting up and down.
6. Add 600 μL of Cell Lysis Solution and resuspend the cells by pipetting up and down or vortex on high speed for 10 s to lyse the cells.
7. Incubate for 10 min at 37° and transfer to a 1.5 mL Eppendorf tube. Cool to room temperature.
8. Add 3 μL of RNase A Solution, and mix by inverting 25 times. Incubate for 15 min at 37 °C. Then incubate at room temperature for 3 min to quickly cool the sample.
9. Add 200 μL of Protein Precipitation Solution, and vortex vigorously for 20 s at high speed.

10. Centrifuge for 3 min at maximum speed and transfer the supernatant by carefully pouring into a clean 1.5 mL tube containing 600 μL of 100% isopropanol. Be sure not to dislodge the protein pellet during pouring.
11. Mix by inverting gently 50 times until the DNA is visible as threads or a clump (*see* **Note 10**).
12. Centrifuge for 1 min at maximum speed. The DNA may be visible as a small white pellet.
13. Carefully discard the supernatant, and drain the tube by inverting on a clean piece of absorbent paper, taking care that the pellet remains in the tube.
14. Add 600 μL of 70% ethanol and invert several times to wash the DNA pellet.
15. Centrifuge for 1 min at maximum speed.
16. Carefully discard the supernatant. The pellet might be loose and easily dislodged. Drain the tube on a clean piece of absorbent paper, taking care that the pellet remains in the tube.
17. Air dry the pellet for at least 15 min. Avoid over-drying the DNA pellet, as the DNA will be difficult to dissolve.
18. Add TE buffer and vortex for 5 s at medium speed to mix (*see* **Note 11**).
19. Measure the DNA using any type of UV spectrophotometer (*see* **Notes 5–8**).

3.4 DNA Extraction from Cell Free Amniotic Fluid

1. Bring samples to room temperature.
2. Bring total volume to 5 mL with PBS if necessary.
3. Set up the QIAvac 24 plus vacuum manifold as shown in Fig. 1.
4. Heat water bath to 60 °C and Heat block to 56 °C.
5. Bring buffer AVE to room temperature.
6. Add reconstituted carrier RNA to Buffer ACL (this will vary depending on number of samples being processed—Follow the manufacturer's instructions).
7. Pipet 500 μL Proteinase K into a 50 mL tube.
8. Add 5 mL of amniotic fluid to the tube.
9. Add 4 mL buffer ACL containing the carrier RNA.
10. Pulse vortex for 30 s.
11. Immediately incubate the tube in the preheated water bath (60 °C) for 30 min.
12. Add 9 mL Buffer ACB (add isopropanol to the buffer when using for the first time according to the manufacturer's instruction) to the lysate in the tube.
13. Pulse vortex for 30 s.

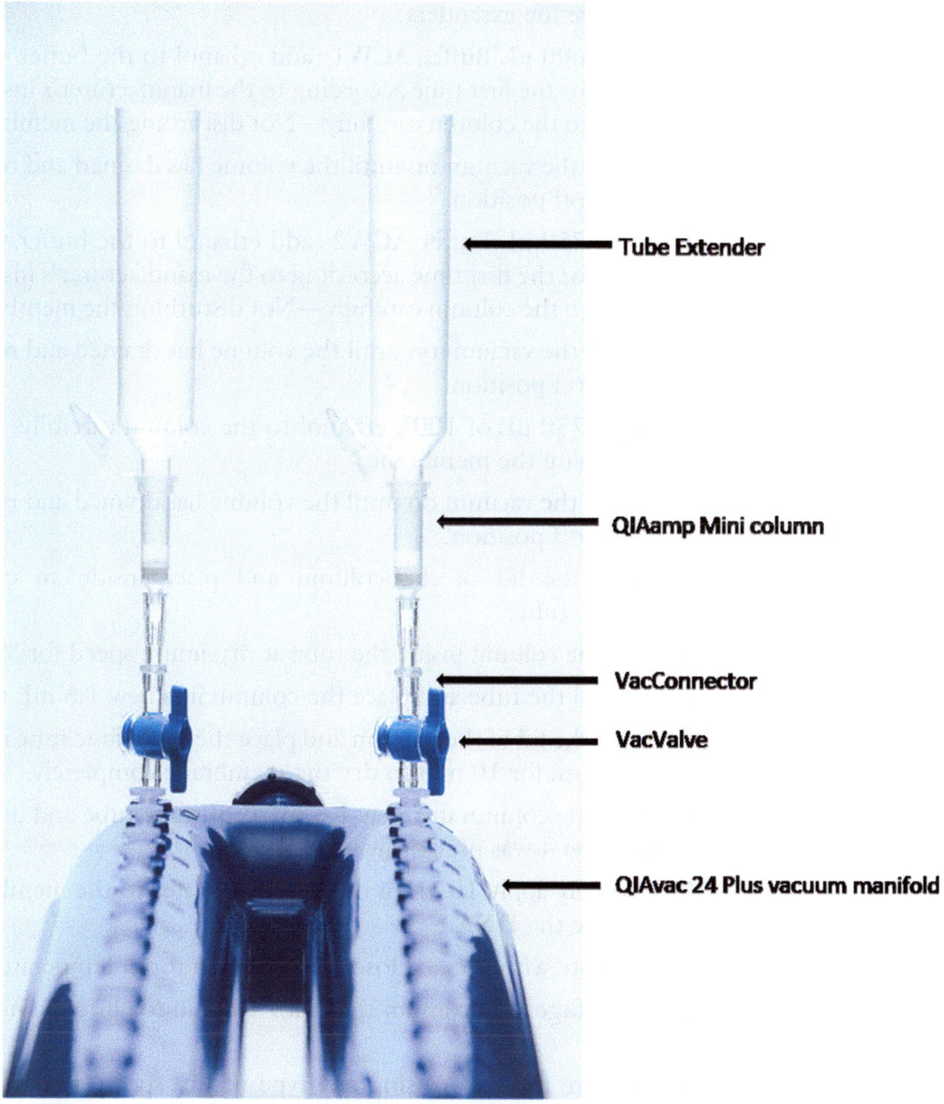

Fig. 1 Setting up the QIAvac 24 plus with the QIAamp mini columns

14. Incubate the mixture on ice for 5 min.
15. Set up the vacuum with the columns according to the instructions with the 20 mL extension tubes (*see* Fig. 1).
16. With the vacuum in the off position, carefully free pour the mixture into the extension tube, and then turn the value to approximately 5/6 of the way. Adjust if the solution is draining too quickly (should be around 10–15 min for the entire solution to drain).
17. Once the solution has entirely drained, switch off the vacuum immediately so the membrane does not dry out.

18. Remove the extenders.
19. Apply 600 μL Buffer ACW1 (add ethanol to the buffer when using for the first time according to the manufacturer's instructions) to the column carefully—Not disturbing the membrane.
20. Switch the vacuum on until the volume has drained and return to the off position.
21. Apply 750 μL Buffer ACW2 (add ethanol to the buffer when using for the first time according to the manufacturer's instructions) to the column carefully—Not disturbing the membrane.
22. Switch the vacuum on until the volume has drained and return to the off position.
23. Apply 750 μL of 100% ethanol to the column carefully—Not disturbing the membrane.
24. Switch the vacuum on until the volume has drained and return to the off position.
25. Close the lid of the column and place inside an empty 1.5 mL tube.
26. Spin the column inside the tube at maximum speed for 3 min.
27. Discard the tube and place the column in a new 1.5 mL tube.
28. Open the lid of the column and place the centrifuge tube in the hot block for 10 min to dry the membrane completely.
29. Place the column in a new 1.5 mL centrifuge tube and discard the tube it was previously in.
30. Carefully apply 10 μL of nuclease free water to the membrane to elute the DNA.
31. Incubate with the lid closed for 5 min at room temperature.
32. Centrifuge at maximum speed for 1.5 min to elute the nucleic acids.
33. Measure the DNA using any type of UV spectrophotometer (*see* **Notes 5–8**).

4 Notes

1. We recommend working with at least 10 mL of amniotic fluid. The greater the volume of fluid, the higher the likelihood of obtaining a sufficient DNA yield.
2. To maximize the quantity of fetal DNA, further DNA extraction from the supernatant of the cell free DNA can be performed (see Subheadings 2.4 and 3.4). This is especially helpful when a low volume of amniotic fluid is received or if the cell pellet is very small. For those laboratories that store the supernatant, the cell free DNA can be extracted at a later date if

necessary. We have had success extracting DNA from supernatant that was frozen for greater than 4 months.

3. If necessary, the extraction procedure can be stopped at this point and continued the next day, keeping the tube at room temperature overnight.
4. Some commercially available kits suggest elution in provided buffer or other salt containing solution. We prefer to elute using molecular biology grade H_2O, as this enables further concentration of DNA if necessary.
5. We recommend using the Nanodrop ONE to measure the DNA concentration.
6. The 260/280 ratio should be between 1.8 and 2.0 and the 260/230 ratio should be above 1.5.
7. Given the precious nature of the DNA, it may still be worth using the DNA even when the 260/280 ration is above 2.1 and/or if the 260/230 ratio is below 1.0. Quality control metrics should be established for each downstream assay that you perform.
8. We highly recommend performing maternal cell contamination studies on all DNA extracted for prenatal studies (*see* Chapter 8).
9. We recommend starting with at least 3 mg of tissue. However, we have obtained successful results for SNP microarray analysis using less than 3 mg. As with amniotic fluid, the greater the starting quantity of villi, the higher the likelihood of obtaining a sufficient DNA yield.
10. A DNA pellet is not always visible after the next centrifugation step, so it is a good idea to position the tubes in the centrifuge in such a way that the location of the pellet will be consistent. We suggest placing all tubes with the hinge pointed out.
11. Adjust the TE volume according to the size of the pellet. If the DNA pellet can be easily seen, we recommend adding at least 100 μL of TE buffer.

References

1. Rebello MT, Hackett G, Smith J et al (1991) Extraction of DNA from amniotic fluid cells for the early prenatal diagnosis of genetic disease. Prenat Diagn 11(1):41–46
2. Williamson R, Eskdale J, Coleman DV et al (1981) Direct gene analysis of chorionic villi: a possible technique for first-trimester antenatal diagnosis of haemoglobinopathies. Lancet 2 (8256):1125–1127
3. Old JM (2011) Prenatal diagnosis of the hemoglobinopathies. In: Milunsky AMJ (ed) Genetic disorders and the fetus: diagnosis, prevention, and treatment, 6th edn. John Wiley & Sons, Ltd, Oxford, UK
4. Winsor EJ, Silver MP, Theve R et al (1996) Maternal cell contamination in uncultured amniotic fluid. Prenat Diagn 16(1):49–54. https://doi.org/10.1002/(SICI)1097-0223(199601)16:1<49::AID-PD808>3.0.CO;2-U
5. Saura R, Roux D, Taine L et al (1994) Early amniocentesis versus chorionic villus sampling

for fetal karyotyping. Lancet 344 (8925):825–826

6. Bianchi DW, LeShane ES, Cowan JM (2001) Large amounts of cell-free fetal DNA are present in amniotic fluid. Clin Chem 47 (10):1867–1869
7. Hui L, Bianchi DW (2011) Cell-free fetal nucleic acids in amniotic fluid. Hum Reprod Update 17(3):362–371. https://doi.org/10.1093/humupd/dmq049
8. Larrabee PB, Johnson KL, Pestova E et al (2004) Microarray analysis of cell-free fetal DNA in amniotic fluid: a prenatal molecular karyotype. Am J Hum Genet 75(3):485–491. https://doi.org/10.1086/423288
9. Lapaire O, Johnson KL, Bianchi DW (2008) Method for extraction of high-quantity and -quality cell-free DNA from amniotic fluid. Methods Mol Biol 444:303–309. https://doi.org/10.1007/978-1-59745-066-9_24
10. Shaw KJ, Thain L, Docker PT et al (2009) The use of carrier RNA to enhance DNA extraction from microfluidic-based silica monoliths. Anal Chim Acta 652(1–2):231–233. https://doi.org/10.1016/j.aca.2009.03.038

Chapter 8

Assessment of Maternal Cell Contamination in Prenatal Samples by Quantitative Fluorescent PCR (QF-PCR)

Christie M. Buchovecky, Odelia Nahum, and Brynn Levy

Abstract

When biopsying a fetal tissue like chorionic villi or amniotic fluid, there is a chance of getting some maternal material that could contaminate the fetal specimen and might lead to a misdiagnosis. Thus, all prenatal samples should be subjected to testing for maternal cell contamination. This is done using quantitative fluorescent PCR (QF-PCR) of short tandem repeat (STR) markers.

Key words Maternal cell contamination, Prenatal diagnosis, Microsatellite markers, Short tandem repeats, Genotyping, Sample identity

1 Introduction

Prenatal sampling procedures pose a risk of including maternal cells alongside the intended fetal sample. This risk has been empirically calculated as approximately 0.5% in amniotic fluid sampling, 1–2% in chorionic villi sampling, and has the potential to be much higher in products of conception depending on the method by which the sample was obtained [1, 2]. Although best practices for obtaining and processing samples can limit the amount and frequency of contamination, misdiagnosis due to maternal cell contamination (MCC) remains a concern in all prenatal diagnosis arenas [3–5]. For this reason, the American College of Medical Genetics and Genomics (ACMG) and the Association for Molecular Pathology (AMP) recommend MCC testing as the standard of care for each prenatal specimen obtained for molecular diagnosis [6, 7].

The method described herein employs DNA genotyping by quantitative fluorescent PCR (QF-PCR), followed by capillary electrophoresis, on 15 highly polymorphic microsatellite or short tandem repeat (STR) markers, and an X–Y specific marker (amelogenin). This allows distinction between maternal and fetal

Brynn Levy (ed.), *Prenatal Diagnosis*, Methods in Molecular Biology, vol. 1885, https://doi.org/10.1007/978-1-4939-8889-1_8,

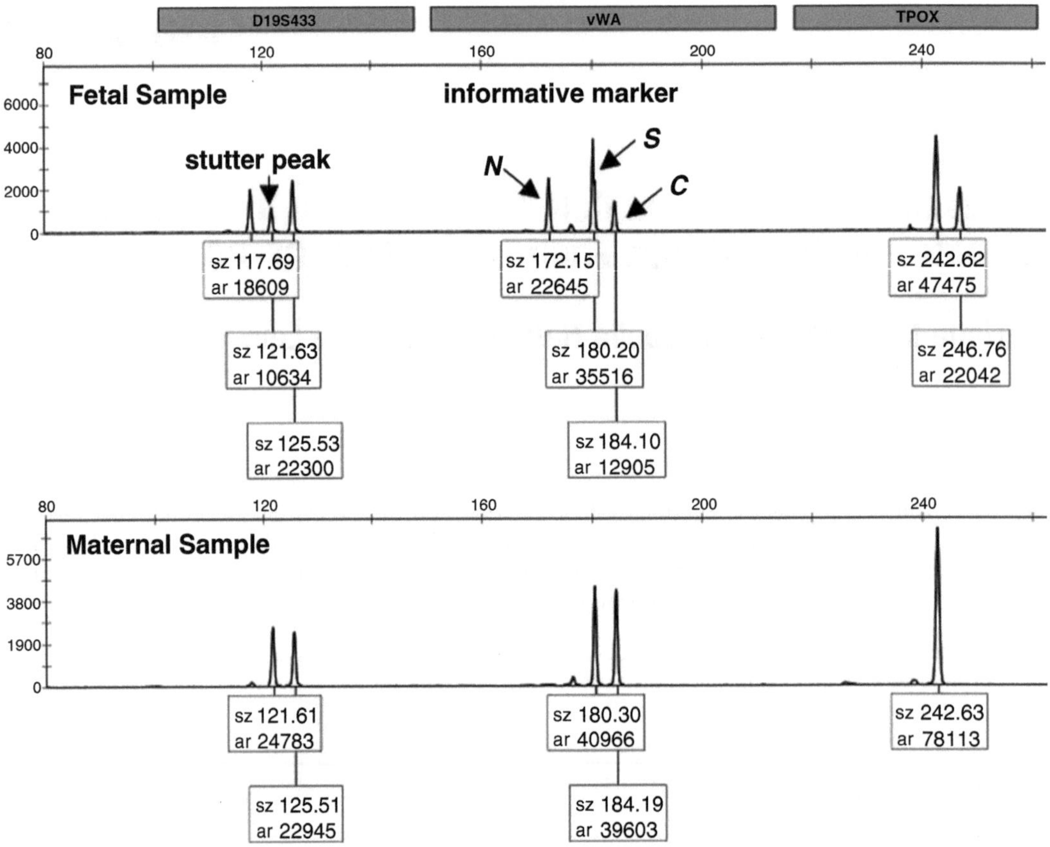

Fig. 1 Prenatal Sample with 36.3% Maternal Cell Contamination. Marker D19S433 is not informative, as the maternal allele that is not shared with the fetus overlaps a stutter peak from the fetal peak at size 125. Marker TPOX is not informative because all maternal peaks are shared with the fetus. Marker vWA is informative, with a shared peak (S) at 180, a non-shared, non-contaminating peak (N) at 172, and a contaminating peak (C) at 184 in the prenatal sample. Using the equation for determining MCC with heterozygous fetal alleles (*see* Subheading 3.1), the MCC calculated from this marker is 36.3%. Note that the allele pattern in a prenatal sample with 100% MCC would match the exact maternal allele pattern, with no unshared peaks

DNA to estimate the presence and level of MCC in prenatal samples. The markers present in the putative fetal DNA sample (derived from cultured or uncultured cells from amniotic fluid, chorionic villi, cord blood, or products of conception) are compared to those in a maternal DNA sample (typically from a blood or buccal specimen). By examining these samples in parallel and comparing the relative ratios of alleles at each marker, it is possible to estimate the presence and level of contaminating maternal cells in the fetal sample (*see* Fig. 1).

Prevention of misdiagnosis, especially of falsely reporting normal or wild-type results, is the primary reason for undertaking MCC testing for each prenatal diagnostic sample obtained, including for gene sequencing and microarray testing. If MCC is not detected, the diagnostic test result can be considered accurate at the level of detection of the MCC assay (which is 5% when following this protocol). Because each instance of sampling includes a risk for MCC, it is important that this testing be performed on DNA extracted from the same sample or culture used for diagnostic testing. In addition to this routine use in diagnostic tests, ruling out MCC is vital when products of conception show a normal female karyotype (46, XX), prenatal karyotyping or FISH studies suggest XX/XY mosaicism, or cytogenetic specimens show discordant results between direct and cultured samples.

Prenatal samples are considered precious as each sampling procedure is associated with a small but definitive risk of miscarriage [8]. The finding of MCC does not automatically dictate that a repeat invasive sampling procedure be recommended/performed. The mere presence of MCC does not preclude diagnostic testing, so long as the test employed is robust to the level of contamination observed. Common cutoffs include 10% for SNP oligonucleotide analysis (SOMA) and 15% for direct sequencing-based tests. For other assays, the MCC cutoff to reject a sample for diagnostic testing should be calculated based on the experimentally ascertained effect of MCC on the sensitivity and specificity of the diagnostic test. If the level of MCC in a sample is anticipated to interfere with diagnostic testing, the availability of a cultured specimen presents an opportunity for further analysis. Culturing of amniotic fluid is especially amenable to reduction of MCC, as culture conditions favor growth of amniocytes over maternal blood cells [9]. On the other hand, culturing can increase levels of MCC in chorionic villi or product of conception samples where maternal decidua remained present in the culture setup, making careful processing of these samples imperative [4]. In cases where clinically significant MCC persists in cultured samples, a request for repeat sampling may be warranted.

In rare instances, a prenatal sample may be negative for MCC, but produce an unexpected result in this assay. Discordance of alleles between the fetal and maternal samples at multiple loci could represent an egg donor, surrogate pregnancy, or laboratory error. If the origin of this discordance is confirmed to be either an egg donor or a surrogate pregnancy by the clinical team, the MCC assay should be used to check for contamination with alleles unique to the gestational carrier. In another scenario, additional, non-maternal contaminating peaks may be observed when there are multiple gestational pregnancies (*see* Fig. 2). In multiple gestation pregnancies, the presence of fetus-to-fetus contamination should be noted as potentially impacting the accuracy of results, but typically does not prevent diagnostic testing. If this pattern occurs without a clinical record of a multiple gestational pregnancy, the possibilities of a vanishing twin or fetal chimerism should be considered. Chromosomal aneuploidy is suggested when a pattern of three fetal alleles at one or more loci is observed on a single chromosome; When observed on multiple chromosomes, triploidy

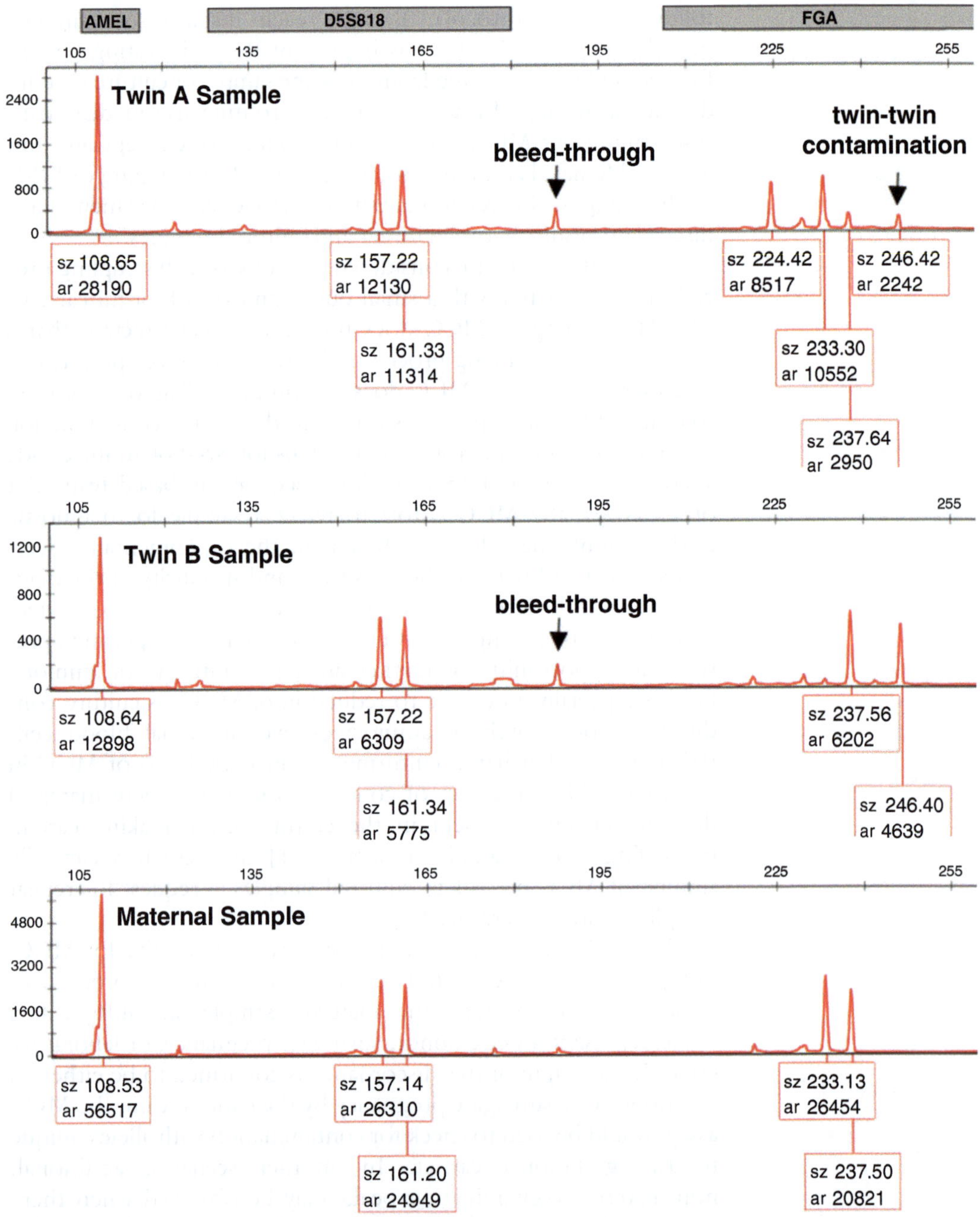

Fig. 2 Twin-Twin Contamination. Marker AMEL indicates the sex of each sample as female. Marker D5S818 is not informative because both alleles are shared between all samples. Marker FGA shows Twin A contaminated with cells from Twin B. The Twin B sample appears non-contaminated. Although the contaminating peak at size 237 is shared with both the maternal sample and twin B, the peak at 246 is found only in twin B. From the relative sizes of these two peaks and similar observations at other markers, we can conclude most of the contamination is of co-twin, rather than maternal origin. Additionally, this figure shows an example of a non-biological peak between the ranges for markers D5S818 and FGA; this is due to bleed-through of signal from another fluorescent channel

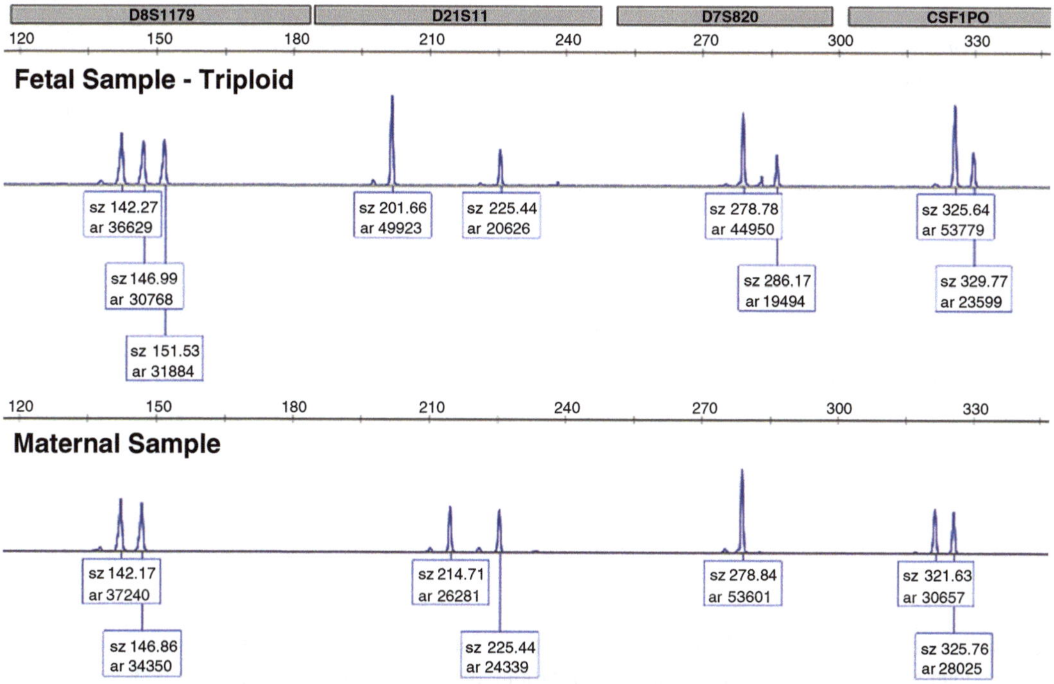

Fig. 3 A Prenatal Sample with Triploidy. In the fetal sample, marker D8S1179 shows three peaks of roughly equal area, while the other three markers each show two peaks with one double the area of the other, indicating three alleles at each marker. A similar pattern could be seen with high MCC. However, this can be excluded in this sample based on marker D21S11, where the larger peak is not shared with the maternal sample, suggesting that the mechanism of triploidy in this fetus was likely caused by dispermy. If a similar pattern of 3 equal peaks or a 2:1 ratio of peaks occurs at a single marker in a sample without MCC, the possibility of trisomy should be considered

is the likely explanation (*see* Fig. 3). In instances where allele patterns suggest a chromosome abnormality, appropriate diagnostic testing should be performed to confirm this finding. Rarely, a fetal sample may appear discordant to the maternal sample at a single locus. Explanations for this phenomenon include mutation at the primer site causing allelic dropout or de novo tandem repeat expansion or contraction (*see* Fig. 4). Given a sufficient number of additional markers, the identity of the maternal specimen can still be assured if there is concordance between the maternal fetal samples at all other loci. Frequencies of null and de novo mutation rates among many markers have been ascertained in the literature; data for those used in this assay are provided with the PCR kit.

In conclusion, assessment of maternal cell contamination by QF-PCR is an effective means of quickly assuring the identity and sufficient purity of prenatal samples, thereby preventing a misdiagnosis that may otherwise occur. The permissible level of MCC for a given diagnostic assay should be empirically determined in each laboratory prior to implementation. Additionally, the data obtained from MCC testing can suggest aneuploidy in a fetus, which should

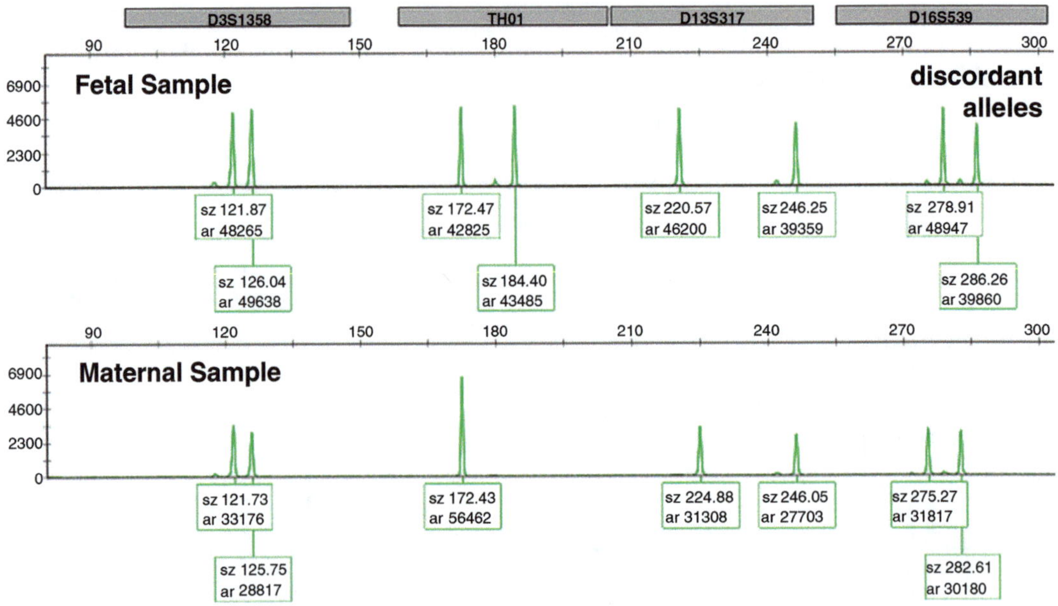

Fig. 4 A prenatal Sample with a Single Discordant Marker. The first three markers (and all other markers from the sample) are consistent with a matched maternal-fetal pair without MCC. However, the fetal sample does not share any alleles with the maternal sample at marker D16S539. In this scenario, it is most likely that the maternal STR allele assessed by this marker expanded or contracted by one repeat between generations as the probability that a sample swap occurred with the mother still matching 14/15 loci is extremely low

then be confirmed by traditional diagnostic means. Lastly, use of this assay prior to performing diagnostic testing reduces costs in a clinical laboratory by allowing a director to avoid testing incorrect or contaminated samples that would require reanalysis.

2 Materials

The protocol described here is for running the AmpFLSTR Identifiler PCR Kit PLUS on the ABI 3130 DNA analyzer (Applied Biosystems, Foster City, CA, USA). The protocol is expected to be similar but not identical using other PCR kits and/or DNA analyzers. Please consider the manufacturers' advice when adapting and optimizing this protocol for use with different equipment and reagents.

2.1 MCC Kit

1. AmpFLSTR Identifiler PCR Kit PLUS (Applied Biosystems, Foster City, CA, USA).
2. HiDi Formamide (Applied Biosystems, Foster City, CA, USA).
3. GeneScan™ 500 LIZ™ dye Size Standard (Applied Biosystems, Foster City, CA, USA).

2.2 DNA Extraction

DNA can be extracted using any commercial kit (*see* Chapter 7).

2.3 ABI 3130

1. POP-7™ Polymer for 3130/3130xl Genetic Analyzers (Applied Biosystems, Foster City, CA, USA).
2. 310 and 31xx Running Buffer, 10× (Applied Biosystems, Foster City, CA, USA).
3. 96-well optical reaction plate (Applied Biosystems, Foster City, CA, USA).

3 Methods

Table 1 shows various troubleshooting solutions when problems are encountered during PCR and electrophoresis.

3.1 Preparation of 5% and 10% Spiked Positive Controls

The spiked positive controls are prepared from DNAs extracted from a mother and fetus pair that is verified as being non-contaminated.

Table 1
PCR & Electrophoresis troubleshooting

Problem	Possible cause	Solution
Weak or no signal at all loci, including controls	Absent/insufficient master mix or primers	Repeat PCR
	Master mix not mixed thoroughly	Vortex master mix thoroughly
	Primer set exposed to too much light	Protect primer set from light
	PCR system malfunction	Check the system
	Incorrect thermal cycler parameters	Check cycler for correct parameters
	Insufficient PCR product injected	Mix 1 μL PCR product, 20 μL Formamide, and 0.5 μL standard
	Degraded Formamide	Avoid multiple freeze/thaw cycles
Positive signal from control DNA but not test samples	Sample DNA is degraded	Evaluate quality. If degraded, re-amplify with more DNA
	Quantity of sample DNA is low	Quantitate DNA and repeat PCR using 1 ng
	Sample DNA contains high amount of PCR inhibitors	Purify DNA and repeat PCR
Not all loci visible	Sample DNA is degraded	Evaluate DNA quality. If degraded, re-amplify with more DNA
	Sample DNA contains high amount of PCR inhibitors	Purify the DNA and repeat PCR
Low peak heights	Incorrect thermocycler parameters	Check parameters

1. Dilute the DNA of both maternal and fetal control samples to approximately 1 ng/μL using molecular grade water (*see* **Note 1**).
2. Prepare the 5% and 10% spiked positive control as follows (*see* **Note 2**):
   - *5%*: Take 1.5 μL of maternal control DNA (1 ng/μL) and add it to 28.5 μL of fetal control DNA (1 ng/μL).
   - *10%*: Take 3 μL of maternal control DNA (1 ng/μL) and add it to 27 μL of fetal control DNA (1 ng/μL).
3. Store the original diluted maternal and original diluted (non-spiked) fetal control samples as well as the spiked control DNAs at −20 °C.

3.2 DNA Extraction

Extract DNA from maternal blood and fetal sample using your standard prenatal DNA extraction methods (*see* Chapter 7).

3.3 PCR Amplification

1. Dilute the DNA of both maternal and fetal samples to approximately 1 ng/μL using molecular grade water.
2. Thaw the AmpFLSTR Identifiler Plus Kit Master Mix and the AmpFLSTR Identifiler Plus Kit Primer Set, then vortex 3 s and centrifuge briefly before opening the tubes (*see* **Note 3**).
3. Prepare the PCR master mix using reagents in the AmpFLSTR Identifiler PCR Plus Kit:

   For each sample use 10 μL of PCR mix and 5 μL of the primer set.
4. Add 2 μL of the diluted DNAs to a well of the 96-well plate (one well per sample) (*see* **Notes 4** and **5**).
5. Aliquot 15 μL of the PCR master mix into each well of the plate.
6. Seal the plate, vortex for 3 s, and short spin (about 20 s) in a tabletop centrifuge to remove bubbles.
7. Place the plate in a pre-warmed thermal cycler and run the following program (approximately 3 h):
   - One cycle: 95 °C for 11 min.
   - Twenty nine cycles: 94 °C for 20 sec, 59 °C for 3 min.
   - One cycle: 60 °C for 60 min.
   - 4 °C hold.
8. Short spin the plate.

3.4 Sizing the DNA Fragments

1. Prepare a master mix using 20 μL of formamide and 0.5 μL of LIZ size standard per sample.
2. In a new 96-well optical reaction plate, add 20.5 μL of master mix and 1 μL of PCR product (*see* **Note 6**).

3. Denature for 3 min at 95 °C and put on ice for another 3 min.
4. Spin the plate and run on the ABI 3130 Genetic Analyzer.

3.5 Analysis and Calculation of Maternal Cell Contamination

1. Import data into a genotyping analysis software according to that software's microsatellite guidelines. Data for a sample will include size, peak height, and area for each identified allele.
2. Identify informative markers for each mother-fetus pair (*see* **Note 7**).
   - *Informative marker*: One maternal allele differs from both fetal alleles for that marker and does not overlap with a fetal stutter peak (stutter peaks occur one microsatellite repeat less than the main allelic peak).
3. For *each* informative allele, determine contamination using the appropriate formula below (*see* **Note 8**):
   - *Informative markers with heterozygous fetal allele*: **% contamination = area(C*)/[area(N**) + area(C*)].**
   - *Informative markers with homozygous fetal allele*: **% contamination = [area(C*) × 2] / [area(S***) + area(C*)].**

   **Contaminating peak (C)*: peak at size of maternal allele that is not shared with the fetus.

   ***Non-shared, non-contaminating peak (N)*: fetal allele that is not shared with mother.

   ****Shared peak (S)*: fetal allele that is common to the mother and fetus.
4. Calculate the mean contamination for all informative markers to determine the maternal cell contamination for that sample (*see* Fig. 1). Informative markers where no contaminating peak is observed should be included as a marker with zero contamination.

3.6 Interpretation of Results

- *100% MCC*: Maternal and fetal samples are identical at all loci tested, indicating the "fetal" specimen likely represents maternal cells. This has been reported in samples from products of conception. Possible diagnostic errors including sample mix-ups, genotyping errors, rare genetic variants which interfere with analysis, and other sources should be excluded.
- *Mid-level MCC (>10%)*: Significant maternal cell contamination is detected in DNA extracted from this fetal specimen. Mutation analysis or SOMA of the fetal sample cannot be interpreted due to the amount of maternal cells detected. Recommend retesting fetal sample from cultured cells, or another direct sample if the current fetal sample was cultured.
- *Low-level MCC (5–10%)*: Low-level maternal cell contamination was detected in DNA extracted from this fetal specimen. Some tests may be amenable to testing despite low-level

contamination. If this is not the case, recommend retesting fetal sample from cultured cells if the current MCC analysis was based on a direct sample, or recommend another direct sample if the current MCC analysis was based on cultured cells.

- *Negative for MCC*: No evidence of maternal cell contamination in the fetal specimen at the level detectible by this assay (*see* **Note 9**).

4 Notes

1. The diluted maternal and non-spiked fetal control samples (1 ng/μL) will also be utilized as control samples with every MCC run (*see* **Note 4**).
2. The 5% and 10% spiked positive controls usually last for about 5 runs. They should be prepared fresh when the final calculations of a clinical run indicate drift from their expected percentage value, i.e., if the 5% appears more like 8% and the 10% appears more like 14%, new spiked control batches should be prepared.
3. Thawing is required only during first use of the kit. After first use, reagents are stored at 2–8 °C and, therefore, they do not require subsequent thawing. Do not refreeze the reagents.
4. For each MCC run, you will be running 6 DNA control samples as follows: (1) Fetal control DNA (*see* **Note 1**), (2) maternal control DNA (*see* **Note 1**), (3) 5% spiked positive control, (4) 10% spiked positive control, (5) non-template control (nuclease-free molecular grade water), and (6) control DNA that comes with the AmpFLSTR Identifiler PLUS PCR Kit.
5. When the total concentration of the entire fetal DNA sample is very low (3–10 ng/μL) it is better to use 3 μL of the diluted fetal DNA sample instead of 2 μL.
6. When the total concentration of the entire fetal DNA sample is very low (3–10 ng/μL) it is better to use 2 μL of the fetal PCR product instead of 1 μL.
7. When the fluorescent signal in a sample is strong, peaks can be seen that represent neither an allele from the individual tested, nor a biological contaminant. These bleed-through peaks occur in neighboring channels because the fluorescent filters do not have perfect specificity for their fluorophores. When an anomalous peak is observed in one channel that matches the size of an intense biological peak in another channel, it is likely a bleed-through peak rather than a sign of contamination.
8. When determining whether a peak is shared between the maternal and fetal sample, the size of the maker may vary by +/−1 due to small differences in capillary electrophoresis runs between samples.

9. At least 2 informative markers must be present to report absence of maternal cell contamination. Peak heights of informative markers should be 1000rfu for heterozygous alleles and 2000rfu for homozygous alleles, to eliminate the possibility of contamination at a 5% level (contaminating allele will then be approximately 50rfu). This minimum does not apply when maternal cell contamination is clearly detected.

References

1. Hsu LY (1992) Prenatal diagnosis of chromosomal abnormalities through amniocentesis. In: Milunsky A (ed) Genetic disorders and the fetus: diagnosis, prevention and treatment, 3rd edn. Johns Hopkins University Press, Baltimore
2. Ledbetter DH, Zachary JM, Simpson JL et al (1992) Cytogenetic results from the U.S. collaborative study on CVS. Prenat Diagn 12(5):317–345
3. Ledbetter DH (1993) Prenatal cytogenetics: indications, accuracy and future directions. In: Simpson JL, Elias S (eds) Essentials of prenatal diagnosis. Churchill Livingstone, New York
4. Saura R, Roux D, Taine L et al (1994) Early amniocentesis versus chorionic villus sampling for fetal karyotyping. Lancet 344 (8925):825–826
5. Weida J, Patil AS, Schubert FP et al (2017) Prevalence of maternal cell contamination in amniotic fluid samples. J Matern Fetal Neonatal Med 30(17):2133–2137. https://doi.org/10.1080/14767058.2016.1240162
6. Nagan N, Faulkner NE, Curtis C et al (2011) Laboratory guidelines for detection, interpretation, and reporting of maternal cell contamination in prenatal analyses a report of the association for molecular pathology. J Mol Diagn 13(1):7–11. https://doi.org/10.1016/j.jmoldx.2010.11.013
7. South ST, Lee C, Lamb AN et al (2013) ACMG standards and guidelines for constitutional cytogenomic microarray analysis, including postnatal and prenatal applications: revision 2013. Genet Med 15(11):901–909. https://doi.org/10.1038/gim.2013.129
8. Akolekar R, Beta J, Picciarelli G et al (2015) Procedure-related risk of miscarriage following amniocentesis and chorionic villus sampling: a systematic review and meta-analysis. Ultrasound Obstet Gynecol 45(1):16–26. https://doi.org/10.1002/uog.14636
9. Winsor EJ, Silver MP, Theve R et al (1996) Maternal cell contamination in uncultured amniotic fluid. Prenat Diagn 16(1):49–54. https://doi.org/10.1002/(SICI)1097-0223(199601)16:1<49::AID-PD808>3.0.CO;2-U

Chapter 9

Rapid Prenatal Aneuploidy Screening by Fluorescence In Situ Hybridization (FISH)

Anja Weise and Thomas Liehr

Abstract

The most common aneuploidies observed in prenatal diagnostics in the second trimester are trisomies of the chromosomes 13, 18 or 21 and gonosomal abnormalities. Rapid detection of these aneuploidies after amniocentesis is possible by fluorescence in situ hybridization (FISH) utilizing centromeric or locus-specific probes. FISH aneuploidy screening results in uncultured amniocytes are available within 24 h or less. Operators should be aware that there are possible pitfalls in connection with the commercially available probe sets and in result interpretation in general and thus proceed with appropriate caution. Here, we explain how rapid prenatal aneuploidy screening is performed using the Food and Drug Administration (FDA-) approved Aneu Vysion kit (ABBOTT/Vysis) and a review is given of drawbacks and opportunities of the method.

Key words Prenatal diagnosis, Molecular cytogenetics, Fluorescence in situ hybridization (FISH), Interphase FISH, Pitfalls

1 Introduction

In the 1980s it took around 3–4 weeks to obtain a fetal karyotype from amniotic fluid cells, mainly due to the necessity for cell culturing [1]. This timeframe was shortened to around 2 weeks [2], due to progress in cytogenetic techniques, i.e., in cell growth media, but also in cell preparation [3]. Even though this is a relatively short time compared to the 3–4 weeks necessary in the 1980s, it was recognized that such moderately long waiting times cause psychological distress for the pregnant women [1].

This was one of the main causes for the introduction of molecular (cytogenetics) methods for prenatal diagnosis of the most common chromosome disorders in the second trimester: trisomy 13, 18, and 21, monosomy X and other gonosomal aberrations, as well as triploidy [4]. Molecular techniques can be performed directly on uncultured fetal cells, obviating the time consuming process of cell culture and allowing for results to be obtained within

Brynn Levy (ed.), *Prenatal Diagnosis*, Methods in Molecular Biology, vol. 1885, https://doi.org/10.1007/978-1-4939-8889-1_9,

24 h. The quantitative fluorescence polymerase chain reaction (QF–PCR), Multiplex ligation-dependent probe amplification (MLPA), or the fluorescence in situ hybridization (FISH) are three popular methods utilized in clinical practice [1]. Despite some key methodological advantages unique to FISH (like single cell analysis and low level mosaicism detection), aneuploidy screening by FISH has virtually been replaced by q-PCR in many places in Europe. However, in the USA, it remains the primary rapid aneuploidy screening method of choice. Nowadays, where chromosomal microarray analysis is fast becoming the first line test in invasive prenatal diagnostics, rapid molecular screening tests (like FISH) still make sense in terms of saving time and resources for the detection of frequent human aneuploidies.

The only Food and Drug Administration (FDA-) approved FISH-test for rapid aneuploidy screening in uncultured amniocytes cells is the Aneu Vysion kit (commercially available at ABBOTT/ Vysis). It consists of two locus-specific probes for 13q14 (LSI 13) and 21q22.13~22.2 (LSI 21) (Fig. 1) and three alpha-satellite DNA-probes for chromosomes X, Y, and 18 (cep X, cep Y, and cep 18) (Fig. 2). The two locus specific and the three centromeric probes are applied in two different hybridization experiments to the samples.

One has to be aware of the fact, that other genetic disorders like (un)balanced structural rearrangements, numerical aberrations beside the five tested chromosomes, microdeletions/microduplications, uniparental disomy, or mutations detectable only by molecular genetics, are not excluded after obtaining a "normal" result for the rapid aneuploidy screening by FISH. To obtain a reliable result 50–100 interphase nuclei have to be evaluated per probe mix; for all five probes cut-off rates of ~10% were suggested recently [4].

Published studies on the use of FISH for rapid aneuploidy screening include tens of thousands of cases and they all show concordance rates in excess of 99% between the results obtained by FISH and those seen by standard G-banded karyotyping [4–10]. However, there are always single case reports of false-positive or false-negative results that are due to centromeric polymorphisms, the presence of small supernumerary marker chromosomes, dicentric chromosomes not detectable in interphase nuclei, or maternal contamination [4–14]. As recently suggested, all the observed pitfalls and reported misdiagnoses (apart from maternal contamination) could easily be prevented by the exclusive use of locus-specific probes [13]. The advantage of such probes, like the LSI 13 and LSI 21 probes in the FDA kit, was proven, e.g., by the fact that the LSI 21 probe is better suited to distinguish between free and translocation trisomy 21 in the interphase [15].

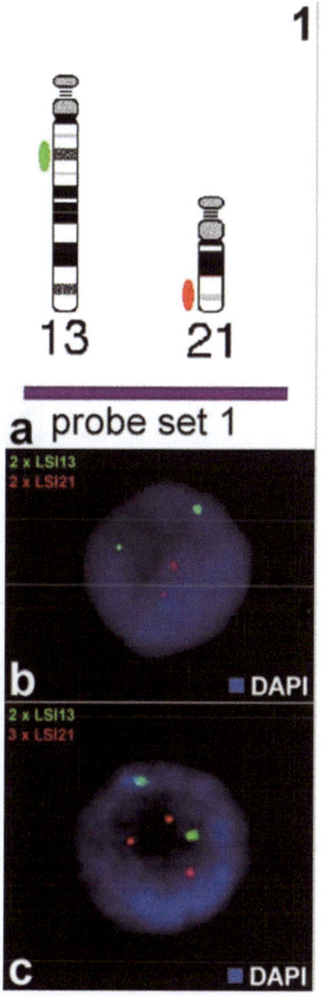

Fig. 1 (**a**) The distribution of the probes LSI13 (SpectrumOrange) and LSI21 (SpectrumGreen) is depicted, which comprise probe set 1. (**b**) A nucleus with normal signal distribution of LSI13 and LSI21 indicating—if present in at least 45 of 50 evaluated nuclei—for the absence of a numerical aberration of chromosomes 13 and 21 within the fetus. The nucleus is counterstained in blue by DAPI. (**c**) In this nucleus there are two signals for LSI13 and three for LSI21 indicative of a (free or translocation) trisomy 21

In summary, the rapid prenatal FISH aneuploidy test is a powerful tool for the clinician in the care for pregnant women. It should be offered to patients with appropriate genetic counseling, discussing the benefits and limitations of the test. This robust rapid prenatal FISH test may also be utilized on preimplantation embryos [16] and prenatal chorionic villi samples [17].

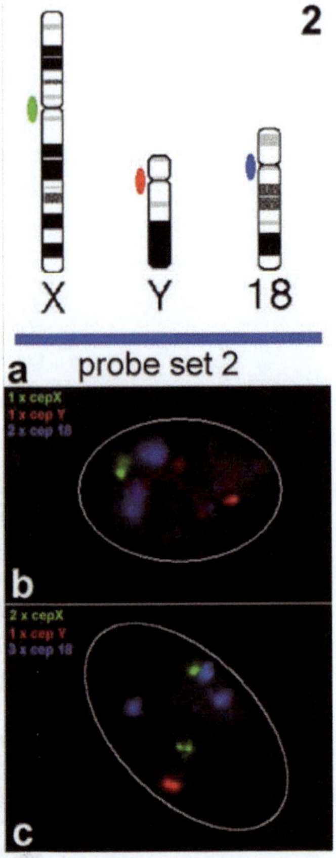

Fig. 2 (**a**) The three centromeric probes cepX, cepY, and cep18 are labeled in SpectrumGreen, SpectrumOrange, and SpectrumBlue, respectively, in probe set 2. (**b**) A nucleus with one signal, each, for cepX and cepY are seen in this cell of a male fetus. Additionally, two signals only are present for the cep18 probe and thus, with high probability a free trisomy 18 is excluded. (**c**) In this case three signals for cep18, but as well two signals for cepX and one for cepY were present in each of the analyzed nuclei. As also three signals, each, for LSI13 and LSI21 were detected (results not shown), a clinically suspected triploidy could be confirmed by FISH and the pregnancy was terminated

2 Materials

2.1 Preparation of Amniotic Fluid Cells

1. Trypsin/EDTA. Pre-warm 3 mL per case (37 °C).
2. Mix 1× PBS with fetal calf serum v/v 4/1. Pre-warm 5 mL per case (37 °C).
3. 0.075 M KCl.
4. Carnoy's fixative: 3:1 Methanol:Glacial acetic acid.

2.2 Slide Pretreatment

1. 20× SSC stock solution: 3.0 M NaCl, 0.3 M Na-citrate; set up with double distilled water, adjust to pH 7.0, autoclave and store at room temperature.
2. Pepsin stock solution 10% (w/v): dissolve 100 mg pepsin in 1 mL of filtered double distilled water at 37 °C; aliquot and store at −20 °C.
3. Pepsin-buffer: Add 1 mL of 1 M HCl to 99 mL of distilled water and incubate at 37 °C for about 20 min; then add 50 μL of the pepsin stock solution 10% (w/v) and leave the coplin jar at 37 °C; make fresh as required.
4. 1× PBS/ $MgCl_2$: 5% (v/v) 1 M $MgCl_2$ in 1× PBS.

2.3 Slide Denaturation

1. Denaturation-buffer: 70% (v/v) deionized formamide, 10% (v/v) filtered double distilled water, 10% (v/v) 20 × SSC, 10% (v/v) phosphate buffer; make fresh as required.
2. Deionized formamide: Add 5 g of ion exchanger Serdolit MB-1 (Serva, Heidelberg, Germany) to 100 mL of formamide, stir for 2 h (room temperature) and filter twice through Whatmann no. 1 filter paper. Aliquot and store at −20 °C.
3. Phosphate buffer: prepare 0.5 M Na_2HPO_4 and 0.5 M NaH_2PO_4, mix these two solutions (1:1) to get pH 7.0, then aliquot and store at −20 °C.

2.4 Hybridization

1. Aneuvision Kit (Abbott Molecular, Des Plaines, IL, USA).

2.5 Posthybridization Washing

1. 20× SSC stock solution: 3.0 M NaCl, 0.3 M Na-citrate; set up with double distilled water, adjust to pH 7.0, autoclave, and store at room temperature.
2. DAPI-solution: Dissolve 5 μL of DAPI (4,6-diamidino-2-phenylindol.2HCl stock-solution) in 100 mL 4× SSC/0.2% Tween; make fresh as required.
3. Vectashield H-1000 Antifade Mounting Medium (Vector Laboratories, Burlingame, CA, USA).

3 Methods

This section describes how amniotic fluid cells are prepared, how the target of the hybridization, i.e., cytogenetic slides with interphase cells, have to be pretreated and how FISH itself is performed and evaluated.

3.1 Preparation of Amniotic Fluid (AF) Cells

For the rapid aneuploidy screening it is necessary to prepare the uncultured amniocytes as recommended in the AneuVysion kit protocol.

1. Place 2–3 mL of AF into a 15 mL reaction tube and centrifuge (175 × *g* for 5 min); discard the supernatant (*see* **Note 1**).
2. Resuspend the pellet in 3 mL trypsine/EDTA and incubate for 15 min at 37 °C.
3. Add 1× PBS/foetal calf serum (4/1), centrifuge (175 × *g* for 5 min—discard the supernatant).
4. Resuspend the pellet in 5 mL 0.075 M KCl and incubate at 37 °C for 20 min.
5. Add 2 mL Carnoy's fixative, centrifuge (175 × *g* for 5 min—discard the supernatant).
6. Add 3 mL Carnoy's fixative, resuspend and incubate at −20 °C for 5 min.
7. Finalize the preparation with one last centrifugation (175 × *g* for 5 min); discard the supernatant and dilute the cells in 200 μL of the remaining supernatant.
8. Dispense the entire remaining suspension on two small regions of a single dry and clean slide and air dry for 10 min at room temperature.
9. Dehydrate in an ethanol series (70%; 90%; 100%, for 3 min each) and air dry.

3.2 Slide Pretreatment

1. Incubate slides in 2× SSC for 1 min at room temperature (in a 100 mL coplin jar on a shaker).
2. Replace 1× PBS with 100 mL pre-warmed pepsin-buffer (37 °C) and incubate the slides for 5 min at 37 °C, without agitation (*see* **Note 2**).
3. Replace pepsin-buffer with 100 mL 1× PBS/$MgCl_2$, incubate at room temperature for 5 min with gentle agitation. $MgCl_2$ will block the enzymatic activity of pepsin.
4. Postfix nuclei on the slide surface by replacing 1× PBS/$MgCl_2$ with 100 mL of formalin-buffer for 10 min (room temperature, with gentle agitation).
5. Formalin-buffer is replaced by 100 mL 1× PBS for 2 min (room temperature, with gentle agitation).
6. Finally, dehydrate slides through an ethanol series (70%, 90%, 100%, 3 min each) and then air dry (*see* **Note 3**).

3.3 Fluorescence In Situ Hybridization (FISH) and Evaluation

The FISH procedure is itself divided into several steps: denaturation, hybridization, posthybridization washing, and evaluation.

3.3.1 Denaturation of Target DNA

1. Add 100 μL denaturation-buffer to the slides and cover with (24 × 50 mm) coverslips.

2. Incubate the slides on a heating plate for 3 min at 75 °C (*see* **Note 2**).
3. Remove the coverslips immediately by forceps and place the slides in a coplin jar filled with 70% ethanol (4 °C) to conserve target DNA as single strands.
4. Dehydrate the slides in ethanol (70%, 90%, 100%, 4 °C, 3 min each) and air dry.

3.3.2 Hybridization

1. For each slide to be hybridized add 8 μL of the probe solution 1 (LSI 13 and LSI 21) on one region of the slide and 8 μL of the probe solution 2 (cep 18, cep X and cep Y) on the dry slide, put 20 × 20 mm coverslips on the drops and seal with rubber cement.
2. Incubate slides overnight at 37 °C in a humid chamber (*see* **Note 4**).

3.3.3 Posthybridization Washing

1. Take the slides out of 37 °C humid chamber and remove rubber cement with forceps.
2. Place slides in 4× SSC/0.2%Tween (room temperature, 100 mL coplin jar) and allow coverslips to slide off (*see* **Note 5**).
3. Postwash the slides 1× 2 min in 0.4× SSC (56–62 °C) followed by 1× 1 min in 4× SSC/0.2% Tween (100 mL, room temperature).
4. Counterstain the slides with DAPI-solution (100 mL in a coplin jar, room temperature) for 8 min.
5. Wash the slides in water for a few seconds and air dry.
6. Add 15 μL of Vectashield H-1000 antifade mounting medium, cover with coverslips, and look at the results in a fluorescence microscope.

3.3.4 Evaluation

1. Evaluate 50 interphase nuclei per case under the fluorescence microscope. This is a semi-statistic evaluation counting 1, 2, 3, or 4 signals for each probe. In case of a questionable result within the cut-off region, enhance evaluated nuclei to 100 or more (*see* **Note 6**).

4 Notes

1. During the whole preparation avoid taking the cells up with a pipette—this would only lead to undesired loss of cells; only mix with supernatant by moving the tube.
2. Pepsin pretreatment conditions, as well as denaturation time of the target DNA should be tested in each laboratory on a single slide first. If pepsin concentration is too stringent, it can result in clean slides without any remaining nuclei.

3. The pretreated slides can be hybridized immediately or stored at room temperature for up to 3 weeks. If longer storage is necessary, the slides are stable at −20 °C for several months.
4. Incubation can be stopped, if necessary, after 3 h. However, this may result in the signals being too weak for evaluation. This is especially true of the LSI-probes.
5. During the washing steps, it is important to prevent the slide surfaces from drying out, otherwise background problems may arise.
6. As long as not more than 7%/10% of the studied cells present with 3 specific signals, no trisomy of the corresponding chromosomal region is suspected and a "normal" report can be issued. Between 7%/10% and 20%, the evaluation can be regarded as an "unclear result," which is with high probability a "normal" result. However, in such cases, try to evaluate 100 or more nuclei for the probe in question to come to a final decision. A value of >20% is indicative at minimum of a mosaic trisomy. We suggest different cut-off rates for female and male fetuses for optimal interpretation of the result [4]. This is due to the fact that maternal cell-contamination is obvious in the amniotic fluid of a male fetus but is not discernible in a female fetus. Thus, the results of female fetuses should be interpreted with slightly more care and the cut-off rates lowered. Similar suggestions are made for the handling of XXX, XYY, or XXY results.

References

1. Hulten MA, Dhanjal S, Pertl B (2003) Rapid and simple prenatal diagnosis of common chromosome disorders: advantages and disadvantages of the molecular methods FISH and QF-PCR. Reproduction 126(3):279–297
2. Held KR (2003) QS Zytogenetik Bericht 2002/2003. Med Genet 15:420–421
3. Claussen U, Ulmer R, Beinder E et al (1993) Rapid karyotyping in prenatal diagnosis: a comparative study of the 'pipette method' and the 'in situ' technique for chromosome harvesting. Prenat Diagn 13(12):1085–1093
4. Liehr T, Ziegler M (2005) Rapid prenatal diagnostics in the interphase nucleus: procedure and cut-off rates. J Histochem Cytochem 53 (3):289–291. https://doi.org/10.1369/jhc.4B6394.2005
5. Caine A, Maltby AE, Parkin CA et al (2005) Prenatal detection of Down's syndrome by rapid aneuploidy testing for chromosomes 13, 18, and 21 by FISH or PCR without a full karyotype: a cytogenetic risk assessment. Lancet 366(9480):123–128. https://doi.org/10.1016/S0140-6736(05)66790-6
6. Eiben B, Trawicki W, Hammans W et al (1999) Rapid prenatal diagnosis of aneuploidies in uncultured amniocytes by fluorescence in situ hybridization. Evaluation of >3,000 cases. Fetal Diagn Ther 14(4):193–197. https://doi.org/10.1159/000020919
7. Leung WC, Waters JJ, Chitty L (2004) Prenatal diagnosis by rapid aneuploidy detection and karyotyping: a prospective study of the role of ultrasound in 1589 second-trimester amniocenteses. Prenat Diagn 24(10):790–795. https://doi.org/10.1002/pd.985
8. Tepperberg J, Pettenati MJ, Rao PN et al (2001) Prenatal diagnosis using interphase fluorescence in situ hybridization (FISH): 2-year multi-center retrospective study and review of the literature. Prenat Diagn 21 (4):293–301
9. Weremowicz S, Sandstrom DJ, Morton CC et al (2001) Fluorescence in situ hybridization

(FISH) for rapid detection of aneuploidy: experience in 911 prenatal cases. Prenat Diagn 21(4):262–269. https://doi.org/10.1002/pd.39

10. Witters I, Devriendt K, Legius E et al (2002) Rapid prenatal diagnosis of trisomy 21 in 5049 consecutive uncultured amniotic fluid samples by fluorescence in situ hybridisation (FISH). Prenat Diagn 22(1):29–33
11. Estabrooks LL, Hanna JS, Lamb AN (1999) Overwhelming maternal cell contamination in amniotic fluid samples from patients with oligohydramnios can lead to false prenatal interphase FISH results. Prenat Diagn 19 (2):179–181
12. Liehr T, Beensen V, Hauschild R et al (2001) Pitfalls of rapid prenatal diagnosis using the interphase nucleus. Prenat Diagn 21 (5):419–421. https://doi.org/10.1002/pd.44
13. Liehr T, Schreyer I, Neumann A et al (2002) Two more possible pitfalls of rapid prenatal diagnostics using interphase nuclei. Prenat Diagn 22(6):497–499. https://doi.org/10.1002/pd.299
14. Skinner JL, Govberg IJ, DePalma RT et al (2001) Heteromorphisms of chromosome 18 can obscure detection of fetal aneuploidy by interphase FISH. Prenat Diagn 21 (8):702–704
15. Liehr T, Starke H, Beensen V et al (1999) Translocation trisomy dup(21q) and free trisomy 21 can be distinguished by interphase-FISH. Int J Mol Med 3(1):11–14
16. Mir P, Rodrigo L, Mateu E et al (2010) Improving FISH diagnosis for preimplantation genetic aneuploidy screening. Hum Reprod 25 (7):1812–1817. https://doi.org/10.1093/humrep/deq122
17. Toutain J, Epiney M, Begorre M et al (2010) First-trimester prenatal diagnosis performed on pregnant women with fetal ultrasound abnormalities: the reliability of interphase fluorescence in situ hybridization (FISH) on mesenchymal core for the main aneuploidies. Eur J Obstet Gynecol Reprod Biol 149(2):143–146. https://doi.org/10.1016/j.ejogrb.2009.12.015

Chapter 10

Prenatal Detection of Chromosome Aneuploidy by Quantitative Fluorescence PCR

Kathy Mann, Erwin Petek, and Barbara Pertl

Abstract

Autosomal chromosome aneuploid pregnancies that survive to term, namely, trisomies 13, 18, and 21, account for 89% of chromosome abnormalities with a severe phenotype identified in prenatal samples. They are traditionally detected by full karyotype analysis of cultured cells. The average reporting time for a prenatal karyotype analysis is approximately 14 days, and in recent years, there has been increasing demand for more rapid prenatal results with respect to the common chromosome aneuploidies, to relieve maternal anxiety and facilitate options in pregnancy. The rapid tests that have been developed negate the requirement for cultured cells, instead directly testing cells from the amniotic fluid or chorionic villus sample, with the aim of generating results within 48 h of sample receipt. Interphase fluorescence in situ hybridization is the method of choice in some genetic laboratories, usually because the expertise and equipment are readily available. However, a quantitative fluorescence (QF)-PCR-based approach is now widely used and reported as a clinical diagnostic service in many studies. It may be used as a stand-alone test or as an adjunct test to full karyotype or array CGH analysis, which scan for other chromosome abnormalities not detected by the QF-PCR assay.

Key words Quantitative fluorescence-polymerase chain reaction (QF-PCR), Chromosome aneuploidies, Rapid prenatal test, Down syndrome

1 Introduction

Autosomal chromosome aneuploid pregnancies that survive to term, namely, trisomies 13, 18, and 21, account for 89% of chromosome abnormalities with a severe phenotype identified in prenatal samples [1]. They are traditionally detected by full karyotype analysis of cultured cells. The average UK reporting time for a prenatal karyotype analysis is approximately 14 days [2], and in recent years, there has been increasing demand for more rapid prenatal results with respect to the common chromosome aneuploidies, to relieve maternal anxiety and facilitate options in pregnancy. The rapid tests that have been developed negate the requirement for cultured cells, instead directly testing cells from the amniotic fluid (AF) or chorionic villus sample (CVS), with the

Brynn Levy (ed.), *Prenatal Diagnosis*, Methods in Molecular Biology, vol. 1885, https://doi.org/10.1007/978-1-4939-8889-1_10,

aim of generating results within 48 h of sample receipt. Interphase-fluorescence in situ hybridization (FISH) [3, 4] is the method of choice in many genetic laboratories, usually because the expertise and equipment are readily available. However, a quantitative fluorescence polymerase chain reaction (QF-PCR)-based approach is more suited to a high throughput diagnostic service. This approach is now widely used and reported as a clinical diagnostic service [5–14]. It may be used as a stand-alone test or as an adjunct test to full karyotype or array CGH analysis, which scan for other chromosome abnormalities not detected by the QF-PCR assay.

1.1 Principle

QF-PCR refers to the amplification of chromosome-specific polymorphic microsatellite markers using fluorescence-labeled primers, followed by quantitative analysis of the products on a genetic analyzer to determine copy number of specific chromosomal material. Tetranucleotide repeat markers are used to minimize PCR-generated "stutter bands" (PCR artifacts that are one to three repeat units smaller than the true allele size). Where a microsatellite marker is heterozygous, the ratio of its allele peak areas represents a disomic (1:1) or trisomic (2:1, 1:2 or 1:1:1) chromosome complement (*see* Fig. 1). A marker is uninformative if only a single peak is observed.

Due to allele size heterogeneity and differences in sample type and quality, the amplification of a single marker relative to other markers in the assay may vary greatly. Thus, a comparison of allele peak areas between markers, as an indicator of chromosome copy number, is not recommended. Furthermore, because only peak areas within a single locus are compared, allele dosage ratios are more resilient to the effects of the plateau phase of the PCR than other dosage assays [15].

The procedure described here uses a "one-tube test," where 17 markers are coamplified in one multiplex reaction (*see* Table 1 and Fig. 1) [9]. Five markers are used for both chromosomes 13 and 21, and seven markers are used for chromosome 18. A separate sex chromosome multiplex can be used for sexing purposes and to diagnose sex chromosome aneuploidy (*see* Table 2 and Fig. 2) [9, 16]. The inclusion of a paralagous marker in the sex chromosome assay is recommended as this adds confidence to a diagnosis of monosomy X. Here, the TAF9L marker is used which amplifies a chromosome 3 and X chromosome sequence with the same primer pair. Comparison of the two peaks is used to determine the copy number of the X chromosome sequence. Markers are located along the length of each chromosome to increase the chance of detecting unbalanced chromosome rearrangements.

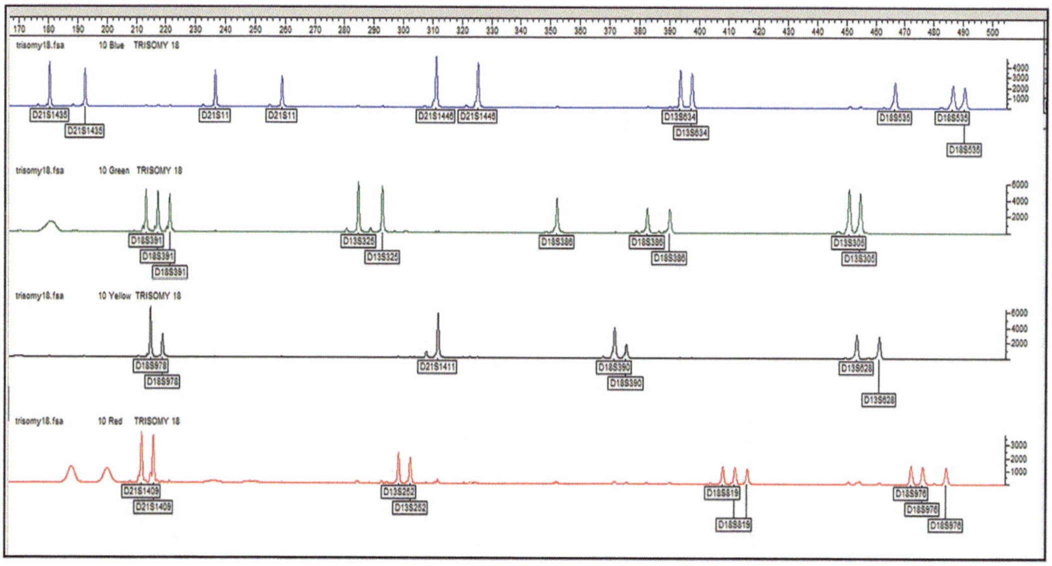

Fig. 1 Genotyper profile (Applied Biosystems CA) depicting the 17 polymorphic markers in the trisomy multiplex. The seven chromosome 18 markers exhibit allele patterns consistent with three copies of chromosome 18. All five chromosome 13 markers and four of five chromosome 21 markers show a normal biallelic profile while the fifth chromosome 21 marker is uninformative. The results are consistent with trisomy 18 and a normal complement for chromosomes 13 and 21

1.2 Potential Problems

1.2.1 Maternal Cell Contamination (MCC)

Evidence of a second genotype, as shown by inconsistent dosage ratios for each chromosome, extra allele peaks, or both, usually indicates contamination of the sample by maternal cells (*see* Fig. 3), although it may represent a twin or chimera. Maternal cell contamination is usually associated with blood-stained AF samples, although the degree of blood staining should not in itself be used as an indicator of maternal cell contamination; blood cells may be fetal or maternal in origin. Usually, samples are accompanied by some degree of blood staining, although this ranges from a pale pink cell pellet and clear liquor to a deep red color of the whole fluid. When the majority genotype shows consistent normal or abnormal results with no inconclusive allele ratios, then the result may be reported, although it may be advisable to confirm the origin of the majority genotype by analysis of a maternal blood sample. We have found the level of blood staining in the AF cell pellet to broadly correlate with the level of maternal genotype; the majority genotype from pellets with fewer red blood cells is consistently fetal in origin. However, when the presence of two genotypes causes allele ratios to skew outside of the normal or abnormal range (*see* Subheading 3.5, **step 1**), it is recommended that the QF-PCR results are not interpreted due to the increased risk of a misdiagnosis. In these cases, if a rapid result is required and one of the genotypes is determined as fetal in origin either by sexing or by genotype analysis of a maternal sample,

Table 1
Details of primers used in the trisomy multiplex. Size ranges given are those used in Genotyper, version 3.7 (Applied Biosystems). Heterozygosity values are based on our cohort and may vary in other populations. Primer concentrations will vary depending on supplier, batch and buffer. All markers are tetranucleotide repeats

Marker Name	Location	Hetero-zygosity	Allele size range (bp)	Primer sequences 5′–3′ (Forward, reverse)	Final conc. (μM) of each primer
D13S252	13q12.1	0.85	260–330	**PET**-GCAGATGTACTGTTTTCCTACCAA AGATGGTATATTGTGGGACCTTGT	0.75
D13S305	13q13.3	0.75	418–482	**VIC**-GCCTGTTTGAGGACCTGTCGTTA TGGTTATAGAGCAGTTAAGGCAC	1
D13S628	13q31.1	0.688	425–474	**NED**- TGGATGAATACGCCACTTTTC TGGTTAAAAGATTGCCAAGGAG	1.5
D13S634	13q21.33	0.812	355–440	**6FAM**-GGCAGATTCAATAGGATAAATAGA GTAACCCCTCAGGTTCTCAAGTCT	0.5
D13S325	13q12.12	0.75	235–315	**VIC**-CTGTGCTATCTCCTCCAACG GTTTGAAAGATAGGCCATGCAG	0.25
D18S386	18q22.1	0.875	320–417	**VIC**-TGAGTCAGGAGAATCACTTGGAAC CTCTTCCATGAAGTAGCTAAGCAG	0.75
D18S390	18q22.3	0.75	340–415	**NED**-GGTCAATAGTGAATATTTGGATAC CTCCAACCTCACTTGAGAGTA	0.25
D18S391	18p11.31	0.75	190–235	**VIC**-GGACTTACCACAGGCAATGTGACT CTGGCTAATTGAGTTAGATTACAA	0.1

D18S535	18q12.3	0.92	450–500	**6FAM**-CAGCAAACTTCATGTGACAAAAGC CAATGGTAACCTACTATTTACGTC	0.5
D18S819	18q11.2	0.78	370–450	**PET**-CTTCTCACCTGAATTACTATGGT TTTGTAATCGATCTACCACAGTT	1
D18S976	18p11.31	0.78	465–495	**PET**- GAGATCCTGAACATGGAGCAG ACACTATTGGCATCCCTTGG	0.5
D18S978	18q12.3	0.667	180–230	**NED**-GTAGATCTTGGGACTTGTCAGA GTCTCCCATGGTCACAATGCT	0.25
D21S11	21q21.1	0.9	220–283	**6FAM**-TTTCTCAGTCTCCATAAATATGTG GATGTTGTATTAGTCAATGTTCTC	1
D21S1437	21q21.1	0.84	283–351	**6FAM**-CTACCACTGATGGACATTTAG GTGGAGGGTGTACCTCCAGAA	0.5
D21S1409	21q21.2	0.81	205–250	**PET**-AAGCGAAGGATTTGGATCAG TTTGCCTCTGAATATCCCTATC	0.5
D21S1411	21q22.3	0.933	256–345	ATAGGTAGATACATAAATATGATGA **NED**-TATTAATGTGTGTCCTTCCAGGC	0.75
D21S1435	21q21.3	0.75	160–200	**6FAM**-CCCTCTCCAATTGTTTGTCTACC ACAAAAGGAAAGCAAGAGATTTCA	0.25

Table 2
Details of primers used in the sex chromosome multiplex. Size ranges given are those used in Genotyper, version 3.7 (Applied Biosystems). Heterozygosity (Het) values are based on our cohort and may vary in other populations. Primer concentrations will vary depending on supplier, batch and buffer. DYS448 is a hexanucleotide repeat, DX6807, DXS981, DXS1187, XHPRT, DXS7423, DXS6803, DXS6809, DXYS267, DXYS218 are tetranucleotide repeats and DXS1283E is a dinucleotide repeat. AMEL, SRY and TAF9L are not polymorphic. TAF9L is present on chromosome 3 and the X chromosome and the ratio of both peaks is used to assess relative X chromosome copy number

Marker Name	Location	Hetero-zygosity	Allele size range (bp)	Primer sequences 5′–3′ (Forward, reverse)	Final conc. (μM) of each primer
DXS6807	Xp22.3	0.7	300–380	**6FAM**- TCTCCCTTATTTGTGGTTTTGC AGCAGTTCTCCCTTATCCAC	1.5
DXS1283E	Xp22.3	0.89	295–340	**NED**-AGTTTAGGAGATTATCAAGCTG CCCATACACAAGTCCTCAAAGTGA	0.75
DXS981	Xq13.1	0.86	225–260	**6FAM**-CTCCTTGTGGCCTTCCTTAAATG TTCTCTCCACTTTTCAGAGTCA	0.25
DXS1187	Xq26.2	0.72	180–220	**VIC**-CAGCTACTCAATGAAAAGCC ATGGGGTAGGGACCAAAAAT	0.25
XHPRT	Xq26.2	0.78	265–300	**VIC**-ATGCCACAGATAATACACATCCCC CTCTCCAGAATAGTTAGATGTAGG	0.5
DXS7423	Xq28	0.74	350–420	**VIC**- TACTGGAGGTGAGGGTTGTG TGGGCTGCCCAGATACAACT	1.5
DXS6803	Xq21.31	0.86	135–152	**6FAM**-AAAATTTTCCTCAAAACAAAAAGG AGAATATTCACCTAGAAATGTGC	0.5

DXS6809	Xq21.33	0.78	399–427	**PET**-TTGCTTTAGGCTGATGTGAGG CAGGTTAATTCAAGATATTTGTCA	0.5
DXYS267	Xq21.31 Yp11.31	0.87	240–280	**PET**-ATGTGGTCTTCTACTTGTGTCA GTG TGT GGA AGT GAA GGA TAG	1.0
AMEL	Xp22.2 Yp11.2	–	106 112	**PET**-CCCTGGGCTCTGTAAAGAATAGTG ATCAGAGCTTAAACTGGGAAGCTG	0.25
SRY	Yp11.31	–	248 bp	**NED**- AGTAAAGGCAACGTCCAGGAT TTCCGACGAGGTCGATACTTA	0.5
DYS448	Yq11.223	–	323–370	**PET**- CAAGGATCCAAATAAAGAACAGAG A GGTTATTTCTTGATTCCCTGTG	0.5
DXYS218	Xp22.33 Yp11.3	0.74	383–411	**6-FAM**- AACTGAGGGGACCTGGAATG GAATCGATTCAACCCGGGAGA	0.5
TAF9L	3p24.2 Xq21.1	–	116 125	AGCATCTCTGTTAAATTTAGAAATG **PET**-CAGGAAACAGCTATGACCTGC TTTTGACAGGTAGTTTTGG	0.5

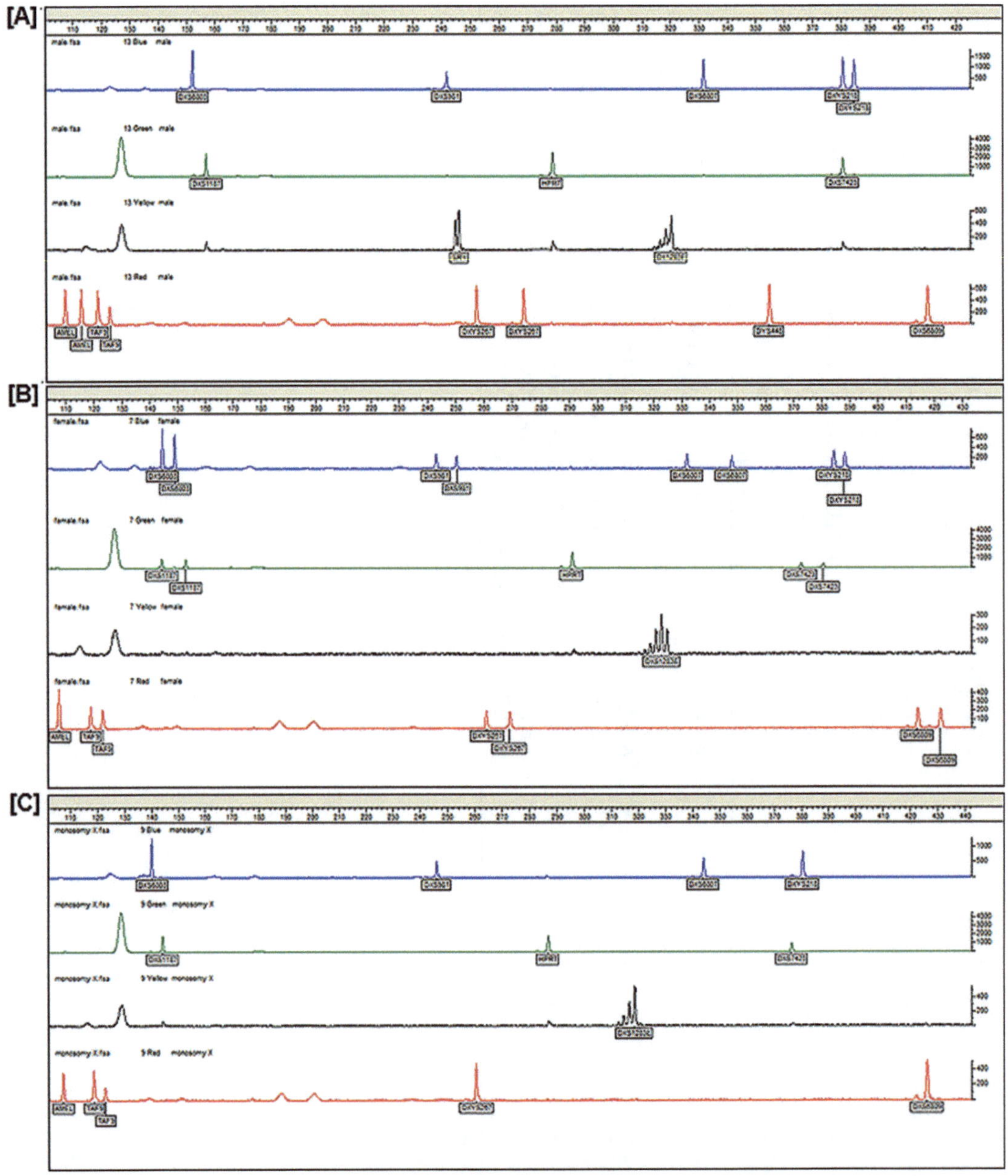

Fig. 2 Three Genotyper Profiles (Applied Biosystems CA) depicting the 14 markers in the sex chromosome multiplex. (**a**) A normal male sample is represented by DXYS267 and DXYS218 which indicate the presence of two sex chromosomes, AMEL which exhibits equal quantities of the X and Y sequences, TAF9 which indicates that there are half as many X chromosome sequences present as chromosome 3 sequences, the presence of Y chromosome-specific sequences (SRY and DYS448) and eight apparently hemizygous polymorphic markers. (**b**) A normal female sample is represented by eight biallelic polymorphic markers indicating two X chromosomes, TAF9 which indicates that X chromosome sequences are present in equal quantities to chromosome 3, and the absence of Y chromosome sequences (AMEL, SRY, DYS448). (**c**) A monosomy X sample is represented by ten apparently hemizygous polymorphic markers, TAF9 which indicates that there are half as many X chromosome sequences present as chromosome 3 sequences, and the absence of Y chromosome sequences (AMEL, SRY, DYS448)

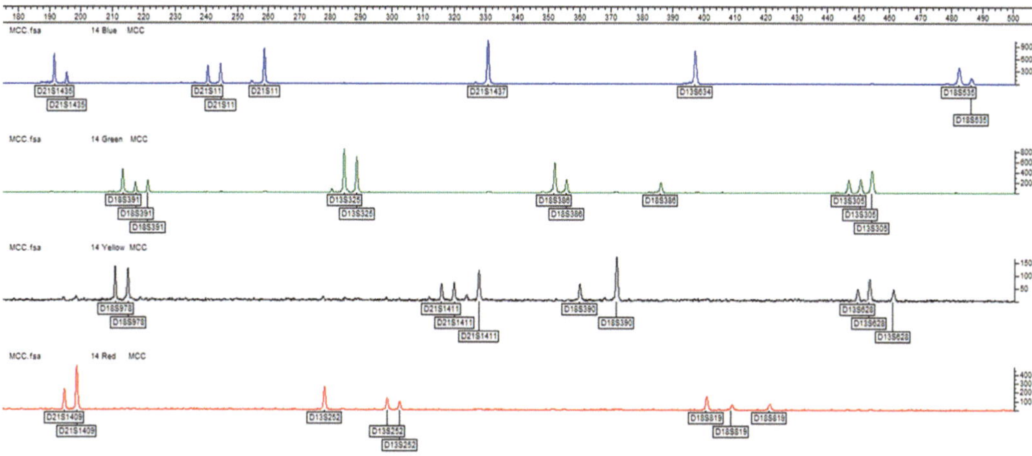

Fig. 3 Genotyper profile of a sample exhibiting a high level of maternal cell contamination. The characteristic triallelic pattern, where the fetal-specific and maternal-specific allele peak areas combine to equal the shared fetal/maternal allele, is observed in markers D21S11, D18S391, D18S386, D13S305, D21S1411, D13S628, D13S252, D18S819

interphase-FISH may then be used if the analysis takes into account the fetal to maternal ratio. The number of analyzed cells can be increased to account for those that are maternal, or a sex chromosome probe can be cohybridized with an autosome probe and only the male cells analyzed.

In our London sample set, approximately 10% of AF samples are found to have two genotypes, although allele ratios vary considerably, proportional to the relative contribution of each cell line. The majority of these samples exhibit a very low level second genotype and can be reported as normal, whereas approximately 2% of AF samples in both the London and Graz cohorts exhibit second genotypes that prevent confident interpretation of allele ratios; therefore, they are reported as unsuitable due to MCC. The detection of maternal cells in an amniotic fluid sample should not discredit the karyotype analysis of cultured cells. Subsequent genotype analysis of cultured cells from samples showing MCC, normally demonstrates a single genotype, consistent with the selection and growth of fetal cells, and loss of maternal cells during the culture process [17]. In those samples with a mixed female/male cell population evident on the direct analysis, a single male genotype is usually detected on the follow-up test. However, the presence of two genotypes in samples where no blood staining is evident may indicate a maternal tissue plug. This may grow in culture and therefore genotype analysis of cultured cells may be useful.

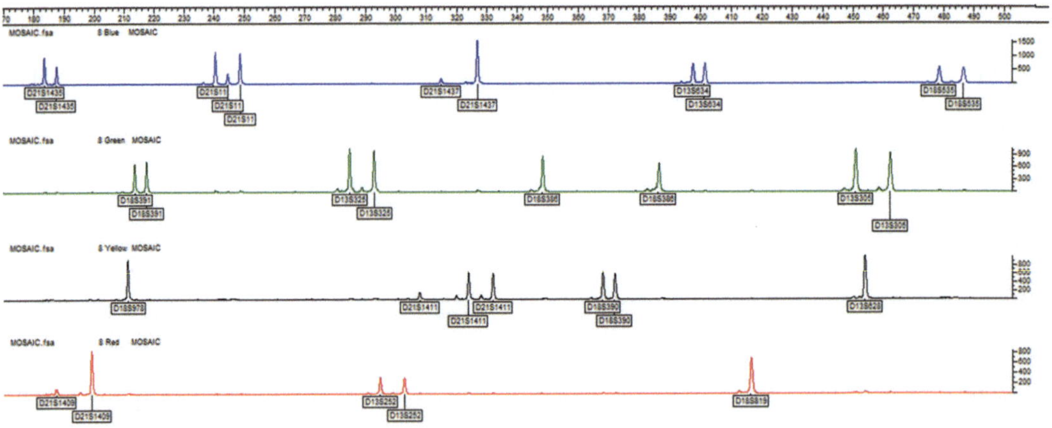

Fig. 4 Genotyper profile of a sample exhibiting trisomy 21 mosaicism. All informative chromosome 21 markers show either an unequal triallelic pattern (D21S11 and D21S1411) or unequal diallelic ratios (D21S1435, D21S1437, and D21S1409). Chromosome 13 and 18 markers are normal. The presence of triallelic chromosome 21 markers is consistent with a meiotic non-disjunction event followed by trisomy rescue to generate the normal cell line

1.2.2 Mosaicism

The problem of mosaic genotypes and karyotypes in prenatal samples is well documented, particularly in CVS (*see* Fig. 4). With respect to QF-PCR, two issues are relevant; the levels of mosaicism detectable by the QF-PCR technique, and the degree of concordance between a direct test result and the fetal genotype.

The first of these can only be determined by the analysis of samples (both postnatal and prenatal) exhibiting mosaicism for one of the tested regions. The generation of "artificial mosaics" by the mixing of two genotypes in known measures represents a chimera rather than a mosaic genotype. The presence of a triallelic result is consistent with a meiotic nondisjunction event generating the trisomy cell line, whereas the absence of a triallelic result is evidence, although not diagnostic, of a normal conception followed by a mitotic nondisjunction event. Analysis of mosaic cases in our sample set found that a minimum level of 15% trisomy mosaicism could be detected if a triallelic allele pattern was observed and 20% trisomy mosaicism if only dialleic ratios were present [18]. Thus, a mitotic error occurring in a disomic fetus may be harder to detect, due to the absence of a third allele. Indeed, QF-PCR identified only one of three trisomy 18 or 21 mosaics described by Pertl et al. [11]; this mosaic case was also triallelic, in this case for chromosome 21.

Discrepancies between the QF-PCR and karyotype result have been described [19, 20]. These have been shown to be due to mosaicism and confinement of cell lines to different regions of the tested sample. To minimize such discrepant results it is recommended that DNA is prepared from dissociated cells prepared from 5 to 15 mg of cleaned villi. Although only a small aliquot of this cell suspension is required, all major cell lines in both the mesoderm and cytotrophoblast should be represented and detected by QF-PCR. Karyotype analysis of cell populations that are subsequently cultured from this cell suspension should minimize discrepancies between the two techniques.

Chorionic villi consist of an outer cytotrophoblast and internal mesoderm layers. The mesoderm layer is derived from a later fetal cell lineage, whereas the cytotrophoblast is derived from a much earlier lineage; thus, it is less representative of fetal tissue [21]. DNA prepared from dissociated cells represents cells from both the cytotrophoblast layer and mesenchymal core [22]. Interphase-FISH results also are thought to represent both cell layers. In contrast, karyotype analysis of direct CVS preparations concerns only the cytotrophoblastic line, whereas culture conditions primarily lead to expansion of the mesoderm cell line, resulting in a final karyotype that is more representative of the fetus. In summary, care should be taken in the interpretation of trisomic prenatal results derived from CVS material, in the absence of a triallelic result demonstrating a meiotic origin to the trisomy cell line.

1.2.3 Submicroscopic Duplications

Partial chromosome duplication may be identified by QF-PCR analysis by the presence of both normal and abnormal marker results on one chromosome. This pattern may indicate a cytogenetically visible abnormality [8] or one that is submicroscopic. If the most distal or proximal markers are duplicated, then this may indicate the unbalanced product of a reciprocal translocation. However, in our experience, the presence of a single abnormal marker result, where all other informative results are normal, is most likely to represent a submicroscopic duplication (SMD) [6]. In the majority of cases, analysis of parental samples shows these SMDs to be inherited. SMDs identified by a single marker that have previously been reported and are flanked by normal markers, require no further investigation and according to Best Practice Guidelines do not have to be reported (http://www.acgs.uk.com/media/765524/acc.cmgs_qfpcr_bp_jan2012_3.01.pdf). A list of SMDs identified to date by markers used in QF-PCR assays is available from Kathy.Mann@viapath.co.uk. For SMDs that have not previously been described, it is necessary to establish the inheritance of the SMD; inherited submicroscopic duplications are unlikely to be clinically significant [23].

1.2.4 Primer Site Polymorphisms (PSPs)

Primer site polymorphisms are a known phenomenon of PCR assays [24]. Sequence differences between the genomic DNA and the primers can result in complete or partial allele dropout (ADO)

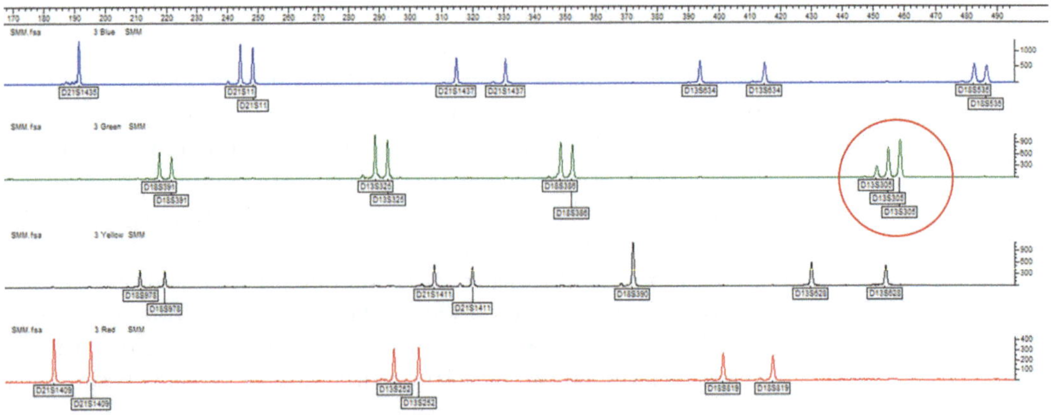

Fig. 5 Genotyper profile of a sample exhibiting a somatic microsatellite mutation (SMM) at marker D13S305. The characteristic triallelic result is evident where the two lowest allele peaks representing the two mosaic cell lines combine to equal the higher allele present in both cell lines. All other informative markers are normal

due to reduced or absent hybridization of the primers to genomic DNA. Partial ADO in a normal sample can either give an abnormal diallelic ratio consistent with trisomy for that region, or an inconclusive ratio (*see* Subheading 3.5). Complete ADO in an abnormal sample can result in a normal diallelic ratio at that locus. In all cases of suspected ADO caused by PSPs, it is recommended to repeat the PCR at a lower annealing temperature (for example, 4 °C lower than the standard temperature). This provides a less stringent environment for primer hybridization, resulting in reduced ADO, as represented by a change in the allele ratio. If the follow-up tests are consistent with the presence of a PSP, the marker result should be failed and not used as part of the QF-PCR analysis, even if it shows a normal ratio; a PSP may cause an abnormal diallelic result to seem normal at a lower annealing temperature.

1.2.5 Somatic Microsatellite Mutations (SMMs)

Somatic changes in the length of a microsatellite sequence, due to DNA replication and proof-reading errors, may be visible as an unequal triallelic result, where the areas of the two lowest alleles combine to equal the highest allele (Fig. 5), or skewed diallelic ratios. The characteristic triallelic pattern represents two cell lines that have one common allele and a second allele of different lengths. QF-PCR analysis of AF samples found <0.1% to have an SMM at a single locus, whereas SMMs were observed at a much higher frequency (4%) in individual whole villi [25]. This high frequency is probably due to the small clonal cell population being analyzed. QF-PCR analysis of digested/chopped villi containing a more diverse cell population (*see* Subheading 3.1.2) therefore results in the identification of fewer SMMs. Interestingly, the majority of SMMs are single repeat unit expansion/contraction events. These somatic changes in repeat length are specific to the microsatellite and are not clinically significant. Thus, a single marker result, showing a characteristic triallelic pattern consistent with a SMM, where all other markers on that chromosome are normal, does not require further clarification. However, it is more difficult to class skewed diallelic results as SMMs; PSPs (*see* Subheading 1.2.4) and SMDs (*see* Subheading 1.2.3) may be alternative explanations. It is important to distinguish between these events if a 1:2 or 2:1 allele ratio is observed, because these ratios may represent a clinically significant imbalance. Once PSPs have been excluded, analysis of cultured cell populations may help to distinguish between an SMD and SMM. In the case of an SMM, the proportion of the two cell lines may change between uncultured and cultured cells thus altering the allele ratio.

2 Materials

2.1 DNA Preparation

1. InstaGene Matrix (Bio-Rad, Hercules, CA). Store at 4 °C.

2.2 PCR

1. T.1E buffer: 10 mM Tris–HCl, pH 7.6, and 0.1 mM EDTA. Filter, sterilizes, and store at room temperature.
2. 10× Multiplex PCR kit (MyTaq, Bioline, London, UK). Store at −20 °C. Once thawed store at 4 °C. Kit contains Taq polymerase and dNTPs.
3. 5′-labeled fluorescent oligonucleotide primers (Thermo Fisher Scientfic, Waltham, MA, USA). We use primers, 5′-labeled with 6-FAM, VIC, NED, or PET. Fluorescence-labeled primers should not be exposed to light for prolonged periods or repeatedly freeze-thawed (see data sheet). These are supplied as precipitates, and are resuspended in T.1E buffer to give a working concentration of 100 μM. The primers are stored at −20 °C. Aliquots in use are stored at 4 °C.
4. Unlabeled oligonucleotide primers (Sigma-Aldrich, Dorset, UK). These primers are supplied as precipitates, and are resuspended in T.1E buffer to a working concentration of 100 μM and stored at −20 °C. Although unlabeled primers are more stable than fluorescent-labeled primers, freeze-thawing should be avoided. Aliquots in use are stored at 4 °C.

2.3 Analysis

1. ABI PRISM 3100 capillary-based genetic analyzer (Thermo Fisher Scientific). All consumables (10× EDTA buffer, POP6 polymer, 36 cm capillaries, plate septa) are purchased from Thermo Fisher Scientific.
2. Deionized formamide (Toxic: refer to the material safety data sheet): HI-DI formamide (Thermo Fisher Scientific) is highly deionized, to minimize the breakdown of the fluorescent label. It is stored at −20 °C in appropriate aliquots.

3. Genescan-500 LIZ size standard (Thermo Fisher Scientific). Standard is designed for 100–500-bp fragment analysis.
4. 96-well plates: We use those recommended for the ABI PRISM 3100 genetic analyzer (Thermo-Fast 96 Detection Plates, ABgene, Epsom, Surrey, UK).
5. Software: For fragment analysis, GeneScan Analysis, version 3.7 was used. For allele size calling and labeling, Genotyper, version 2.5 (Thermo Fisher Scientific) was used. Microsoft Excel (Microsoft, Redmond, WA) is used to calculate and tabulate allele dosage ratios. Other fragment analysis software is available including GeneMapper IDX (Thermo Fisher Scientific) and GeneMarker (SoftGenetics LLC, PA 16803, USA) which include specific aneuploidy analysis modules.

3 Methods

The processing of a number of prenatal samples at one time, and the risk of sample mixup, necessitates stringent quality control procedures (*see* **Note 1**). In addition, care must be taken, as with all PCR-based tests, to avoid contamination of tested material with amplified products of previous reactions and external DNA (*see* **Note 2**).

3.1 Sample Preparation

Sample and DNA preparation procedures are carried out in a class II biological containment cabinet, up to **step 5**, Subheading 3.2. (*see* **Note 3**).

3.1.1 Amniotic Fluid (AF)

Between 10 and 20 mL of AF is normally received in a 20 mL sterile universal container.

1. Centrifuge the sample at 200 × *g* for 10 min.
2. Carefully remove the supernatant fluid using a 20 mL syringe and leave approximately 1 mL of fluid (equal to the top of the conical section of the Universal) in the container.
3. Resuspend the cell pellet in the fluid by using a plastic Pasteur pipette, and transfer approximately 100 μL (2–3 drops) to a 0.5 mL Eppendorf tube. This aliquot (approx 1/10 of the original AF sample) can be stored at 4 °C until processed. The remainder can be cultured for subsequent karyotype analysis, as required.

3.1.2 Chorionic Villus (See **Note 4**) and Tissue Samples (See **Note 5**)

1. Remove the maternal decidua from 5 to 15 mg of chorionic villi.
2. Either finely chop the cleaned villi or digest with collagenase (final concentration 2.5 mg/mL) at 37 °C for 35 min, followed by trypsin digestion (final concentration 2.5 mg/mL) at 37 °C

for 25 min. The addition of 2 mL of medium prevents further digestion.

3. Remove a single drop (approx 100 μL) of the dissociated cell slurry for QF-PCR analysis. This may be stored at 4 °C. The rest of the sample is cultured for karyotype analysis or DNA is extracted for array CGH analysis. For tissues, a small section of whole tissue sample is isolated and can be stored at 4 °C.

3.2 DNA Preparation (See Note 6)

This is a quick and simple procedure and it can be successfully applied to a number of sample types and different sample qualities (*see* **Note 7**). Because it is based on a boiling lysis protocol, aided by vigorous vortexing, the safety issues associated with phenol/chloroform extractions also are avoided. After cell lysis, the InstaGene Matrix commercial resin removes trace metal contaminants that may inhibit the PCR.

Before the DNA extraction, place the InstaGene Matrix on a magnetic stirrer and set at a medium speed for at least 5 min.

1. Pellet the cells/villus/tissue at 12,000 × *g* for 1 min in a microcentrifuge and carefully remove the liquid, leaving enough to resuspend the pellet (approx 10–20 μL). For amniotic fluid samples, any blood staining in the cell pellet is noted as a percentage of whole pellet. If >50% of the pellet is red, follow **steps 2** and **3**. For all other samples, proceed to **step 4**.
2. Vortex to resuspend the cell pellet and add 200 μL of H_2O to wash the sample (*see* **Note 8**).
3. Vortex the sample, pellet the cells, and remove the wash solution as described above. Resuspend the cells in the remaining wash solution by vortexing.
4. Add between 100 and 400 μL (*see* **Note 9**) of InstaGene Matrix to the cells/villus by using a wide-bore pipette tip, e.g., a Gilson p1000 tip and vortex.
5. Incubate at 100 °C for 8 min.
6. Vortex again at high speed for 10 s, and pellet the InstaGene Matrix at 12,000 × *g* for 3 min in a microcentrifuge.
7. Place the samples on ice to cool.
8. The DNA preparation should be stored at −20 °C (*see* **Note 10**).

3.3 PCR Setup

Batches of PCR assays can be prepared in advance, tested and stored at −20 °C. These are 20 μL aliquots of a master mix that contains all components except DNA, which is added immediately before temperature cycling, to give a total volume of 25 μL. The final concentrations of the reaction components are 1× Multiplex PCR kit and 2.5–42.5 pmol of each primer (*see* Tables 1 and 2), in a total volume of 25 μL (Note: DNA is added according to volume rather than concentration, as concentration is not measured).

1. To a thin-walled PCR tube containing 20 μL of the master mix, add 5 μL of DNA solution (*see* **Note 11**), taking care not to disturb the InstaGene Matrix pellet. Mix by pipetting.
2. Add 1 drop of mineral oil, if a heated lid is not being used, and place in the PCR machine.
3. PCR cycling conditions: Taq polymerase activation and initial denaturation at 95 °C for 15 min followed by 25 cycles of 94 °C for 30 s, 58 °C for 90 s, 71 °C for 90 s (*see* **Note 12**). Final synthesis: 72 °C for 20 min followed by storage at 10 °C (*see* **Note 13**).

3.4 Analysis

3.4.1 PCR Product Preparation

Post-PCR cleanup to remove excess primers and free dye molecules is not carried out (*see* **Note 14**). We use the Thermo Fisher Scientific ABI 3100 PRISM genetic analyzers, and conditions specific to this instrument are described. Standard use of this analyzer is not detailed here. Other genetic analyzers capable of fragment resolution, fluorescence detection, and quantification also can be used, and they include Thermo Fisher Scientific ABI capillary-based analyzer model 3130, 3730, and 3500; and Spectrum Compact CE system (Promega Corporation, Madison, WI, USA).

1. Prepare PCR products for analysis by the addition of 3 μL of product to 15 μL of HI-DI formamide in 96-well plates (*see* **Note 15**).
2. Denature at 95 °C for 2 min and snap-chill on ice.

3.4.2 3100 Analysis

Separate PCR products through a 36 cm capillary array filled with POP6 (*see* **Note 16**). A 10-sec injection time is suitable for most samples (*see* **Note 17**). The running conditions are 60 °C for 3000 s.

3.4.3 Genotyper Analysis

Macros are used to label allele peaks with marker name, size, and peak area (Fig. 1) (*see* **Note 18**). The Genotyper table is transferred to an Excel spreadsheet for allele ratio analysis.

3.5 Result Interpretation

The criteria listed below are based on >40,000 QF-PCR prenatal tests (*see* **Note 19**). For additional information, see the UK ACGS Best Practice Guidelines for the Diagnosis of Aneuploidy at (http://www.acgs.uk.com/media/765524/acc.cmgs_qfpcr_bp_jan2012_3.01.pdf).

1. Normal allele dosage ratios range between 0.8 and 1.4 (*see* **Note 20**). For alleles separated by >24 bp, ratios up to 1.5 are acceptable. Trisomy is indicated by an allele ratio of between 1.8 and 2.4 or between 0.65 and 0.45 or by the

presence of three alleles of equal areas (*see* **Note 21**). All of these results are described as informative.

2. Two informative markers per chromosome are required for confident interpretation. This minimizes the risk of misdiagnosis due to primer-site polymorphisms and/or somatic repeat instability (*see* **Note 22**). Single marker abnormal results should not be reported.
3. If both normal and abnormal marker results are obtained for a single chromosome, follow-up studies should be carried out. Such results may represent polymorphisms or a clinically significant partial chromosome imbalance (*see* Subheadings 1.2.3–1.2.5). Single marker assays, additional markers, lowering the PCR annealing temperature and analysis of cultured cell populations and parental samples can clarify these results.

4 Notes

1. To prevent sample mix-up a minimal number of tube-to-tube transfers should be used (three transfers are required for this protocol). Each sample transfer and analysis should be checked by another laboratory member, and the use of two identifiers per tube, such as sample number and name, aids sample tracking.
2. Contamination of a PCR by external DNA or PCR amplicons is evident by the appearance of allele peaks in the negative (no DNA) PCR control; a critical part of any PCR procedure and a reaction that should be set up last in a series of samples. Separation of the PCR setup and post-PCR analysis areas should help to prevent contamination.
3. To ensure that DNA is prepared from the correct sample, it is advisable to prepare the initial sample aliquot (*see* Subheadings 3.1.1 and 3.1.2) one sample at a time in a class II biological containment cabinet, with only one sample in the cabinet during the procedure. Because the subsequent DNA preparation (*see* Subheading 3.2) is carried out without further tube transfers, DNA from a number of samples can be prepared simultaneously. This DNA can then be used for subsequent PCR tests.
4. It is recommended that DNA is prepared from dissociated cells prepared from 5 to 15 mg of cleaned villi. Although only a small aliquot of this cell suspension is required, all major cell lines in both the mesoderm and cytotrophoblast should be represented and detected by QF-PCR. The analysis of whole villi has rarely been associated with discrepant results between QF-PCR and karyotype analysis due to mosaic cell lines

confined to one region of the sample [19, 20]. Analysis of cell populations that are subsequently cultured for karyotype or array CGH analysis should minimize discrepancies between the techniques.

5. The QF-PCR procedure can be applied effectively to solid tissue samples (e.g., skin and cartilage). This is particularly useful for confirming a prenatal diagnosis or for a poor-quality sample where chromosome analysis of cultured cells may not be possible.
6. DNA prepared using the protocols described here also may be used for other molecular prenatal tests. The protocol has benefits over the traditional phenol/chloroform-based approach in terms of labor and time savings and reduced safety risks. However, as the extracted DNA may contain residual contaminants, its suitability for use in other tests should be determined.
7. Although the procedure is generally successful in extracting DNA of sufficient quality for use in the multiplex, in our experience, DNA extracted from bloodstained or discolored AF fluid may contain PCR inhibitors. These inhibitors can be removed by a subsequent extraction (*see* **Note 9**).
8. Deionized water lyses red blood cells, and it also may aid lysis of cells in villus and tissue samples. A deionized water wash is used for blood-stained/discolored AF.
9. It is beneficial to adjust the volume of InstaGene Matrix to balance removal of all cell lysis products with excessive dilution of the DNA. A 300 μL volume of InstaGene Matrix is generally used for CVS and tissue samples and the larger AF cell pellets (those that cover the base of the 0.5 mL microcentrifuge tube). Only 100 μL of InstaGene Matrix is required for average and small AF pellets. It is important that the DNA extraction is not overloaded with too much starting material. This leads to a failure by the InstaGene Matrix to chelate all metal ions and can result in inhibition of the PCR. In particular, the larger sized markers in the multiplex may fail to amplify. If inhibition is observed, a further extraction can be used to remove the contaminants; 100 μL of the DNA extract is added to 100 μL of InstaGene Matrix and treated as per the extraction protocol (*see* Subheading 3.2, **steps 5–8**).
10. Because the DNA prepared here is relatively crude, and cell lysis products that damage DNA may remain, the DNA should be stored at −20 °C. However, the DNA is stable for at least 3 days at room temperature, which allows some flexibility, such as transfer of the sample to another laboratory.
11. As well as the necessary inclusion of the negative (no DNA) PCR control for the reasons given in **Note 2**, the use of a DNA control trisomic for one of the chromosomes and exhibiting

2:1 or 1:2 dosage for at least one marker is recommended. Normal allele dosage is exhibited by the other two nontrisomic chromosomes. The control not only demonstrates that the amplified DNA represents allele copy number for that procedure but also can be used as a standard against which any spurious background bands or free-dye peaks can be compared.

12. Samples that do not generate sufficient amplified sequences for analysis, due to low initial DNA concentration (usually evident by a very small original cell pellet) can be amplified with a greater number of cycles. Any change in PCR cycling conditions should always be accompanied by a trisomy control, to ensure the reaction is still quantitative.

13. The 20-min incubation at 72 °C is necessary, because Taq polymerases lacking exonuclease activity add a template-independent dATP to the 3′ end of amplified sequences [26]. Without the 72 °C incubation, a single base-pair size difference in the amplified sequences can resolve as a "split peak" on the profile and hinder analysis. This is a particular problem here due to the size of the fragments generated (100–500 bp). In this size range, the analysis systems efficiently resolve single base-pair differences especially in smaller alleles.

14. Free-dye peaks are caused by the detachment of the fluorescent molecule from the labeled primer. These molecules are resolved as broad peaks, usually up to 180 bp (*see* **Note 16**); as such, they can be distinguished from allele peaks. The breakdown of fluorescent primers can be minimized by the use of deionized formamide stored at −20 °C and reduced exposure of labeled primers to temperatures above −20 °C. Free-dye molecules can be removed, along with unincorporated primers, by standard post-PCR cleanup protocols if required.

15. Accurate transfer of samples to the wells of a 96-well plate can be difficult. The risk of error can be minimized not only by the use of a multichannel pipette but also by the addition of loading buffer containing dextran blue, which is visible but does not interfere with the fluorescent analysis. Transparent piercable sheets also are available (ABGene) that can be sealed onto the plate, or rubber septa can be placed over wells that are not in use.

16. The POP6 polymer can be used on the 3100 genetic analyzer if greater resolution is required, although this requires longer run times. Resolution of free-dye molecules (*see* **Note 14**) is not linear in respect to fragment size, but it is influenced by both temperature and the separating matrix. A different polymer may be used to resolve free-dye molecules that coincide with allele peaks.

17. Allele peak heights >6000 fluorescent units on the 3100 genetic analyzer are not analyzed. The charge-coupled device camera becomes saturated in this range, and peak fluorescence may be underrepresented. If a sample is overloaded, injection times can be reduced to accommodate differences in DNA concentration and the corresponding amplification. This is one of the advantages of the capillary-based genetic analyzers, where a repeat injection does not require repeat sample preparation.
18. Tetranucleotide alleles demonstrate few visible stutter bands (*see* Subheading 1.2), and only the main allele peak is labeled. However, some microsatellite markers contain a mix of both tetranucleotide and dinucleotide repeats and generate significant stutter bands. For dinucleotide alleles, the larger alleles generally exhibit more significant stutter effects than smaller alleles, due to the longer repeat. It is therefore necessary to recognize and label at least the first stutter peak and include it in the allele peak area measurement.
19. Although there are now several published studies describing the use of QF-PCR as a diagnostic test [5–14], it is important to validate the QF-PCR strategy in the laboratory in which it is to be used. Control samples are required, and a pilot study is recommended before the implementation of a QF-PCR-based aneuploidy diagnostic service, especially if primer sets are used that are not described in the published literature.
20. The large normal range is necessary due to the use of tetranucleotide repeats. These can result in widely spaced alleles (up to 50 bp apart), and marked preferential amplification of the smaller allele, which in turn results in skewed allele dosage ratios. However, closely spaced alleles should exhibit less allele specific preferential amplification and would be expected to have dosage ratios closer to 1.0.
21. As more than one sample is usually processed, the sample identity of abnormal results should be confirmed. This can be done by a repeat QF-PCR test. Alternatively, genotype analysis of a maternal blood sample by using the same markers can be used to confirm sample identification.
22. Polymorphisms in the primer-binding site can result in partial or complete amplification failure of an allele (*see* Subheading 1.2.4). This can result in a misdiagnosis if the result is used in isolation. In addition, SMMs (*see* Subheading 1.2.5) [25] and submicroscopic imbalance (*see* Subheading 1.2.3) [6] also could result in misdiagnosis if a single marker was used independently.

References

1. Lewin P, Kleinfinger P, Bazin A et al (2000) Defining the efficiency of fluorescence in situ hybridization on uncultured amniocytes on a retrospective cohort of 27407 prenatal diagnoses. Prenat Diagn 20(1):1–6
2. Waters JJ, Waters KS (1999) Trends in cytogenetic prenatal diagnosis in the UK: results from UKNEQAS external audit, 1987–1998. Prenat Diagn 19(11):1023–1026
3. Klinger K, Landes G, Shook D et al (1992) Rapid detection of chromosome aneuploidies in uncultured amniocytes by using fluorescence in situ hybridization (FISH). Am J Hum Genet 51(1):55–65
4. Spathas DH, Divane A, Maniatis GM et al (1994) Prenatal detection of trisomy 21 in uncultured amniocytes by fluorescence in situ hybridization: a prospective study. Prenat Diagn 14(11):1049–1054
5. Cirigliano V, Voglino G, Ordonez E et al (2009) Rapid prenatal diagnosis of common chromosome aneuploidies by QF-PCR, results of 9 years of clinical experience. Prenat Diagn 29(1):40–49. https://doi.org/10.1002/pd.2192
6. Hills A, Donaghue C, Waters J et al (2010) QF-PCR as a stand-alone test for prenatal samples: the first 2 years' experience in the London region. Prenat Diagn 30(6):509–517. https://doi.org/10.1002/pd.2503
7. Levett LJ, Liddle S, Meredith R (2001) A large-scale evaluation of amnio-PCR for the rapid prenatal diagnosis of fetal trisomy. Ultrasound Obstet Gynecol 17(2):115–118. https://doi.org/10.1046/j.1469-0705.2001.00340.x
8. Mann K, Fox SP, Abbs SJ et al (2001) Development and implementation of a new rapid aneuploidy diagnostic service within the UK National Health Service and implications for the future of prenatal diagnosis. Lancet 358 (9287):1057–1061. https://doi.org/10.1016/S0140-6736(01)06183-9
9. Mann K, Hills A, Donaghue C et al (2012) Quantitative fluorescence PCR analysis of >40,000 prenatal samples for the rapid diagnosis of trisomies 13, 18 and 21 and monosomy X. Prenat Diagn 32(12):1197–1204. https://doi.org/10.1002/pd.3986
10. Pertl B, Kopp S, Kroisel PM et al (1997) Quantitative fluorescence polymerase chain reaction for the rapid prenatal detection of common aneuploidies and fetal sex. Am J Obstet Gynecol 177(4):899–906
11. Pertl B, Kopp S, Kroisel PM et al (1999) Rapid detection of chromosome aneuploidies by quantitative fluorescence PCR: first application on 247 chorionic villus samples. J Med Genet 36(4):300–303
12. Pertl B, Yau SC, Sherlock J et al (1994) Rapid molecular method for prenatal detection of Down's syndrome. Lancet 343 (8907):1197–1198
13. Schmidt W, Jenderny J, Hecher K et al (2000) Detection of aneuploidy in chromosomes X, Y, 13, 18 and 21 by QF-PCR in 662 selected pregnancies at risk. Mol Hum Reprod 6 (9):855–860
14. Verma L, Macdonald F, Leedham P et al (1998) Rapid and simple prenatal DNA diagnosis of Down's syndrome. Lancet 352 (9121):9–12. https://doi.org/10.1016/S0140-6736(97)11090-X
15. Lubin MB, Elashoff JD, Wang SJ et al (1991) Precise gene dosage determination by polymerase chain reaction: theory, methodology, and statistical approach. Mol Cell Probes 5 (4):307–317
16. Donaghue C, Roberts A, Mann K et al (2003) Development and targeted application of a rapid QF-PCR test for sex chromosome imbalance. Prenat Diagn 23(3):201–210. https://doi.org/10.1002/pd.569
17. Stojilkovic-Mikic T, Mann K, Docherty Z et al (2005) Maternal cell contamination of prenatal samples assessed by QF-PCR genotyping. Prenat Diagn 25(1):79–83. https://doi.org/10.1002/pd.1089
18. Donaghue C, Mann K, Docherty Z et al (2005) Detection of mosaicism for primary trisomies in prenatal samples by QF-PCR and karyotype analysis. Prenat Diagn 25(1):65–72. https://doi.org/10.1002/pd.1086
19. Waters JJ, Mann K, Grimsley L et al (2007) Complete discrepancy between QF-PCR analysis of uncultured villi and karyotyping of cultured cells in the prenatal diagnosis of trisomy 21 in three CVS. Prenat Diagn 27 (4):332–339. https://doi.org/10.1002/pd.1675
20. Waters JJ, Walsh S, Levett LJ et al (2006) Complete discrepancy between abnormal fetal karyotypes predicted by QF-PCR rapid testing and karyotyped cultured cells in a first-trimester CVS. Prenat Diagn 26 (10):892–897. https://doi.org/10.1002/pd.1519
21. Gardner RJM, Sutherland GR (1996) Chromosome abnormalities and genetic counseling.

Oxford monographs on medical genetics No. 29, 2nd edn. Oxford University Press, New York

22. Mann K, Kabba M, Donaghue C et al (2007) Analysis of a chromosomally mosaic placenta to assess the cell populations in dissociated chorionic villi: implications for QF-PCR aneuploidy testing. Prenat Diagn 27(3):287–289. https://doi.org/10.1002/pd.1663
23. Sharp AJ, Locke DP, McGrath SD et al (2005) Segmental duplications and copy-number variation in the human genome. Am J Hum Genet 77(1):78–88. https://doi.org/10.1086/431652
24. Andrew SE, Whiteside D, Buzin C et al (2002) An intronic polymorphism of the hMLH1 gene contributes toward incomplete genetic testing for HNPCC. Genet Test 6(4):319–322. https://doi.org/10.1089/10906570260471868
25. Mann K, Donaghue C, Ogilvie CM (2003) In vivo somatic microsatellite mutations identified in non-malignant human tissue. Hum Genet 114(1):110–114. https://doi.org/10.1007/s00439-003-1032-3
26. Clark JM (1988) Novel non-templated nucleotide addition reactions catalyzed by procaryotic and eucaryotic DNA polymerases. Nucleic Acids Res 16(20):9677–9686

Chapter 11

Multiplex Ligation-Dependent Probe Amplification (MLPA) for Prenatal Diagnosis of Common Aneuploidies

Jan Schouten, Paul van Vught, and Robert-Jan Galjaard

Abstract

Multiplex Ligation-dependent Probe Amplification (MLPA) is a method to determine the copy number of up to 60 genomic DNA sequences in a single multiplex PCR based reaction.

MLPA probes consist of two oligonucleotides that can hybridize next to each other on a certain DNA sequence of interest, where they are ligated. All ligated probes are subsequently amplified by PCR using a single set of primers. Each amplified MLPA probe has a unique length and can be visualized and quantified by capillary electrophoresis. As the primers are almost 100% consumed in the PCR reaction, the quantity of each PCR amplicon is proportional to the number of copies of each probe target sequence in the DNA sample. A trisomy 21 can therefore be detected by an approximately 50% increased signal of each chromosome 21 specific probe relative to reference samples.

MLPA with the P095 Aneuploidy probemix for chromosomes 13, 18, 21, X and Y has been used as a rapid detection method on large numbers of samples from uncultured amniotic fluid or from chorionic villi. As compared to FISH and karyotyping, MLPA is more rapid, has a higher throughput, and is less expensive. MLPA however cannot detect low grade mosaicism, female triploidies, and copy number neutral chromosome abnormalities such as inversions and translocations.

Key words Aneuploidy, Multiplex ligation-dependent probe amplification (MLPA), Trisomy, Multiplex polymerase chain reaction (PCR), Amniotic fluid, Chorionic villi, Gene dosage

1 Introduction

Multiplex Ligation-dependent Probe Amplification (MLPA) is a multiplex method to detect abnormal copy numbers of up to 60 different genomic DNA sequences [1]. MLPA reactions are easy to perform, require little hands-on time and results can be obtained within 24 h. Furthermore, it requires only standard equipment that is present in most DNA diagnostic laboratories.

In contrast to normal multiplex PCR, in MLPA not the sample DNA is amplified, but the probes that are hybridized to the target DNA (Fig. 1). Each single probe initially consists of two oligonucleotides (left probe oligo [LPO] and right probe oligo [RPO]), which are designed to hybridize immediate adjacent to each other

Brynn Levy (ed.), *Prenatal Diagnosis*, Methods in Molecular Biology, vol. 1885, https://doi.org/10.1007/978-1-4939-8889-1_11,

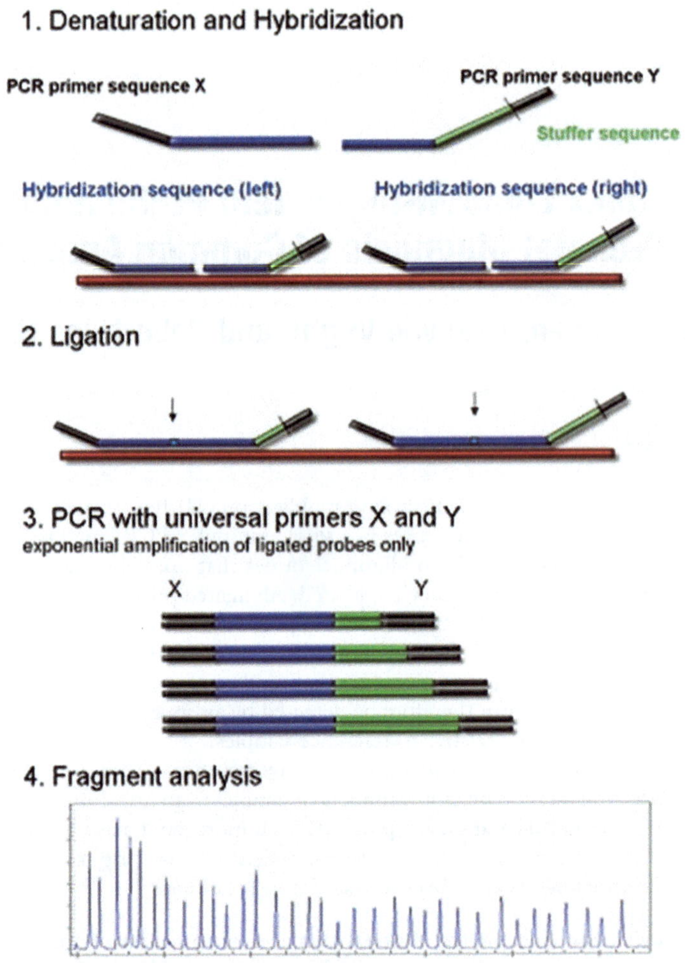

Fig. 1 Outline of the MLPA technique. After hybridization to their target sequence in the sample DNA, the probe oligonucleotides are enzymatically ligated. One probe oligonucleotide contains a non-hybridizing stuffer sequence of variable length. Ligation products can be amplified using PCR primer sequences X and Y, amplification product of each probe has a unique length (90–500 nt). Amplification products are separated by capillary electrophoresis. Relative amounts of probe amplification products, as compared to a reference DNA sample, reflect the relative copy number of target sequences. Adapted from www.mlpa.com

on the target DNA. After hybridization, the two oligonucleotides can be ligated by a specific ligase enzyme, thereby creating a single molecule, but only when both probe oligonucleotides are perfectly hybridized to adjacent sites of the sample DNA. The ends of this probe molecule contain two sequences recognized by a PCR primer pair. After ligation, all probes are amplified by a single PCR primer pair, of which one is fluorescently labeled. Since all probes have a unique length, the resulting MLPA amplified products have a size that ranges from 90 to up to 500 nucleotides, and can be visualized by capillary electrophoresis.

MLPA probes that do not find a target sequence cannot be amplified by PCR, and do not have to be removed. The protocol for an MLPA reaction is therefore very simple (Fig. 1):

1. Denature 20–500 ng DNA by heating to 98 °C in a thermocycler, followed by addition of the MLPA probes and buffer. Leave overnight at 60 °C for hybridization.
2. Add the Ligase and ligase buffers and ligate at 54 °C for 15 min.
3. Inactivate the Ligase by heating to 98 °C. Add PCR primers, dNTPs and polymerase and start the PCR.
4. Analyze the products by capillary electrophoresis.

In MLPA, it is important that all fragments are amplified with the use of only one pair of PCR primers that is present in limited amounts. This abolishes differences in PCR efficiencies, which is normally observed in multiplex PCRs, as well as the difference in DNA input among multiple reactions. As a result, the relative signal strength of each amplification product is determined primarily by the copy number of the target sequence in a DNA sample. By comparing these probe signals with those obtained from reference samples, a decrease or increase in signal intensity can be observed, reflecting a deletion or duplication, respectively (Fig. 2).

The MLPA technique allows discrimination of sequences that differ only in a single nucleotide. MLPA can therefore also be used for the detection of known mutations. A variation on the MLPA technique can be used to determine the methylation status of DNA sequences [2]. MLPA products for more than 400 different

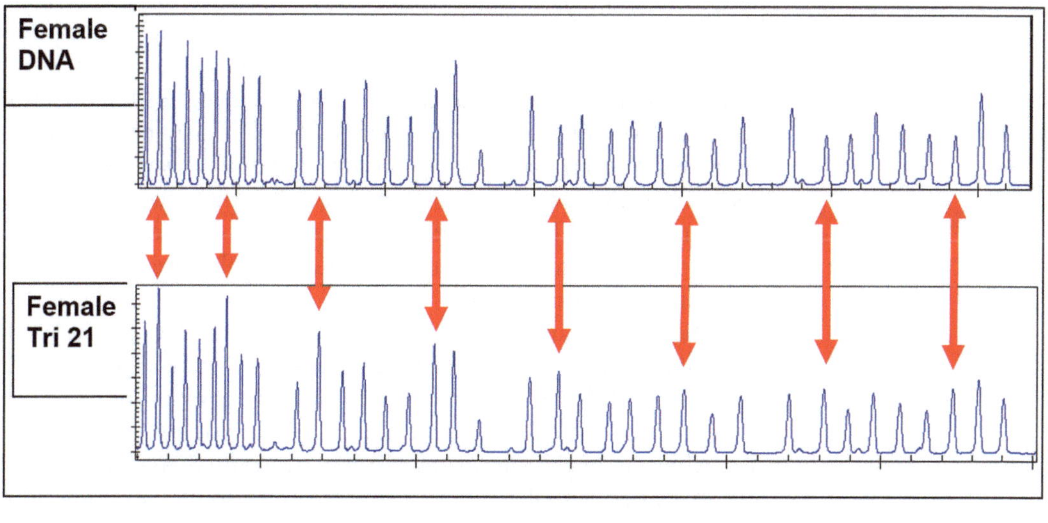

Fig. 2 Detection of trisomy 21 with MLPA. Arrows indicate alterations. An increase of the signal from the chromosome 21 specific probes is seen

applications are commercially available from the MRC-Holland company (www.mlpa.com).These include MLPA probemixes for the detection of:

1. Aneuploidy of chromosomes 13, 18, 21, X, and Y (P095 probemix).
2. Deletions or duplications of specific chromosomal areas, e.g., the P250 probemix for the 22q11 region involved in DiGeorge syndrome.
3. Copy number changes of all 41 unique subtelomeric regions (P036 and P070 probemixes), all centromeric regions (P181, P182 probemix) or 23 different microdeletion syndromes, in a single reaction (P245 probemix).
4. Deletions or duplications involving only one or more exons of a gene (e.g., DMD, BRCA1 or BRCA2). Small chromosomal rearrangements can be detected as the sequences analyzed by MLPA probes are only 60 nucleotides in length. Probemixes for more than 100 different genes are available.

For aneuploidy testing on capillary electrophoresis systems, the SALSA P095 probe mix is available. This probemix contains eight independent probes for each of the chromosomes 13, 18, 21 and X, as well as four Y-specific probes, and is used as a rapid test for aneuploidies of these chromosomes. Extensive tests, several of which included more than 4000 samples, indicated a diagnostic accuracy of MLPA for the detection of common trisomies that is statistically similar (non-inferior) to that of karyotyping or FISH [3–10].

MLPA is not able to detect all chromosomal abnormalities seen with karyotyping. It is designed for detection of specific copy number changes of chromosomes 13, 18, 21 and the sex chromosomes. MLPA analysis is expected to detect high level of chromosomal mosaicism since it will give the average copy number per cell. The P095 probemix is able to detect male triploidies but will not detect cases of 69,XXX [3–6]. Cases of 69,XXY may be difficult to discriminate from maternal DNA contamination as was shown for a case of 69,XXY which was assigned as a sample contaminated by maternal DNA [4]. However we have correctly diagnosed two cases [6]. It should be noted, though, that many triploidies result in fetal ultrasound abnormalities.

The MLPA aneuploidy kit is not designed for detection of balanced chromosomal rearrangements like translocations and inversions. MLPA however provides several opportunities that are not possible with other techniques such as karyotyping. For example, when a quick diagnostic result is warranted in case of fetal abnormalities visualized by advanced ultrasound examination, amniotic fluid samples can first be rapidly tested for the copy number of the most common occurring aneuploidies. If normal, further selective testing based on clinical preselection could be done for using MLPA probemixes for all subtelomeric regions and the most common microdeletion syndromes.

2 Materials

2.1 Contents of SALSA MLPA Probemix and Reagents

1. SALSA Probemix: Mixture of up to 60 pairs of probe oligonucleotides.
2. SALSA MLPA buffer: Contains 1.5 M salt + additives. Does not always freeze at −20 °C.
3. Ligase-65 enzyme solution. Does not freeze at −20 °C.
4. Ligase-65 Buffer A: Contains cofactor NAD required for the Ligase-65 enzyme.
5. Ligase-65 Buffer B: Contains the salts required by the Ligase-65 enzyme.
6. SALSA PCR Primer mix: Contains one fluorescently labeled and one unlabeled PCR primer + dNTPs.
7. SALSA Polymerase enzyme solution. Does not freeze at −20 °C.

SALSA MLPA kits are stable for at least 1 year when stored in the dark at −20 °C.

All enzymes, nucleic acids, and buffer constituents are non-hazardous.

In addition to standard lab equipment, such as pipettors and water, a thermocycler with heated lid and capillary electrophoresis instrument is required.

2.2 DNA Extraction from Amniotic Fluid

1. PBS .
2. QIAamp DNA Mini Kit (QIAGEN, Hilden, Germany).

2.3 Separation and Quantification of the MLPA Amplification Products by Capillary Electrophoresis Using the Beckman CEQ Apparatus

1. Beckman D1-labeled 60–600 size standard (Beckman Coulter, Brea, CA, USA).
2. Deionized formamide.

3 Methods

3.1 Amniotic Fluid Sample Preparation Protocol: DNA-Isolation

1. Mix the amniotic fluid gently, just before a sample is removed. Most cells might be at the bottom of the tube.
2. Centrifuge a 2 mL sample of amniotic fluid for 5 min at 10,000 × *g*. Remove the supernatant carefully. Wash the pellet

with 1 mL of PBS and centrifuge for 5 min at 10,000 × *g*. Remove the supernatant carefully and resuspend the pellet in 200 μL of PBS. DNA-isolation is done according to the Qiagen Blood and Body Fluid Spin Protocol. DNA is eluted with 50 μL buffer AE instead of 200 μL to increase the DNA concentration. Transfer 5 μL DNA to a 0.2 mL vial tube for the MLPA reaction. Store the remainder at −20 °C.

3.2 DNA Denaturation and Hybridization of the SALSA Probes

1. Heat 5 μL DNA-sample (20–500 ng DNA) (*see* **Notes 1** and **2**) for 5 min at 98 °C in a 0.2 mL vial in a thermocycler with heated (105 °C) lid.
2. Cool to 25 °C before opening the thermocycler.
3. Prepare a mixture of equal volumes SALSA Probemix and MLPA buffer at room temperature. Mix well.
4. Add 3 μL of this mixture to each sample. Mix with care by repeated pipetting.
5. Incubate for 1 min at 95 °C, followed by a 16 h incubation (*see* **Note 3**) at 60 °C (*see* **Note 4**).

3.3 Ligation Reaction

1. Prepare a Ligation master mix containing 3 μL Ligase-65 buffer A, 3 μL Ligase-65 buffer B, 25 μL water, and 1 μL Ligase-65 enzyme for each reaction (*see* **Note 5**). Mix well by repeated pipetting.
2. Reduce the temperature of the thermocycler to 54 °C.
3. Add 32 μL Ligase master mix to the MLPA reaction, while the samples are in the thermocycler, and mix by repeated pipetting.
4. Incubate for 15 min at 54 °C, than heat 5 min at 98 °C for Ligase inactivation. Remove vials from the thermocycler.

3.4 PCR

1. Prepare a Polymerase master mix for each reaction containing 2 μL of SALSA PCR-primer mix, 7.5 μL of water, and 0.5 μL of SALSA Polymerase. Mix well but do not vortex. Store on ice until used (*see* **Note 5**).
2. While the vials are at room temperature, add 10 μL of Polymerase master mix to each vial. Mix by pipetting up and down, place the vials in the thermocycler, and start the PCR reaction (*see* **Note 6**).

3.4.1 PCR Conditions

- 30 s 95 °C.
- 30 s 60 °C.
- 60 s 72 °C; 35 cycles.

End with 20 min incubation at 72 °C (*see* **Note 7**).

3.5 Separation and Quantification of the MLPA Amplification Products by Capillary Electrophoresis

The amount of the MLPA PCR reaction required for analysis by capillary electrophoresis depends on the apparatus and fluorescent label used. As an example, conditions for the Beckman CEQ apparatus are shown:

1. Following the PCR reaction, mix 0.7 μL of the PCR reaction, 0.2 μL of the Beckman D1-labeled 60–600 size standard, 32 μl deionized formamide.
   - Settings: Capillary temperature 50 °C. Denaturation 90 °C for 120 s. Injection time: 1.6 KV for 30 s. Runtime: 60 min at 4.8 KV. Analysis settings: Include peaks >3%; Size standard-600. Slope threshold 1.

3.6 Thermocycler Program for the Complete MLPA Reaction

- 5 min 98 °C; 25 °C pause.
- 1 min 95 °C; 60 °C pause.
- 54 °C pause; 15 min 54 °C.
- 5 min 98 °C; 20 °C pause.
- 30 s 95 °C; 30 s 60 °C; 60 s 72 °C, 35 cycles.
- 20 min 72 °C; 15 °C pause.

N.B. Heated lid is at 105 °C during all steps.

3.7 Data Analysis

For data analysis of an MLPA experiment, Coffalyser.Net software with the appropriate lot specific MLPA product sheet must be used and is available free of charge on MRC-Holland's website. Although Coffalyser.Net uses a more sophisticated algorithm, this section describes the basic principles.

Analysis of MLPA data consists of roughly three different parts:

First, Coffalyser.Net starts with raw data analysis (baseline correction, peak identification) and extensive quality control (e.g., DNA quantity used; complete DNA denaturation, degree of sloping).

Next, MLPA data is normalized and peak signals are translated to probe ratios. The absolute fluorescence measured by capillary electrophoresis cannot be used directly for copy number calculations as it is affected by many variables. First, each probe's measured fluorescence must be normalized within each sample to get meaningful data (intra-sample normalization).

In the third step, the relative probe signals are then used in the inter-sample normalization; final probe ratios are determined by comparing the relative probe peak in the DNA sample of interest to all reference samples. Reference DNA samples are expected to have a normal copy number for both the reference and target probes.

This final probe ratio is also called Dosage Quotient (DQ). Coffalyser.Net calculates the DQ for each probe in each sample.

The MLPA peak pattern of a DNA sample without genomic abnormalities will be identical to that of reference samples: final

Table 1
P095 Dosage Quotients expected in aneuploidy and normal cases when using 46, XY as reference samples. Note that the P095 MLPA probemix cannot make distinction between 69, XXX and 46, XX samples (*)

Sample type	chr. 13 probes	chr. 18 probes	chr. 21 probes	chr. X probes	chr. Y probes
46, XY	1	1	1	1	1
46, XX *	1	1	1	2	0
47, XY,+13	1.5	1	1	1	1
47, XY,+18	1	1.5	1	1	1
47, XY,+21	1	1	1.5	1	1
45, X0	1	1	1	1	0
47, XXX	1	1	1	3	0
47, XXY	1	1	1	2	1
47, XYY	1	1	1	1	2
69, XXX *	1	1	1	2	0
69, XXY	1	1	1	1.33	0.67
69, XYY	1	1	1	0.67	1.33

probe ratios will be ~1.0, reflecting 2 copies for autosomal regions. For heterozygous deletions, probe ratios of ~0.5 are expected, while heterozygous duplications will have a DQ-value of ~1.5. Probes should be arranged based on chromosomal location for correct interpretation; this will also aid in detecting subtle changes such as mosaicism.

3.8 Interpretation of Results

Once the correct DQ values of each probe are established, the relative copy number of each sample can be determined. In theory, all probes located on a certain chromosome should give approximately the same DQ-value, also in cases of aneuploidy (Table 1). In practice, however, certain variables such as SNPs, sample impurities etc., can affect the DQ-value obtained for a certain probe. Also, partial chromosome gains or losses may occur.

Based on Van Opstal and colleagues [6], the following rules are recommended for determination of copy number status in aneuploidy cases:

1. When the DQ-values of at least 4 of the 8 probes for a certain chromosome are equal to or higher than 1.30, and the values for the remaining four probes are close to 1.30, a trisomy for that chromosome should be considered.

2. A monosomy X should be considered if the relative probe signals of probes on the X chromosome are within the normal ranges of those for normal males, and Y signals are absent.
3. A 47, XXY should be considered if the relative probe signals of probes on the Y chromosome are within the normal ranges of those for normal males, and those of the chromosome X probes are within the normal range for normal females.
4. A 47, XYY should be considered if the relative probe signals of probes on the Y chromosome are ~1.8 times those for normal males, and those of the chromosome X probes are within the normal range for normal males.
5. A 47, XXX should be considered if the relative probe signals of probes on the X chromosome are ~2.5 times those for normal males, and Y signals are absent.
6. We recommend follow-up study of samples in which several probes for a certain chromosome are marked as having a statistically abnormal probe value by Coffalyser.Net analysis. The use of a 1.30 cut-off value to distinguish a normal from a trisomy result does not allow detection of mosaic samples. As an example, all chromosome 21 specific probes may have a ratio between 1.10 and 1.20 in a mosaic sample with 30% trisomy 21 cells. Coffalyser.Net analysis may identify such mosaic samples when the experiment was performed well.

4 Notes

1. If necessary, dilute DNA with TE (10 mM Tris–HCl pH 8.0; 0.1 mM EDTA).
2. The volume of the reaction is important for the hybridization speed, which is probe and salt concentration-dependent. Do not use more than 5 μL sample DNA.
3. Minimum recommended hybridization period 14 h. Maximum 20 h.
4. Evaporation may occur during (A) overnight hybridization or (B) pipetting the ligation reaction at 54 °C. In case you suspect evaporation problems, the following may help: (A): Test evaporation by incubating 8 μL H_2O overnight at 60 °C; >5 μL H_2O should remain, or (B): Reduce handling time by using multi-channel pipettes. To reduce evaporation: (1) ensure heated lid works well; (2) increase/decrease pressure of lid on tubes; (3) try different tubes (e.g., Thermo Fischer ABgene AB-0773, AB-0451); (4) use mineral oil (Vapor-lock, Qiagen 981611): add small drop of oil to DNA sample, just enough to cover it. There is no need to remove oil. After addition of MLPA buffer-probemix mixture or polymerase mix, centrifuge

very briefly. After addition of ligase mix, gently pipet up and down.

5. Ligase and polymerase master mixes can be stored at 4 °C for at least 1 h.
6. Never use micro-pipettes for performing MLPA reactions that have been used for handling MLPA PCR products! Following PCR, the tubes should not be opened in the vicinity of the thermocycler.
7. PCR products can be stored in the dark at 4 °C for at least 4 days.
8. An extensive trouble shooting section is present on the www.mlpa.com website.

References

1. Schouten JP, McElgunn CJ, Waaijer R et al (2002) Relative quantification of 40 nucleic acid sequences by multiplex ligation-dependent probe amplification. Nucleic Acids Res 30(12):e57
2. Nygren AO, Ameziane N, Duarte HM et al (2005) Methylation-specific MLPA (MS-MLPA): simultaneous detection of CpG methylation and copy number changes of up to 40 sequences. Nucleic Acids Res 33(14):e128. https://doi.org/10.1093/nar/gni127
3. Slater HR, Bruno DL, Ren H et al (2003) Rapid, high throughput prenatal detection of aneuploidy using a novel quantitative method (MLPA). J Med Genet 40(12):907–912
4. Gerdes T, Kirchhoff M, Lind AM et al (2005) Computer-assisted prenatal aneuploidy screening for chromosome 13, 18, 21, X and Y based on multiplex ligation-dependent probe amplification (MLPA). Eur J Hum Genet 13 (2):171–175. https://doi.org/10.1038/sj.ejhg.5201307
5. Hochstenbach R, Meijer J, van de Brug J et al (2005) Rapid detection of chromosomal aneuploidies in uncultured amniocytes by multiplex ligation-dependent probe amplification (MLPA). Prenat Diagn 25(11):1032–1039. https://doi.org/10.1002/pd.1247
6. Van Opstal D, Boter M, de Jong D et al (2009) Rapid aneuploidy detection with multiplex ligation-dependent probe amplification: a prospective study of 4000 amniotic fluid samples. Eur J Hum Genet 17(1):112–121. https://doi.org/10.1038/ejhg.2008.161
7. Gerdes T, Kirchhoff M, Lind AM et al (2008) Multiplex ligation-dependent probe amplification (MLPA) in prenatal diagnosis-experience of a large series of rapid testing for aneuploidy of chromosomes 13, 18, 21, X, and Y. Prenat Diagn 28(12):1119–1125. https://doi.org/10.1002/pd.2137
8. Kooper AJ, Faas BH, Kater-Baats E et al (2008) Multiplex ligation-dependent probe amplification (MLPA) as a stand-alone test for rapid aneuploidy detection in amniotic fluid cells. Prenat Diagn 28(11):1004–1010. https://doi.org/10.1002/pd.2111
9. Kooper AJ, Faas BH, Feuth T et al (2009) Detection of chromosome aneuploidies in chorionic villus samples by multiplex ligation-dependent probe amplification. J Mol Diagn 11(1):17–24. https://doi.org/10.2353/jmoldx.2009.070140
10. Boormans EM, Birnie E, Oepkes D et al (2010) Comparison of multiplex ligation-dependent probe amplification and karyotyping in prenatal diagnosis. Obstet Gynecol 115 (2 Pt 1):297–303. https://doi.org/10.1097/AOG.0b013e3181cbc652

Chapter 12

Chromosomal Microarray Analysis Using Array Comparative Genomic Hybridization on DNA from Amniotic Fluid and Chorionic Villus Sampling

Ankita Patel

Abstract

Chromosomal Microarray analysis offers an objective high resolution view of copy number changes in the genome that contribute to genomic disorders in various clinical setting such as postnatal, prenatal, and oncology. Here, we describe a fast and reliable method of using chromosomal microarray analysis in detection of genomic imbalances that may be associated with congenital malformations in a prenatal setting. Results can be obtained in 4–5 days using direct amniotic fluid (AF) or chorionic villus samples (CVS).

Key words Array CGH, Microarray, Prenatal diagnosis, Comparative genomic hybridization

1 Introduction

Comparative genomic hybridization (CGH) was initially developed for analysis of tumors with complex chromosomal imbalances and low mitotic index [1]. Differentially labeled tumor and normal DNA were applied to normal metaphase chromosomes and therefore the resolution of the analysis was still dependent on chromosome length. Crucial advancement in CGH technology came with the replacement of normal metaphase chromosomes with arrays of BAC or PAC (Bacterial or P1 artificial chromosome) clones immobilized on glass slides for hybridization targets and later oligonucleotide probes. This enabled the detection of copy number changes throughout the genome at a higher resolution and therefore, provided a basis for high throughput analysis of genomic imbalances for clinical diagnostics [2–6]. Clinical implementation of **Chromosomal Microarray Analysis (CMA)** using BAC-based comparative genomic hybridization was initially for the purpose of diagnosing genomic imbalances primarily in individuals with development delay, multiple congenital anomalies, and neuropsychiatric

Brynn Levy (ed.), *Prenatal Diagnosis*, Methods in Molecular Biology, vol. 1885, https://doi.org/10.1007/978-1-4939-8889-1_12,

disorders. The CMA arrays includes probes for virtually all known microdeletion/duplication syndromes, pericentromeric and subtelomeric regions, as well as probes for some single gene disorders that may occur due to gain or loss of large DNA segments. Probes distributed randomly along all chromosome arms are also included to identify any full trisomies. Therefore, with a single test, CMA will detect almost all of the disorders detected by standard multiple FISH tests and provides a major advance in the diagnosis of patients in which a genetic cause of disability is strongly suspected but not observed by traditional cytogenetic analysis. In an extensive review of 33 studies including 22,698 patients overall, the International Standard Cytogenomic Array Consortium found that CMA offered a diagnostic yield of 15–20% as compared to 3% for G-banded chromosome analysis in patients with intellectual disability or congenital anomalies [7]. Consequently, CMA is now recommended by the American College of Medical Genetics as the first tier genetic test for the evaluation of individuals with multiple anomalies and nonsyndromic developmental delay/intellectual disability [8]. CMA was then applied to prenatal studies and a large prospective NIHD study was initiated which showed the advantage of CMA over karyotyping for detection of submicroscopic microdeletion and microduplication syndromes [9]. In this chapter, we describe the methods for extracting DNA from amniotic fluid and CVS samples for microarray analysis on oligonucleotide arrays manufactured by Agilent Technologies. Included are methods of whole genome amplification for when the DNA yield is low especially from lower gestation samples.

2 Materials

2.1 DNA Extraction of Direct Amniotic Fluid (AF) and CVS Samples

1. Phosphate Buffered Saline, 1×.
2. Qiagen DNA extraction kit (Midi) (Qiagen, Germantown, MD, USA).
3. Isopropanol (Molecular Grade, 99.5%).
4. Ethanol (Molecular Grade, 99.5%).
5. DNA Clean Concentrator ™-5 (Zymo Research, Irvine, CA, USA).

2.2 Genomic DNA Concentration and Integrity

1. NanoDrop (NanoDrop Technologies, Wilmington, DE, USA).
2. Water (Molecular Grade).

2.3 Sample Digestion for Hybridization (Optional Is Using Agilent SNP Arrays)

1. RsaI (10.0 U/μl) (Promega, Madison, WI, USA).
2. AluI (10.0 U/μl) (Promega, Madison, WI, USA).

2.4 Sample Labeling

1. SureTag complete DNA labeling kit (Agilent Technologies, Santa Clara, CA, USA).
2. Human Cot-1 DNA (1.0 mg/ml) (Promega, Madison, WI, USA).

2.5 Hybridization of Patient Samples

1. Human Cot-1 DNA (1.0 mg/ml) (Promega, Madison, WI, USA).
2. 10× Blocking Agent (Agilent Technologies, Santa Clara, CA, USA).
3. 2× Hybridization Buffer (Agilent Technologies, Santa Clara, CA, USA).
4. SureHyb Chambers (Agilent Technologies, Santa Clara, CA, USA).
5. CustomHD-CGH Microarray (Agilent Technologies, Santa Clara, CA, USA).
6. Hybridization Chamber gasket slides (Agilent Technologies, Santa Clara, CA, USA).

2.6 Array Washing

1. Distilled, deionized water (Millipore Sigma, Burlington, MA, USA).
2. 100% Acetonitrile.
3. Agilent Oligo aCGH/ChIP-on-Chip Wash Buffer 2 (Agilent Technologies, Santa Clara, CA, USA).
4. Agilent Oligo aCGH/ChIP-on-Chip Wash Buffer 1 (Agilent Technologies, Santa Clara, CA, USA).

2.7 Scan Slides

1. Agilent Laser Scanner (Agilent Technologies, Santa Clara, CA, USA).
2. Agilent Feature Extraction Software (Agilent Technologies, Santa Clara, CA, USA).

3 Methods

3.1 DNA Extraction from Direct Amniotic Fluid

1. Preparing the starting material.
2. Spin 3–10 cc amniotic fluid in a 15.0 ml tube in the Eppendorf 5810 (swinging bucket table top), centrifuge at 3500 rpm (2465 × *g*) for 15 min at room temperature.
3. Remove the supernatant with a sterile transfer pipet, leaving the cell pellet with approximately 50.0 μl of media.

4. Tap the tube to resuspend the pellet in the remaining media. Ensure that the pellet is completely resuspended with no visible clumps.
5. Add 500.0 μl 1× Phosphate Buffered Saline (PBS) to the cells in the 15.0 ml tube with micropipettor taking care to wash down the sides of the tube.
6. Transfer the sample using a Pasteur pipet to a new labeled 1.5 ml screw-top tube.
7. Add 500.0 μl PBS to the empty tube and transfer to the 1.5 ml screw-top tube to transfer any remaining cells.
8. Centrifuge the tube at maximum speed in an Eppendorf 5415D benchtop microcentrifuge for 30 s.
9. Remove the PBS with an SL1000 micropipettor and transfer into a second, new labeled 15.0 ml conical tube, leaving approximately 20.0 μl. Vortex and resuspend the pellet.
10. Wash the cells with 1 ml of 1× PBS and centrifuge at maximum speed for 30 s. Remove the PBS with a Pasteur pipet, leaving ~20 μl and repeat **step 10**.
11. Remove the PBS with a Pasteur pipet, leaving ~20 μl. Vortex the tube vigorously to resuspend the pellet.
12. Add 600.0 μl of Cell Lysis Solution to the resuspended pellet.
13. Add 100.0 μl of Proteinase K (20.0 mg/ml) to the tube.
14. Screw on the top, place parafilm around the top, and invert 25 times to mix. Put the sample(s) in the "Shake and Bake" oven at 37 °C ± 2 °C overnight with the rocker turned on.
15. Remove the tube(s) from the 37 °C ± 2 °C "Shake and Bake" oven.
16. Add 3.0 μl of RNase A solution (100.0 mg/ml) to the cell lysate. Screw on the top and place parafilm around it.
17. Invert the tube 25 times and then incubate at 37 °C ± 2 °C in the "Shake and "Bake" oven for 15 min.
18. Remove the samples from the oven, briefly spin and place the sample(s) on ice for 5 min. Add 200.0 μl of Protein Precipitation Solution to the sample. Vortex vigorously for 20 s to uniformly mix the sample.
19. Centrifuge at maximum speed in the Eppendorf 5415D tabletop centrifuge for 5 min.
20. Pipet 600.0 μl of 100% Isopropanol into a new 2.0 ml labeled tube. Place on ice for at least 5 min to cool.
21. Transfer the supernatant to the tube containing the ice-cold isopropanol.
22. Mix the sample by gently inverting 50 times.

23. Centrifuge at maximum speed in the Eppendorf 5415D table-top centrifuge for 2 min.
24. Carefully pour off the isopropanol into a waste container, being careful to leave the pellet undisturbed.
25. Spin for an additional 30 s. Pipet to remove residual isopropanol.
26. Add 600.0 μl of 70% ethanol to the tube. Replace the top and invert several times to wash the pellet.
27. Centrifuge at maximum speed in the Eppendorf 5415D table-top centrifuge for 1 min.
28. Carefully pour off the ethanol into an ethanol waste container being careful to leave the pellet undisturbed.
29. Spin for an additional 30 s. Pipet to remove residual ethanol.
30. Invert the tube on a clean absorbent paper for 10–15 min. Make sure that all of the ethanol has evaporated before proceeding.
31. Add 50.0 μl of DNA Hydration Buffer to the DNA pellet.
32. Incubate the tube at 55 °C ± 2 °C for 2 h to rehydrate the pellet, tapping the tube periodically.
33. If possible, leave the tube overnight at room temperature to further rehydrate the DNA.
34. Mix the sample by tapping the tube and briefly spin the sample.
35. Take and record the concentration using the NanoDrop (protocol Genomic DNA Concentration and Integrity).
36. Concentrate and clean up the DNA with Zymo column (Subheading 3.3).

3.2 DNA Extraction of Direct Chorionic Villus Sample (CVS)

1. Centrifuge the tubes containing the cleaned CVS (3 mg–10 mg) at maximum speed for 2–5 s. Remove as much of the media as possible using a sterile transfer pipet.
2. The supernatant should be transferred to a new labeled 1.5 ml screw top tube. It should be kept until you are sure that sufficient DNA was isolated in this protocol and it should then be immediately bleached and discarded.
3. If received in a 15 ml tube, transfer villi to a labeled 1.5 screw top tube.
4. Add 1.0 ml 1× Phosphate Buffered Saline (PBS) to the villi in the tube.
5. Centrifuge the tube at maximum speed in a benchtop microcentrifuge for 15 s.
6. Remove the PBS with an SL1000 micropipettor, leaving approximately 20.0 μl.

7. Flick the tube gently to resuspend the pelleted villi and repeat **steps 4** and **5**.
8. Add 600.0 μl of Cell Lysis Buffer and 20.0 μl of Proteinase K (20 mg/ml) to the microfuge tube. Parafilm the tube and invert 25 times to mix. Place on rocking platform at 37 °C ± 2 °C overnight.
9. Remove the sample from the rocking platform (*see* **Note 1**).
10. Add 3.0 μl of RNaseA (100.0 mg/ml) to the cell lysate. Invert the tube 25 times and incubate in a 37 °C ± 2 °C incubator for 15 min.
11. Add 600.0 μl of room-temperature 100% isopropanol to a new, labeled 2.0 ml empty tube and place on ice for at least 2 min before **step 12**.
12. Quickly spin the tube and place the sample on ice for 5–10 min.
13. Add 200 μl of protein precipitation solution and vortex vigorously for 20 s.
14. Spin at maximum speed in a tabletop centrifuge for 5 min.
15. If the pellet is not tight, place on ice for another 5 min and centrifuge again for 3 min.
16. Transfer the Supernatant to the tube containing ice-cold isopropanol.
17. Mix the sample by gently inverting 50 times.
18. Centrifuge at maximum speed in the tabletop centrifuge for 5 min.
19. Pour off the isopropanol into a clean labeled waste tube, being careful to leave the pellet undisturbed. Spin for an additional 30 s to remove any residual isopropanol and pipet out.
20. Add 600.0 μl of 70% ethanol to the tube. Replace the top and invert several times to wash the pellet.
21. Centrifuge at maximum speed in the tabletop centrifuge for 5 min.
22. Pour off the ethanol into a labeled waste tube, being careful to leave the pellet undisturbed. Spin for an additional 30 s to remove any residual ethanol and pipet out.
23. Leave the tube to air dry for 10–15 min for the remaining ethanol to evaporate off.
24. Add 50.0 μl of DNA Hydration Buffer (or more for a large pellet) to the DNA pellet.
25. Incubate the tube at 55 °C ± 2 °C for 2 h to rehydrate the pellet, tapping the tube periodically. If possible, leave the tube overnight at room temperature to further rehydrate the DNA.

26. Mix the sample by tapping the tube and briefly spin the sample. Measure the concentration using the Nanodrop and then clean a maximum of 5 μg of DNA on a Zymo column.
27. If the concentration prior to cleanup is more than 500 ng/μl, parafilm the sample and let it sit overnight at room temperature.

3.3 DNA Clean Up Using Zymo Columns

1. Add 100 μl of Binding buffer to 5 μg of DNA sample. Vortex and let it sit for 5 min at room temperature.
2. Add the sample to the zymo mini filter sitting in a collection tube. Spin for 30 s. Discard the waste.
3. Add 200 μl of wash buffer to the zymo mini filter. Spin for 30 s. Discard the waste. Repeat.
4. For elution A, transfer the mini filter to a new labeled 1.7 ml tube.
5. Add 18 μl of water to the filter. Let it sit for 10 min and spin for 30 s into the first labeled tube.
6. For elution B, transfer the mini column to another new labeled 1.7 ml tube.
7. Add 10 μl of water to the filter. Let it sit for 5 min. Spin for 30 s into a second labeled tube.
8. Determine the concentration of each elution using the Nanodrop.

3.4 Genomic DNA Concentration and Integrity

1. Determine the DNA concentration and quality using any standard DNA measuring technique. 260/280 ration should be between 1.75 and 2.00 and the 260/230 ratio should be above 1.5.
2. If the 260/280 ratio is below 1.75 or above 2.00, or the 260/230 ratio is below 1.5, or the concentration is below 66 ng/μl, purify the sample by again by using the Zymo column.
3. At this point an aliquot may be taken for maternal cell contamination studies before proceeding further.

3.5 Sample Digestion for Hybridization

1. If using Agilent CGH + SNP arrays, then digestion of the DNA with AluI and RsaI is necessary since the SNP probes on the array are AluI/RsaI restricted. If the non-SNP Agilent arrays are used or the SNP probes are not to be evaluated the DNA can be processed for labeling (Go to DNA labeling method).
2. Place top labels on closed 1.7 ml microfuge tubes for both the patients and the controls.
3. Add the appropriate amount of nuclease-free water and genomic DNA to make 1.0 μg genomic DNA in 20.0 μl to a labeled

Table 1
Digestion master mix for each single tube reaction (prepare in order)

Reagent		Volume (μl)	Final concentration
1	Nuclease-free water	2.50	
2	10× Buffer C	2.10	
3	Acetylated BSA (10.0 μg/μl)	0.40	0.67 μg/μl
4	AluI (10.0 U/μl)	0.50	0.83 U/μl
5	RsaI (10.0 U/μl)	0.50	0.83 U/μl
	Total volume	6.00	

tube for each reaction, following the volumes stated on the worksheet.

4. Add 1.0 μg final volume of 20 μl genomic gender-matched control DNA to a separate labeled 1.7 ml microfuge tube.
5. The gender control should be thoroughly mixed by tapping or inverting before use. DNA should not be vortexed regularly, as this will shear it.
6. Prepare the digestion master mix on ice with the components listed in Table 1, in the order indicated.
7. Add 6.0 μl of the Digestion Master Mix to each reaction tube.
8. Each tube should now have a total volume of 26.0 μl. Place the tubes on ice as soon as you have added the Master Mix.
9. Mix well by flicking the bottom of the tubes and spin them at maximum speed for 2–10 s.
10. Place the sample tubes at 37 °C ± 2 °C (either in a floating rack in a water bath or in a standard rack in an oven) and incubate from 2 to 17 h (approximately overnight).
11. Transfer the sample tubes to a floating rack in a water bath at 65 °C ± 2 °C and incubate for 20 min to inactivate the enzymes. Place tubes on ice for at least 5 min.
12. Proceed to the Sample Labeling protocol.

3.6 Sample Labeling

3.6.1 Fluorescent Labeling of Genomic DNA

1. If samples were stored at −20 °C ± 2 °C after enzyme digestion (Sample Digestion for Hybridization protocol), thaw at room temperature for 5 min.
2. Centrifuge the tubes at maximum speed for 2–10 s.
3. Add 5.0 μl of 10× Random Primers to each reaction tube containing 26.0 μl of digested genomic DNA.
4. Flick to mix. Centrifuge the tubes at maximum speed for 2–10 s.

Table 2
Labeling master mix set up for Single Tube Reaction

Reagent		Volume (μl)
1	Nuclease-free water	2.0
2	5× Reaction buffer	10.0
3	10× dNTP	5.0
4	dCTP labeled dye (Cy3—1.0 mM or Cy5—1.0 mM)	3.0
5	Klenow (Exo-)	1.0
	Total volume	21.00

5. Denature the DNA in a 105 °C ± 2 °C heat block for 3 min.
6. Immediately place the tubes on ice for 5 min, and then spin the tubes at maximum speed for 2–10 s. Return the tubes to ice.
7. Make a master mix for each dye (Cy5 for the sample DNA and Cy3 for the control DNA) using the volumes in Table 2, which list volumes for one labeling reaction. Add the components on ice in the order indicated. Mix by tapping and spin at maximum speed for 2–10 s.
8. Add 19.0 μl of Labeling Master Mix to each reaction tube. Flick to mix. Centrifuge the tubes at maximum speed for 2–10 s.
9. Place the sample tubes in a floating rack in a water bath at 37 °C ± 2 °C and incubate for 2 h.
10. Transfer the sample tubes to a water bath at 65 °C ± 2 °C and incubate for 10 min to inactivate the enzyme. Place tubes on ice for at least 5 min (*see* **Note 2**).

3.6.2 Clean-Up of Labeled Genomic DNA

1. Unincorporated dyes and dNTPs are removed by using Millipore Microcon Columns provided in the SureTag labeling kit.
2. Add 430.0 μl of 1× TE (pH 8.0) to each reaction tube, bringing the total volume to 480.0 μl.
3. Place a Microcon YM-30 filter into the supplied labeled 1.7 ml microfuge tube and load the correct labeled DNA sample onto the filter. Spin for 10 min at 9300 RPM (8000 × *g*) in a microcentrifuge at room temperature. Discard the flow-through in a labeled Cy-3 / Cy-5 waste container.
4. Add 480.0 μl of 1× TE (pH 8.0) to each filter. Spin for 10 min at 9300 RPM (8000 × *g*) in a microcentrifuge at room temperature. Discard the flow-through in the labeled Cy-3 / Cy-5 waste container.

5. Invert the filter into a fresh supplied labeled 1.7 ml microfuge tube. Spin for 1 min at 9300 RPM (8000 × *g*) in a microcentrifuge at room temperature to collect the purified sample.
6. Measure and record the volume of each eluate in μl. If the sample volume is more than 21 μl, return the sample to its filter and spin for 1 min at 9300 RPM (8000 × *g*) in a mirocentrifuge at room temperature. Discard the flow-through in a labeled Cy-3/Cy-5 waste.
7. Repeat **steps 5** and **6** until each sample volume is less than or equal to 21.0 μl.
8. Bring the total sample volume to 21.0 μl with 1× TE (pH 8.0) if necessary.
9. Proceed to Subheading 3.6.3 (*see* **Note 3**).

3.6.3 Quantitate the Yield and Specific Activity of the Labeling

1. Open program "ND-1000 v3.30" on the desktop of a computer attached to a NanoDrop Spectrophotometer.
2. Select "MicroArray" from the first screen.
3. Place 1.5 μl of Nuclease-Free water on the pedestal. Lower the arm. Click OK. Wait for reading.
4. Select "DNA-50" for "Sample Type" from the next screen.
5. Wipe off pedestal with a Kimwipe.
6. Place 1.5 μl of 1× TE (pH 8.0) on the pedestal.
7. Click "Blank" or press F3. All readings should go to 0.0.
8. Wipe off the sample with a Kimwipe and replace with a fresh 1.5 μl of 1× TE (pH 8.0).
9. Click "Measure" or press F1.
10. If the concentration reading is between 0.0 ng and 1.0 ng, proceed to the next step.
11. Measure the absorbance at A260nm (DNA), A550nm (cyanine 3), and A650nm (cyanine 5).
12. Calculate DNA (μg) = $(A_{260}–A_{320})$ × 50 μg/ml × volume in ml

    Dye Incorporation:

    Cy3™ (pmole) = $(A_{550}–A_{650})/0.15$ × volume in μl

    Cy5™ (pmole) = $(A_{650}–A_{750})/0.25$ × volume in μl
13. Match each patient sample with the gender-matched control that most closely matches its concentration. The concentration must be above 4 μg and the pmole >100.
14. Proceed to Hybridization of Patient Samples to Agilent Arrays protocol (*see* **Note 4**).

3.7 Hybridization

1. Add the components listed in Table 3, in the order listed, to a nuclease-free labeled tube.

Table 3
Hybridization volumes for different Agilent array formats

Component	2×400K array (μl)	4×180K array (μl)	2×105K array (μl)	8×60K array (μl)
1 Cyanine 5-labeled sample	19.5	19.5	19.5	19.5
2 Cyanine 3-labeled sample	19.5	19.5	19.5	19.5
3 1× TE	40.0	0.0	40.0	0.0
4 CoT-1 DNA (1.0 mg/ml)	25.0	5.0	25.0	2.5
5 Agilent 10× blocking agent	26.0	11.0	26.0	4.5
6 Agilent 2× hybridization buffer	130.0	55.0	130.0	22.5
Final hybridization sample volume	260.0	110.0	260.0	68.5

2. Mix the sample by pipetting it up and down several times. Flick the bottom of the tube to mix. Centrifuge the tubes at 8000 × *g* for 2–10 s.
3. Place sample tubes in a heat block at 105 ± 2 °C and incubate for 3 min.
4. Immediately transfer sample tubes to a water bath at 37 ± 2 °C and incubate for 30 min.
5. Remove sample tubes from the water bath. Spin for 1 min at 8000 × *g* in a microcentrifuge.
6. Load a clean gasket slide into the Agilent SureHyb chamber base with the gasket label facing up and aligned with the rectangular section of the chamber base. Ensure that the gasket slide is level and seated properly within the chamber base.
7. Slowly dispense the hybridization sample mixture into the gasket well. Load all gasket wells, being extremely careful to dispense each sample into the correct well.
8. After checking the Hybridization Worksheet to be sure that you have the correct slide, place the slide microarray-side down onto the SureHyb gasket slide, so the numeric barcode side is facing up and the "Agilent"-labeled barcode is facing down. The label on the gasket slide should be lined up with the label on the array slide.
9. Gently place the SureHyb chamber cover onto the sandwiched slides and slide the clamp assembly onto both pieces.
10. Hand-tighten the clamp onto the chamber. Experience will show how to get the chambers tight enough, but not too tight to break the slide.

11. Vertically rotate the assembled chamber to wet the slides and assess the mobility of the bubbles. Tap the assembly on the palm of your hand if necessary to move bubbles.
12. Place the assembled slide chamber in the rotator rack in a hybridization oven set to 65 °C ± 2 °C. Be sure that the rotator is balanced both side-to-side and front-to-back. Set the hybridization rotator to 20 rpm.
13. Hybridize at 65 ± 2 °C for 20–68 h.
14. Proceed to Array Washing protocol.

3.8 Array Washing

1. Place at least 250 ml of Agilent Oligo aCGH/ChIP-on-Chip Wash Buffer 2 in a 37 ± 2 °C water bath and a dish labeled "Wash BF2" in a 37 ± 2 °C incubator overnight, or at least 3 h before washing.
2. Fill a slide-staining dish labeled "Wash BF1" with approximately 350 ml of room-temperature Agilent Oligo aCGH/ChIP-on-Chip Wash Buffer 1 and place it in a fume hood.
3. Place a slide rack into another slide-staining dish labeled "Wash BF1." Add a magnetic stir bar. Fill this dish with enough room-temperature Oligo aCGH Wash Buffer 1 to cover the slide rack (~250 ml). Place this dish on a magnetic stir plate in the hood.
4. Place the dish labeled "Acetonitrile" in the fume hood and fill with approximately 300 ml with room-temperature acetonitrile (*see* **Note 5**).
5. The procedure of washing is conducted as depicted in Table 4.
6. Remove the hybridization chambers to be washed from the 65 ± 2 °C incubator.
7. Place the first slide into the wash buffer. Place the hybridization chamber assembly on a flat surface and disassemble it. Loosen the thumbscrew, turning counter-clockwise. Slide off the clamp assembly and remove the chamber cover. Remove the array-gasket sandwich from the chamber base by grabbing the slides from their ends.
8. Keep the microarray slide numeric barcode facing up and submerge the array-gasket sandwich into the first dish containing Oligo aCGH Wash Buffer 1. Do not let go of the slides.
9. With the sandwich completely submerged in Oligo aCGH Wash Buffer 1, pry the sandwich open from the barcode end. Insert one end of the plastic forceps between the slides and gently turn the forceps to separate the slides. Let the gasket slide drop to the bottom of the staining dish. Remove the microarray slide and place it into the slide rack in the second dish containing Oligo aCGH Wash Buffer 1, being very careful not to touch the array. Minimize exposure of the slide to air.

Table 4
Procedure of microarray slide washing

Procedure	Wash Buffer	Temperature	Time
Disassembly	Oligo aCGH Wash Buffer 1	Room temperature	Depends on the total number of slides
1	Oligo aCGH Wash Buffer 1	Room temperature	5 min
2	Oligo aCGH Wash Buffer 2	37 ± 2 °C	1 min
3	Acetonitrile	Room temperature	1 min

10. Repeat **steps** 7 and **8** for up to four additional slides, leaving a blank space between each pair of slides. No more than five slides can be washed in each wash batch. Larger dishes can be used for a maximum of 10 slides.
11. When all slides in the batch are placed into the slide rack in the second dish, stir using a setting between 110 and 130 for 5 min (Table 4).
12. When there is 1 min left on the previous wash, remove a pre-warmed dish and the Oligo aCGH Wash Buffer 2 from the 37 °C ± 2 °C incubator and water bath. Place the dish on a stir plate, add a magnetic stir bar, and fill the dish with Oligo aCGH Wash Buffer 2 to the top of the label.
13. When the time is up, transfer the slide rack to the dish containing the Oligo aCGH Wash Buffer 2 and stir on a setting between 110 and 130 for 1 min (Table 4).
14. Remove the slide rack from the dish and tilt the rack slightly to minimize wash buffer carry-over. Transfer the slide rack to the dish containing Acetonitrile and leave for 1 min (Table 4).
15. Remove the slide rack very slowly to minimize droplets on the slides. It should take about 10 s to remove the slide rack.
16. Scan slides immediately to minimize the impact of air oxidation on signal intensities, or store slides in slide boxes in a desiccator.
17. If necessary, repeat **steps 6–16** for the next group of five slides using fresh Oligo aCGH Wash Buffer 1 and pre-warmed Oligo aCGH Wash Buffer 2. The Oligo aCGH Wash Buffer 1 in the dish used to open the array-gasket assembly can be used throughout the day and should be discarded after all of the day's washing has been completed. The Oligo aCGH Wash Buffer 1 (on the stir plate) and Oligo aCGH Wash Buffer 2 can be used for up to 5 slides (*see* **Notes 5** and **6**).
18. When all washing for the day has been completed, wash all of the dishes, the slide rack, and the stir bars. Pour used Oligo aCGH Wash Buffer 1 and Oligo aCGH Wash Buffer 2 down

the lab sink. Rinse the dish and lid with tap water, and then fill the dish several times with Millipore water and empty. Rinse the lid with Millipore water. Air dry the Oligo aCGH Wash Buffer 1 dishes. The Oligo aCGH Wash Buffer 2 dish can be placed directly in the incubator. Discard the acetonitrile in the acetonitrile waste container in the hood. Air dry the dishes in the hood.

3.9 Scanning Slides and Analysis

1. Open the "Feature Extraction" software by double-clicking its icon on the desktop. Select the appropriate project. Start Extracting, or click the "start extracting" icon. Minimize the "Feature Extraction" window.
2. Open the "Scan Control" software by double-clicking its shortcut on the desktop.
3. Place the slides in the Agilent slide carriers.
4. Place the slide carrier on a flat surface. Use your thumb to slide the ridged end of the cover toward the open rectangle at one end. Open the hinged cover.
5. Holding a slide with the array side up and with the word "Agilent" toward the open rectangle. Place the one end of the slide on the ledge inside the slide holder. Gently lower the slide into place. Make sure that it is seated flush on the support ledges.
6. Gently lower the hinged cover. If it does not close easily, make sure that the slide is seated properly on the ledge. Push down the cover gently and slide the locking tabs in place.
7. Place the slide carriers into the carousel. Open the hinged chamber of the scanner.
8. Place each slide carrier into the carousel.
9. Do not place a carrier in the slot marked "H." Place the first carrier in position one and continue to load all of the carriers. Do not skip any slots otherwise this will cause the run to stop. The slides should be placed with the word "Agilent" at the center and facing toward lower numbers, i.e., the open back of the slide showing the barcode should be facing out.
10. Close the chamber door.
11. Enter the position of the first slide to be scanned in the "Start slot:" field of the software. This will normally be "1."
12. Enter the position of the last slide to be scanned in the "End slot:" field.
13. Select the appropriate scanner profile.

14. Select the proper resolution. The current settings are 5 μm for standard resolution arrays and 3 μm for high resolution arrays.
15. Press the "Scan slot 1—X" button, where "X" is the number you entered for the last slide to be scanned.
16. Scanning will take approximately 10–15 min per slide depending on the resolution.
17. The .tiff images will be automatically output to the folder "D: \Scanner Output Location."
18. The .tiff files will be automatically extracted as they are completed. The software will automatically detect new .tiff files as they are created.
19. The software will remain active until it has not detected a new file generation in X min (X can be a number you can preset on the Feature Extraction program). The program can be stopped by the user by selecting the "Project/Stop" icon from the menu bar.
20. Only the slides with barcodes will be automatically extracted.
21. After scanning the text files can be uploaded into the Agilent CytoGenomics software. After normalization and subtraction of background noise the data are to log ratios and plotted.

4 Notes

1. DNA isolation can stop here for continuation the next day. Samples may also be left at this point over the weekend. Keep the cell lysate at room temperature if extraction is to be continued later.
2. Samples can be stored at −20 °C for a day before proceeding to the clean-up step.
3. Cleaned, labeled DNA can be stored overnight or over the weekend at −20 °C ± 2 °C, either before or after quantitating.
4. Subheading 3.7 is adapted with modification from Agilent manual "Agilent Oligonucleotide Array-Based CGH for Genomic DNA Analysis".
5. If fewer than 5 slides are washed and more are to be washed later the same day, leave the Oligo aCGH Wash Buffer 1 in the hood and place the Oligo aCGH Wash Buffer 2 in its tray in the 37 ± 2 °C incubator until ready for use.
6. Acetonitrile can be used for up to 20 slides. Leave in the hood if it will be used later for another wash.

References

1. Kallioniemi A, Kallioniemi OP, Sudar D et al (1992) Comparative genomic hybridization for molecular cytogenetic analysis of solid tumors. Science 258(5083):818–821
2. Solinas-Toldo S, Lampel S, Stilgenbauer S et al (1997) Matrix-based comparative genomic hybridization: biochips to screen for genomic imbalances. Genes Chromosomes Cancer 20 (4):399–407
3. Snijders AM, Nowak N, Segraves R et al (2001) Assembly of microarrays for genome-wide measurement of DNA copy number. Nat Genet 29 (3):263–264. https://doi.org/10.1038/ng754
4. Cai WW, Mao JH, Chow CW et al (2002) Genome-wide detection of chromosomal imbalances in tumors using BAC microarrays. Nat Biotechnol 20(4):393–396
5. Ylstra B, van den Ijssel P, Carvalho B et al (2006) BAC to the future! or oligonucleotides: a perspective for micro array comparative genomic hybridization (array CGH). Nucleic Acids Res 34(2):445–450. https://doi.org/10.1093/nar/gkj456
6. Cheung SW, Shaw CA, Yu W et al (2005) Development and validation of a CGH microarray for clinical cytogenetic diagnosis. Genet Med 7 (6):422–432. https://doi.org/10.109701.GIM.0000170992.63691.32
7. Miller DT, Adam MP, Aradhya S et al (2010) Consensus statement: chromosomal microarray is a first-tier clinical diagnostic test for individuals with developmental disabilities or congenital anomalies. Am J Hum Genet 86 (5):749–764. https://doi.org/10.1016/j.ajhg.2010.04.006
8. Manning M, Hudgins L, Professional P et al (2010) Array-based technology and recommendations for utilization in medical genetics practice for detection of chromosomal abnormalities. Genet Med 12(11):742–745. https://doi.org/10.1097/GIM.0b013e3181f8baad
9. Wapner RJ, Martin CL, Levy B, et al (2012) Chromosomal microarray versus karyotyping for prenatal diagnosis. The New England journal of medicine. 367(23):2175–2184. https://doi.org/10.1056/NEJMoa1203382

Chapter 13

Prenatal Diagnosis Using Chromosomal SNP Microarrays

Mythily Ganapathi, Odelia Nahum, and Brynn Levy

Abstract

Chromosomal microarray is a high resolution genomic technology to diagnose genetic conditions associated with losses or gains of the human genome. This technology is currently routinely used in numerous clinical settings, including postnatal diagnosis of disorders with genetic etiologies such as intellectual disability, developmental delay, neurocognitive phenotypes, congenital anomalies, and prenatal diagnosis wherein the referral could be ultrasound anomalies, advanced maternal age, and normal course of pregnancy. We describe the use of Chromosomal SNP microarrays for prenatal diagnosis of genetic disorders which result from both copy number or copy neutral changes in the genome.

Key words Chromosomal microarray analysis, Chromosomal SNP microarray, Prenatal diagnosis, Ultrasound abnormalities

1 Introduction

Chromosomal microarray analysis offers a high resolution approach to diagnose disease conditions which occur due to losses and gains in the human genome which are denoted as copy number variants (CNVs). They include whole chromosomal aneuploidies as well as submicroscopic gains or losses that are too small to be detected by conventional karyotyping. For chromosomal microarray analysis, patient's DNA is fluorescently labeled and hybridized to a solid support containing thousands of oligonucleotide-based DNA probes. The copy number of a probe on the microarray is determined by comparative hybridization of the labeled patient DNA to an in silico reference set. Oligonucleotide probes can be designed to detect copy number changes in a sequence compared with a control, additionally, they may be designed to identify a specific genotype or allele of a single nucleotide polymorphism (SNP). Chromosomal microarray platforms with copy number as well as SNP probes additionally provide clinically relevant information about copy neutral changes such as long continuous stretches of

Brynn Levy (ed.), *Prenatal Diagnosis*, Methods in Molecular Biology, vol. 1885, https://doi.org/10.1007/978-1-4939-8889-1_13,

homozygosity, uniparental disomy and will also identify ploidy changes.

Chromosomal microarray analysis is particularly useful in the diagnosis of genetic abnormalities in the prenatal setting as a direct CVS/amniocentesis/POC sample can be assayed obviating the need for a cultured specimen, resulting in faster turnaround times. However, if DNA amounts from a direct sample are insufficient, then a cultured sample can be used for the assay. Targeted chromosomal microarrays wherein known regions of interest are analyzed are the preferred choice of most laboratories offering prenatal testing to avoid the calling of VOUS variants which can be a source of anxiety and distress for the parents. The American College and the Society for Maternal-Fetal Medicine in 2013 recommended chromosomal microarray analysis as the First-tier prenatal test in case of abnormal ultrasound findings [1]. Further, CNVs identified by chromosomal microarray analysis such as microdeletions and microduplications are not associated with advanced maternal age [2]; hence it was recommended to offer this test to all pregnant women and not restrict it to those aged 35 years and older. In cases of intrauterine fetal demise or stillbirth chromosomal microarray analysis on fetal tissue (i.e., amniotic fluid, placenta, or products of conception) was recommended because of its improved detection of causative abnormalities.

The microarray platform we currently use is the Affymetrix Cytoscan HD array which has a total of 2.67 million markers and includes 1.9 million non-polymorphic copy number probes and 750,000 SNPs for genotype calls. The described method can be applied to direct or cultured prenatal specimens (amniotic fluid or chorionic villi) as well as for products of conception from miscarriages. On the day of sample receipt, DNA can be extracted, restriction enzyme digested and ligated with adaptors. Extraction is performed by a lysis procedure using a commercial extraction kit (Qiagen DNA mini kit cat, QIAGEN, Germantown, MD, USA). The DNA is then PCR amplified, fragmented by DNAse digestion, and labeled by Terminal Deoxynucleotidyl transferase reaction. DNAse digestion is performed to fragment the genomic DNA into segments approx 25 bp to 125 bp. After labeling, the DNA is denatured and then loaded on to the array. The arrays are hybridized overnight, washed to remove any unbound genomic DNA, stained, scanned and analyzed. Herein, we report common chromosomal SNP microarray procedure used to take a sample from receipt to results in a clinical diagnostic setting.

2 Materials

Unless otherwise specified, reagents are provided with the Affymetrix Cytoscan HD kit (Thermo Fisher Scientific, Waltham, MA, USA) (*see* **Note 1**).

2.1 Restriction Enzyme Digestion

1. 100× BSA.
2. 10× NspI Buffer.
3. NspI Enzyme.
4. Chilled Affymetrix Nuclease-free water.

2.2 Ligation Reaction

1. 10× T4 DNA Ligase Buffer.
2. 50 μM Adaptor, NspI.
3. T4 DNA Ligase.

2.3 PCR

1. Affymetrix Nuclease-free water.
2. PCR Primer 002 (100 μM).
3. dNTPs (2.5 mM each).
4. Titanium DNA Amplification Kit (Clontech Laboratories, Mountain View, CA, USA): Contains GC-Melt (5 M), TITANIUM™ Taq DNA Polymerase (50×), TITANIUM™ Taq PCR Buffer (10×).

2.4 Checking the PCR Reaction Results

1. Affymetrix Nuclease-free water.
2. DNA Marker (USB/Thermo Fisher Scientific, Waltham, MA, USA): PCR Markers, 50–2000 bp.
3. E-Gel EX 2% Agarose Gels (Invitrogen, Carlsbad, CA, USA).
4. 6× DNA loading buffer (USB/Thermo Fisher Scientific, Waltham, MA, USA).
5. Strip Tubes (Bio-Rad Laboratories, Hercules, CA, USA).

2.5 PCR Product Purification

1. Elution Buffer.
2. Purification Wash Buffer.
3. Magnetic beads.

2.6 PCR Product Quantitation of Purified PCR Products

1. Affymetrix nuclease-free water.

2.7 Fragmentation

1. Fragmentation Buffer.
2. Fragmentation Reagent (enzyme; DNase I).
3. Affymetrix Nuclease-free water.

2.8 Checking the Fragmentation Reaction by Running a Gel

1. 4% E-Gel EX agarose gel (Invitrogen, Carlsbad, CA, USA).
2. DNA Marker (TrackIt-25 bp) (Invitrogen, Carlsbad, CA, USA).
3. 6× DNA loading buffer (USB/Thermo Fisher Scientific, Waltham, MA, USA).
4. Strip Tubes (Bio-Rad Laboratories, Hercules, CA, USA).

2.9 Labeling

1. DNA Labeling Reagent (30 mM).
2. Terminal Deoxynucleotidyl Transferase (TdT; 30 U/μL).
3. Terminal Deoxynucleotidyl Transferase Buffer (TdT Buffer; 5×).

2.10 Hybridization

1. Hybridization buffer Part 1.
2. Hybridization buffer Part 2.
3. Hybridization buffer Part 3.
4. Hybridization buffer Part 4.
5. Oligo Control Reagent (OCR), 0100.

2.11 Washing, Staining and Scanning the Arrays

1. Stain Buffer 1.
2. Stain Buffer 1.
3. Affymetrix GeneChip Array holding buffer.
4. Affymetrix GeneChip Wash A.
5. Affymetrix GeneChip Wash B.

3 Methods (*See* Notes 2–5)

1. Include Affymetrix Nuclease-free water as a negative control and REF 103 DNA (supplied in the kit) in every batch of samples to be set up for microarray analysis.
2. The duration of the assay can take between 3 and 4 days. We usually do it in 4 days as described below, however it can be shortened to 3 days:
   - Day 1: Digestion + Ligation.
   - Day 2: PCR + Purification.
   - Day 3: Fragmentation + Labeling + Hybridization (overnight).
   - Day 4: Washing and Staining + Scanning.

3.1 DNA Dilution

A starting concentration of 50 ng/μL (range: 45–64 ng/μL) of DNA is needed for samples that have to be run on the Affymetrix Cytoscan HD protocol (*see* **Note 6**).

1. Thaw the genomic DNA (gDNA).

2. Vortex the gDNA samples at high speed for 3 s and short spin it.
3. If sample concentration is unknown, take an OD measurement of the sample.
4. Based on OD measurements, dilute each sample to 50 ng/μL using molecular biology grade water/TE (depending upon the original solution that the DNA was eluted in) (*see* **Note 6**).

3.2 Restriction Enzyme Digestion

During this stage, one aliquot of each sample is digested by the NspI restriction enzyme. This assay has to be conducted in a Pre-PCR clean area (preferably in a hood).

1. Thaw the Buffers and BSA on ice.
2. Leave the enzymes at −20 °C until ready to use.
3. Using a marker, label one 1.5 mL Eppendorf tube as NspI.
4. Put tube on ice. Vortex the gDNA and controls at high speed for 3 s, spin down the DNA, and place in the cooling chamber on ice.
5. Vortex the buffers and BSA three times, 1 s each time.
6. Pulse spin for 3 s and place in the cooling chamber on ice.
7. Power on the thermal cycler to preheat the lid.
8. Make a master mix by adding the following to the labeled Eppendorf tubes (*see* **Notes 7** and **8**): For *each sample* add 5 μL of the diluted genomic DNA (250 ng), 11.55 μL Affymetrix Nuclease-free water, 2 μL 10× NspI Buffer, 0.2 μL 100× BSA and 1 μL NspI. Scale quantities according to the number of samples to be processed. Place the master mix on the cooling chamber between adding reagents.
9. Vortex the master mix at high speed three times, 1 s each time.
10. Pulse spin for 3 s and place in the cooling chamber.
11. Return any remaining enzyme to the freezer.
12. Using a single channel P20 pipette, add 14.75 μL of the Digestion Master mix to each well containing the genomic DNA. The total volume in each well is now 19.75 μL.
13. Seal the plate tightly with a microseal film.
14. Vortex the center of the plate and all corners at 75% speed for 1 s. Spin the plate at 650 × *g* for 1 min.
15. Ensure that the lid of thermal cycler is preheated.
16. Load the plate onto the thermal cycler and run the CytoScan Digest program as follows: 37 °C for 120 min, 65 °C for 20 min, 4 °C hold (*see* **Note 9**).
17. When the program is finished, remove the plate and spin it down at 650 × *g* for 1 min.
18. If proceeding directly to the ligation assay, place the plate on a cooling chamber on ice. Otherwise, store the plate at −20 °C.

3.3 Ligation Reaction

During this stage, the NspI digested samples are ligated using the NspI Adaptor.

This assay should be conducted in a Pre-PCR clean area (preferably in a hood).

1. Allow the following reagents to thaw on ice: Adaptor NspI (50 μM), T4 ligase buffer (10×)—mix it thoroughly before use to ensure precipitate is resuspended.
2. Turn the Power on the thermal cycler to preheat the lid.
3. Make a master mix by adding the following to a 500 μL Eppendorf tube (*see* **Notes 7** and **8**): For *each sample* add 0.75 μL Adaptor NspI/Sty (50 μM), 2.5 μL T4 DNA Ligase buffer (10×), 2 μL T4 DNA ligase (400 U/μL). Scale quantities according to the number of samples to be processed. Place the master mix on the cooling chamber between adding reagents.
4. Vortex the master mix at high speed three times, 1 s each time then spin for 3 s and place in the cooling chamber.
5. Using a single channel P100 pipette, add 5.25 μL of the Ligation Master mix to each well containing the digested genomic DNA. The total volume in each well is now 25 μL.
6. Seal the plate tightly with microseal film.
7. Vortex the center and the corners of the plate at 75% speed for 3 s.
8. Spin the plate at 650 × *g* for 1 min.
9. Ensure that the lid of thermal cycler is preheated.
10. Load the plate onto the thermal cycler and run the Ligation program as follows: 16 °C for 180 min, 70 °C for 20 min, 4 °C hold (*see* **Note 9**).
11. When the program is finished, remove the plate and spin at 650 × *g* for 1 min.
12. Place the plate on a cooling chamber if PCR assay is going to be set up immediately. Otherwise, store the plate at −20 °C.

3.4 PCR

The assay should be set up in a Pre-PCR clean area (preferably in a hood). The PCR should be run on the thermal cycler in a post PCR area.

1. Add 75 μL of Affymetrix Nuclease-free water to each DNA ligation reaction, in order to dilute the DNA (*see* **Note 10**).
2. Tightly seal the plate. Vortex at 75% speed power for 1 s; then spin the plate at 650 × *g* for 1 min.
3. Allow the following reagents to thaw on ice: G-C Melt (5 M), dNTP (2.5 mM each), PCR Primer (100 μM), Taq buffer (10×).

4. Turn the Power on the thermal cycler to preheat the lid.
5. Label a fresh 96-well plate in such way that each sample will be added in 4 wells. In a case where you process 8 samples (a whole column) the new plate should have 4 columns labeled, so each sample will now have 4 wells. To each well, add 10 μL of the diluted ligated DNA.
6. Make a master mix by adding the following to a 1.5 mL Eppendorf tube (*see* **Notes 7**, **8**, and **11**): For *each* reaction add 39.5 μL Affymetrix nuclease-free water, 10 μL Taq buffer (10×), 20 μL, G-C melt (5 M), 14 μL dNTP, 4.5 μL PCR primer, 2 μL Taq polymerase. Scale quantities according to the number of reactions to be processed. Place the master mix on the cooling chamber between adding reagents.
7. Vortex the master mix at 75% speed power three times, 1 s each time.
8. Using a multi-channel P100 pipette, add 90 μL of the PCR Master mix to each well containing the diluted genomic DNA to obtain a total volume of 100 μL (*see* **Note 10**).
9. Seal the plate tightly with microseal film.
10. Vortex the center of the plate at high speed for 3 s.
11. Spin the plate at 650 × *g* for 1 min.
12. Ensure that the lid of thermal cycler is preheated.
13. Load the plate onto the thermal cycler and run the *Cyoscan PCR* program as follows:
    - One cycle: 94 °C for 3 min.
    - Thirty cycles: 94 °C for 30 s, 60 °C for 45 s, 68 °C for 15 s.
    - Once cycle: 68 °C for 7 min.
    - 4 °C hold (*see* **Note 9**).
14. When the program is finished, remove the plate and perform a short spin.
15. If proceeding immediately to the purification step, put the plate in a cooling chamber on ice. Otherwise, store the samples at −20 °C.

3.5 Checking the PCR Reaction by Running a Gel

This step serves as the first quality control (QC) checkpoint. Gel should be run in the post PCR area. Never bring in amplified PCR products into the Pre-PCR Clean room.

1. Label a fresh set of strip tubes.
2. Aliquot 0.6 μL of 6× Gel Loading Dye and 5 μL water to each well in the strip to be used.
3. Load 5 μL DNA marker to the first lane of the gel.

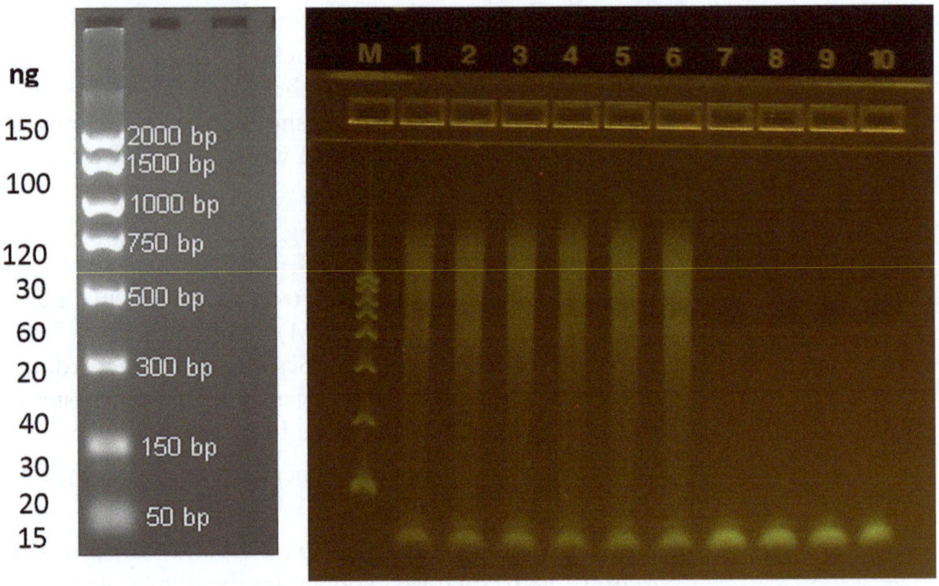

Fig. 1 Example of PCR products run on 2% agarose gel at 120 V for 10 min

4. Using a multichannel pipette transfer 3 μL of NspI PCR product from each well in **one column only** (no need to run all 4 duplicates) to the corresponding wells of the gel plate.
5. Load 8 μL from each well of the gel plate onto a 2% agarose gel. Load all 4 wells of the negative control.
6. Run the gel program: "E-Gel EX 1-2%" for 10 min.
7. Verify that the majority of the PCR product is between ~150 bp to 200 bp (compare to Fig. 1).
8. The lanes with the negative control should be empty as shown in Fig. 1 (*see* **Note 12**).

3.6 PCR Product Purification

This assay should be performed in post PCR area.

1. If frozen, thaw the PCR products in a plate holder on the bench top to room temperature.
2. Spin the plate at 650 × *g* for 1 min.
3. Add 45 mL of absolute Ethanol to the Purification wash buffer prior to use. Cap the bottle tightly and shake. Enter the preparation date on the bottle label and put a check mark in the check box.
4. Using a P200 single channel pipet, transfer all 4 aliquots of each sample to a 2.0 mL round bottom tube: Mark each 2.0 mL microcentrifuge tube with the appropriate sample number (such as A, B, C, D) after the sample was transferred.
5. Cut the seal of only one row at a time so only one sample will be transferred at a time. Do not pool the negative control. Be very careful to avoid cross-contamination while pooling the PCR products.

6. When finished, examine the PCR plate and ensure that the total volume in each well has been transferred and pooled.
7. Thoroughly mix the magnetic bead stock by vigorously shaking the bottle. Examine the bottom and the sides of the bottle and ensure that the solution appears homogenous.
8. Aliquot 720 mL of magnetic beads to each pooled sample. Securely cap each tube and mix well by inverting 10 times.
9. Incubate at room temperature for 10 min. During incubation, the DNA binds to the magnetic beads.
10. Load the tubes—cap hinge facing out—onto the microcentrifuge and spin for 3 min at maximum speed.
11. Place the tubes on the magnetic stand. Leaving the tubes in the rack, pipet off the supernatant without disturbing the bead pellet and discard.
12. Using a P1000 pipet, add 1 mL of washing buffer to each tube (be sure to add 45 mL of absolute ethanol to the purification wash buffer prior to use).
13. Cap the tubes and load them into the foam tube adaptor. Fully insert tubes into the foam to ensure they are secure. Space tubes adequately to balance. Vortex at maximum settings for 2 min.
14. Centrifuge the tubes for 3 min at maximum speed (hinges facing out).
15. Place the tubes on the magnetic stand. Leaving the tubes in the rack, pipet off the supernatant without disturbing the bead pellet and discard.
16. Spin the tubes for 30 s at maximum speed (hinges facing out).
17. Place the tubes back on the magnetic stand. Using a P20 pipet, remove remaining drops of purification wash buffer from the bottom of each tube. Transfer the tubes to a different rack and allow the remaining purification wash buffer to evaporate by leaving the tubes uncapped at room temperature for10 min.
18. Using a P100 pipet, add 52 μL of Elution buffer to each tube.
19. Cap the tubes and load them into the foam tube adaptor. Vortex at maximum power for 10 min. Vortexing will resuspend the magnetic beads. Examine each tube to ensure that the beads are resuspended in homogeneous slurry. If needed you can flick the pellet to ensure full resuspension.
20. Centrifuge the tubes for 3 min at maximum speed (hinges facing out).
21. Place the tubes on the magnetic stand for 10 min. The magnetic beads are pulled to the side of the tube. Check that all of the beads have been pulled to the side in each tube. If all of the

beads have not been pulled to the side of the tubes, leave the tubes on the stand an additional 3 min.

22. Transfer 47 μL of eluted sample to the appropriate well on a fresh 96-well plate. Open one tube at each time of transfer, and make sure the order of the samples matches the one in the plate. Presence of some brown residue on pipet tips is fine. Tightly seal the plate.
23. Vortex the plate at high speed in all corners and in the center, and spin down at 650 × *g* for 1 min.

3.7 Quantitation of Purified PCR Products on a Nanodrop

This assay should be performed in the post PCR area.

1. Label 500 μL tubes as A, B, C, D according to your plate layout.
2. Using a P20 pipet, aliquot 18 μL of water to the corresponding 500 μL tube. Place the dilution tube in a separate rack.
3. Using a P2 pipet, transfer 2 μL of each purified sample to the corresponding tube. Make sure to open only the tube of the sample that is being diluted. Dilute one sample at a time.
4. Vortex and spin the diluted samples. The result is a tenfold dilution.
5. Blank the NanoDrop with water.
6. Take 1.5 μL of the diluted sample and measure the OD of each sample at 260 and 280 nm.
7. The average purification yield for seven or more samples should be ≥3 μg/μL (*see* **Notes 13–15**).
8. PCR products can be stored at −20 °C if not proceeding to the fragmentation assay.

3.8 Fragmentation

This assay should be performed in the post PCR area on ice.

1. Thaw the Fragmentation Buffer (10×) on ice.
2. Vortex the buffer three times, 1 s each time. Pulse spin for 3 s and place in the cooling chamber.
3. Preheat the thermal cycler.
4. The Fragmentation Reagent must be diluted to 0.1 U/μL in the master mix. Read the Fragmentation Reagent tube label and record the concentration.
5. Prepare fragmentation mastermix in an eppendorf tube on ice, as per Table 1 (*see* **Note 16**).
6. Vortex the master mix at high speed for 5 s. Pulse spin for 3 s and immediately place on ice.
7. Add 10 μL of the fragmentation mastermix to each sample. The total volume of each sample should be 55 μL.

Table 1
Mastermix volumes for Fragmentation

Reagent	Volume (μL)
Chilled nuclease free water	271.2
Fragmenation buffer	343.8
Fragmentation reagent	10

8. Cover the plate with microseal and pulse vortex five times 1 s each.
9. Spin down at 650 × *g* for 1 min in a prechilled centrifuge.
10. Place in the preheated thermal cycler (at 37 °C) and run the Fragmentation program as follows: 37 °C for 35′, 95 °C for 15′, 4 °C hold.
11. Take the plate out and spin briefly.

3.9 Check the Fragmentation Reaction by Running a Gel

This step serves as the second QC checkpoint.

1. Add 28 μL of affymetrix nuclease-free water, to the appropriate wells in the strip.
2. Add 4.0 μL of each sample to the wells containing the water.
3. Take an 8 μL aliquot out and add to a strip tube.
4. Add 0.6 μL gel loading dye to each sample.
5. Load 8 μL of each sample onto the gel.
6. Dilute the DNA marker as follows: 1 μL of marker with 9 μL of water.
7. Load 10 μL of DNA marker to the first lane.
8. Run the gel program: "E-Gel Ex 4%" for 15 min.
9. Inspect the gel and compare it against the Fig. 2. Average fragment size should be between 25 and 125 bp (*see* **Note 17**).

3.10 Labeling

1. Thaw the buffer and labeling reagent on ice.
2. Vortex each reagent three times on high speed, 1 s each time. Pulse spin for 3 s, then place on cooling chamber on ice.
3. Preheat the thermal cycler.
4. Make a master mix by adding the following to a 1.5 mL Eppendorf tube (*see* **Notes 7** and **8**): For *each sample* add 14 μL 5× TdT buffer, 2 μL DNA Labeling reagent (30 mM), 3.5 μL TdT (30 U/μL). Scale quantities according to the number of samples to be processed. Place the master mix on the cooling chamber between adding reagents.

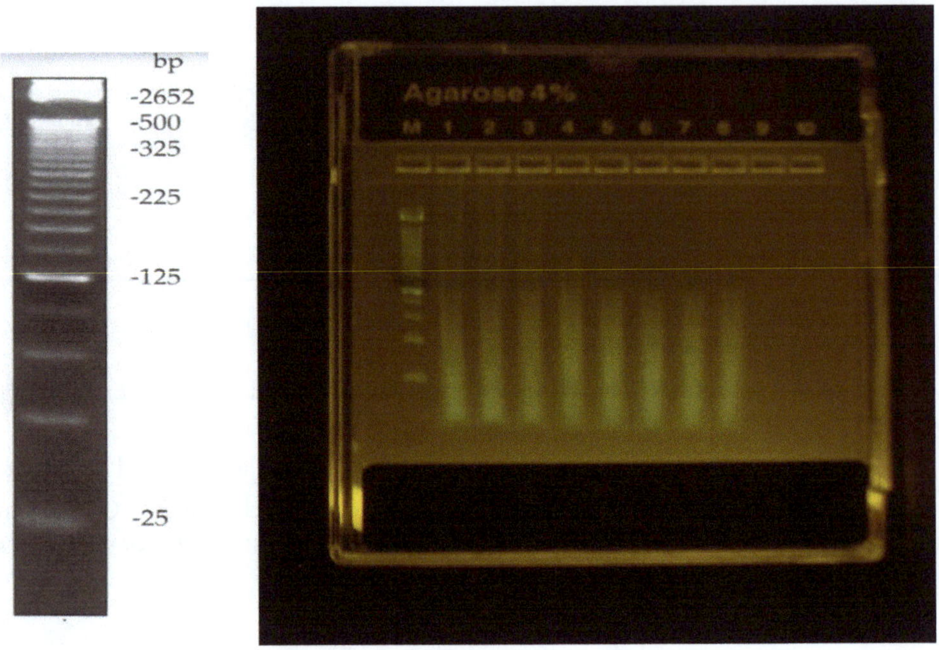

Fig. 2 Typical example of fragmented PCR products

5. Vortex the master mix at high speed three times, 1 s each time. Pulse spin for 3 s.
6. Using a P20 pipet, add 19.5 μL of the master mix to each fragmented sample. Pipet up and down to ensure that all of the mix is added to the samples.
7. Tightly seal the plate. Vortex at high speed for 3 s; then spin the plate at 650 × *g* for 1 min.
8. Place on the preheated thermal cycler block and run the Labeling program as follows: 37 °C for 4 h, 95 °C for 15 min, 4 °C hold (*see* **Note 9**).
9. When the Labeling program is finished, remove the plate from the thermal cycler and spin down for 30 s.
10. If not proceeding with the hybridization assay, freeze the labeled samples at −20 °C.

3.11 Preparation of Arrays for Hybridization

1. Unwrap the arrays and place on the bench top, septa-side up.
2. Mark the front of each array with the sample number (A, B, C).
3. Allow the arrays to warm to room temperature on the bench top 10–15 min.
4. Log in the arrays in AGCC. The sample information is stored in a Sample file with an ARR extension. The arrays used in analysis and the data files produced by analysis are linked to this sample file.

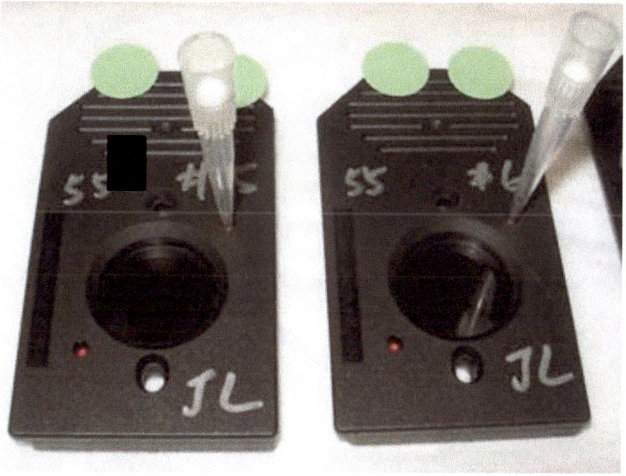

Fig. 3 Arrays prepared for sample loading

5. Insert a 200 μL pipet tip into the upper right septum of each array (*see* Fig. 3).
6. Preheat the thermal cycler.
7. Preheat the hybridization oven to 50 °C at least 1 h before hybridization.
8. Make a master mix by adding the following to a tube (15 mL falcon tube or 1.5 mL/2 mL amber tube. The choice of the tube depends on the number of samples to be hybridized): For *each sample* add 165 μL Hyb Buffer part 1, 15 μL Hyb Buffer part 2, 7 μL Hyb Buffer part 3, 1 μL Hyb Buffer part 4, 2 μL Oligo Control Reagent. Scale quantities according to the number of samples to be processed.
9. Vortex the master mix at high speed three times, 1 s each time. Pulse spin for 3 s and place in the cooling chamber.
10. Using a single channel P200 pipette, add 190 μL of the Master mix to each well containing the labeled DNA, pipette up and down to mix. The total volume in each well is now 260 μL.
11. Seal the plate tightly with microseal film. Vortex and spin the plate at 650 × *g* for 1 min.
12. Ensure that the lid of thermal cycler is preheated.
13. Load the plate onto the thermal cycler and run the Hybridization program as follows: 95 °C for 10 min, 49 °C hold.
14. Allow the samples to incubate at 49 °C for at least 1 min before loading.
15. Open the thermocycler lid, and load 200 μL of each sample in the bottom left septa of the corresponding array. Make sure that another technician is watching so that all the samples are hybridized to the right labeled array. It is critical that the

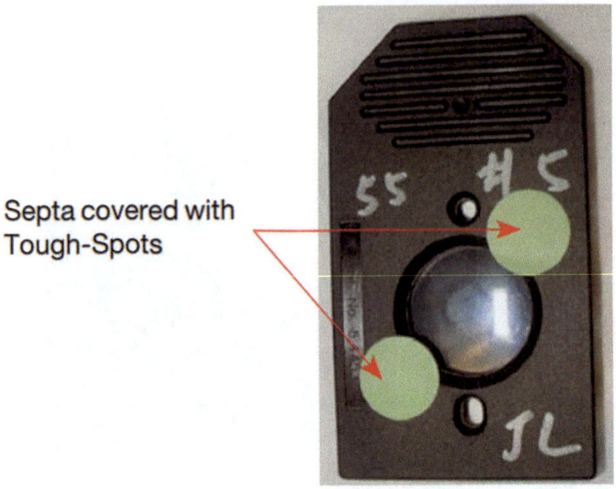

Fig. 4 Covering the array septa with Tough-Spots

samples remain on the thermal cycler at 49 °C after denaturation and while being loaded onto arrays.

16. Take out the tip, and apply Tough-Spot on both septae of the array (Fig. 4).
17. Load the arrays into hybridization oven (50 °C and 60 rpm) for 16–18 h. Ensure that the oven is balanced as the trays with the arrays are loaded.

3.12 Priming the Fluidics Station for Washing and Staining

Priming ensures the lines of the fluidics station are filled with the appropriate buffers and the fluidics station is ready to run fluidics station protocols. Priming should be done:

- When the fluidics station is first started.
- When wash solutions are changed.
- Before washing, if a shutdown has been performed.
- If the LCD window instructs the user to prime.

1. Turn on the Fluidics station using the switch on the lower left side of the machine.
2. Pour wash solutions A and B into the appropriate bottles, and fill the water bottle with DI water.
3. Place all the bottles including the waste in the right place on the side of the machine, and insert the corresponding tubing.
4. Turn on the computer.
5. Click on Affy Launcher icon, and hit Fluidics from the menu bar.
6. In the experiment name field choose "no probe array."
7. In the protocol field choose "Prime_450."

8. Check "all modules" when using all four modules, otherwise choose the Prime_450 protocol for the respective modules.
9. Click run for each module to begin priming, and follow the LCD instructions (*see* **Note 18**).

3.13 Washing and Staining the Arrays

The staining protocol is a three-stage process: (1) A Streptavidin Phycoerythin (SAPE) stain, (2) An antibody amplification step, and (3) A final stain with SAPE. Once stained, each array is filled with Array Holding Buffer prior to scanning.

1. After 16–18 h of hybridization, remove the arrays from the oven.
2. Remove the Tough-Spot from both septae of the array (*see* **Note 19**).
3. Select your sample name on the computer. The Probe Array Type and the corresponding protocol appear automatically (i.e., "CytoScanHD_Array_450" protocol for Cytoscan arrays).
4. Start the protocol and follow the instructions in the LCD on the fluidics station.
5. Insert an array into the designated module of the fluidics station while the cartridge lever is in the Down or Eject position.
6. When finished, verify that the cartridge lever is returned to the Up or Engaged position.
7. Remove any vials remaining in the positions of the fluidics station module(s) being used.
8. When prompted to "Load Vials 1-2-3," place the three vials into positions 1, 2, and 3 on the fluidics station.
   - Place one amber tube containing 500 μL stain buffer 1 in position 1.
   - Place one clear tube containing 500 μL stain buffer 2 in position 2.
   - Place one amber tube containing 800 μL Array Holding Buffer in position 3.
   - Press down on the needle lever to snap needles into position and to start the run.
9. Once these steps are complete, the fluidics protocol begins. The Fluidics Station dialog box at the workstation terminal and the LCD window displays the status of the washing and staining steps (*see* **Notes 20** and **21**).
10. When staining is finished, Remove the arrays from the fluidics station by first pressing down the cartridge lever to the eject position.

11. Check the array window for large bubbles or air pockets. If large bubbles are present, insert the array back into the module and follow the instructions on the LCD panel.
12. Remove all 3 microcentrifuge vials containing stain and buffer and replace with three empty vials as prompted.
13. Check the array window for dust or glue spots and wipe it off with kimwipes wet with DI water or non-abrasive towel.
14. If the array has no large bubbles, it is ready for scanning. Pull up on the cartridge lever to engage wash block and proceed to scanning.
15. If the arrays cannot be scanned promptly, store the arrays at 4 °C in the dark until ready for scanning. Scan must be performed within 24 h.
16. When finished washing and staining, insert all wash lines (except the waste one) to the DI bottle.
17. In the fluidics station dialog box (on the computer), select "no probe array."
18. In the protocol field choose "Shutdown_450."
19. Check "all modules" when using all four modules, otherwise choose the "Shutdown_450" protocol for the respective modules.
20. Hit run to begin shutdown.
21. Shutdown takes about 10–15 min. After the protocol is over, shut down the machine with the switch located on the lower left side of the machine (*see* **Note 22**).

3.14 Scanning the Arrays

1. Turn on the scanner at least 10 min before use.
2. If the arrays were stored at 4 °C, allow them to warm to room temperature before scanning.
3. If necessary, clean the glass surface of the array with a non-abrasive towel or tissue before scanning. Do not use alcohol to clean the glass.
4. On the back of the array cartridge, clean excess fluid from around the septa.
5. Carefully cover both septa with Tough Spots. Press to ensure the spots remain flat.
6. Open the scanner lid and place the arrays in the carousel starting with position # 1.
7. Close the lid.
8. Click on Affymetrix Launcher icon on the computer, and hit Scanner control from the menu bar.
9. Hit "Start" from the scanner menu bar.

10. If you re-scan some of the chips, check the "allow rescan" box and then hit ok. Otherwise, uncheck it and just hit ok.
11. If you need to add additional arrays to the scanner in the middle of a run, hit "add chips"-> "add arrays after scan." Once scanning of the current array is completed, the lid of the scanner will become "unlocked" and more arrays can be added. After you close the lid hit" resume."
12. In case there is an error during scan and the array wasn't scanned (usually "fousuing error") cleaning again the array's glass might help (*see* **Note 23**).
13. When scanning, the green light is flashing. The light is stable when it's switching between arrays.
14. After scanning is done (green light is stable) take the arrays out of the carousel, and turn off the scanner.

4 Notes

1. Some of the Affymetrix reagents can be substituted with the following:
   - NspI enzyme and NspI 10× buffer (New England Biolabs, Ipswich, MA, USA).
   - T4 DNA Ligase enzyme and buffer (New England Biolabs, Ipswich, MA, USA).
   - Agencourt AMPure XP magnetic beads (Beckman Coulter, Brea, CA, USA).
   - Qiagen elution (EB) buffer (Qiagen, Germantown, MD, USA).
   - 75% Ethanol solution can be used instead of the Affymetrix wash buffer in the purification step.
2. Perform assays in designated areas (DNA extraction, Pre- PCR and Post- PCR areas).
3. Never bring amplified products into the Pre-PCR Clean Area.
4. Keep dedicated equipment in each room or area used for this protocol. To avoid contamination, do not move pipets between the Pre-PCR Clean Area and the Post-PCR Area.
5. It is essential to set up the digestion, ligation, and PCR reactions in the Pre-PCR clean room. This helps prevent contamination.
6. Prenatal samples, particularly, uncultured amniotic fluid, usually do not yield much DNA. We found that for these samples we can use a lower concentration than what is recommended by the manufacturer. We have used DNA concentrations as low as 2 ng/μL and the data was still good.

7. Preparing master mixes with a 15% excess ensures consistency in reagent preparation by minimizing pipetting errors and reducing handling time of temperature sensitive reagents. The success of this assay depends on the accurate pipetting and subsequent thorough mixing of small volumes of reagents.
8. Before making the mastermix, remove the enzyme from the freezer and immediately place in a cooler. Spin the enzyme for 3 s before adding to mastermix and then immediately add the enzyme to the master mix. Place the remaining enzyme back in the cooler.
9. If necessary, sample may be left in the PCR machine at 4 °C overnight.
10. When processing more than four samples, you should use a reservoir to aliquot the water and later the PCR mastermix to the samples, using a multichannel pipette.
11. 1 sample in this table represents one well of this sample. Since each sample is being multiplied by 4, the calculation should be × 4 plus the 15% excess.
12. In case where all four lanes of the negative show some DNA contamination, it is better to start the assay from the digestion step using new vials of reagents. However, if only one lane of the four shows contamination, it is most likely due to a splash during vortexing and it does not necessarily mean that there is an actual contamination.
13. Remember that each sample is diluted ×10, so the measurements should be multiplied by 10 in order to get the right yield.
14. If the sample yield is between 2.5 and 3 μg, it is still worth continuing with the sample to see if it passes the second QC point (which is the fragmentation gel electrophoresis). In situations where the sample is lower than 2.5 μg, it is better to re-PCR the sample.
15. If the sample fails any of the QC checks after PCR, before repeating the entire assay from scratch, you could try re-PCR the sample using the remaining diluted ligated DNA and then recheck the QC metrics.
16. Before making the mastermix, remove the fragmentation enzyme from the freezer and vortex it vigorously for 10 s. Immediately place in a cooler. Spin the enzyme for 3 s before adding to mastermix and then immediately add the enzyme to the master mix. Place the remaining enzyme back in the cooler.
17. It is very important to get the right sizing after fragmentation. If the samples show a "tail" as seen in the first three samples in the image, it is ok to proceed as long as most of the DNA is between 25 and 125 bp. Samples that look too fragmented or under fragmented should not be taken to the next step and should be re-amplified by PCR. Also samples that look faint

compared to the other samples on the gel should not be taken to the next step and should be re-amplified by PCR.

18. The priming takes about 10–15 min. In the meantime, prepare the staining solutions.
19. Forgetting to do so might not interfere with the washing process, but can damage the needle of the fluidics that needs to go through the septae.
20. The washing and staining takes about 1.5 h. Ten minutes before it ends, turn on the scanner for it to warm up (orange light is on). Once the scanner is ready the green light will be on.
21. It is very important to check the computer every once in a while during the wash for an error message. When there is fluid missing, an error message pops up. In this case, check the level of wash A and B in the bottle and make sure the tube is in the fluid. Make sure to hit "resume" so the wash will continue from where it stopped.
22. A cleaning protocol using sodium hypochlorite bleach should be performed on the Fluidics Stations biweekly or as needed. This is designed to eliminate any residual SAPE- antibody complex that may be present in the fluidics station tubing and needles. This protocol runs a bleach solution through the system followed by a rinse cycle with DI water.
23. Sometimes there are glue stains on the array glass. Simply use wet kimwipes with DI water to try and remove the stain.

Acknowledgments

We thank the technical staff at Affymetrix, who developed and standardized these protocols for use in a clinical laboratory. The members of clinical chromosomal array laboratory at Columbia University Medical Center are also acknowledged for setting up and fine-tuning these protocols.

References

1. American College of O., Gynecologists Committee on G (2013) Committee Opinion No. 581: the use of chromosomal microarray analysis in prenatal diagnosis. Obstet Gynecol 122 (6):1374–1377. https://doi.org/10.1097/01.AOG.0000438962.16108.d1
2. Wapner RJ, Martin CL, Levy B et al (2012) Chromosomal microarray versus karyotyping for prenatal diagnosis. N Engl J Med 367 (23):2175–2184. https://doi.org/10.1056/NEJMoa1203382

Chapter 14

Rapid Detection of Fetal Mendelian Disorders: Thalassemia and Sickle Cell Syndromes

Joanne Traeger-Synodinos, Christina Vrettou, and Emmanuel Kanavakis

Abstract

The inherited disorders of hemoglobin synthesis constitute the most common monogenic diseases world-wide. The clinical severity of β-thalassemia major and the sickle cell syndromes targets them as priority genetic diseases for prevention programs, which incorporates population screening to identify heterozygotes, with the option of prenatal diagnosis for carrier couples. Rapid genotype characterization is fundamental in the diagnostic laboratory, especially when offering prenatal diagnosis. The application of real-time PCR provides a means for rapid and potentially high throughput assays, without compromising accuracy. It has several advantages over end-point PCR analysis, including the elimination of post-PCR processing steps and a wide dynamic range of detection with a high degree of sensitivity. Although there are over 200 mutations associated with the β-thalassemia and sickle cell syndromes, the relatively small size of the β-, *HBB* gene (less than 2000 base-pairs) and the close proximity of most mutations facilitates the design of a minimal number of real-time PCR assays using the LightCycler™ system, which are capable of detecting the majority of most common β-gene mutations world-wide. These assays are highly appropriate for rapid genotyping of parental and fetal DNA samples with respect to β-thalassemia and sickle cell syndromes.

Key words Prenatal diagnosis, β-thalassemia and sickle cell syndromes, Real-time PCR

1 Introduction

Prenatal diagnosis (PND) aims to provide an accurate, rapid result as early in pregnancy as possible. A prerequisite involves obtaining fetal material promptly and safely. In addition, for monogenic diseases the parental mutation(s) have to be characterized prior to analysis of the fetal sample. The majority of methods currently used for genotyping parental samples and performing prenatal diagnosis are based on the polymerase chain reaction (PCR) (e.g., allele-specific oligonucleotide (ASO) hybridization analysis of PCR amplicons, amplification refractory mutation system (ARMS) PCR, restriction endonuclease analysis of PCR amplicons, and direct DNA sequencing). Most of these techniques are relatively simple, fairly quick and inexpensive (with the possible exception of

Brynn Levy (ed.), *Prenatal Diagnosis*, Methods in Molecular Biology, vol. 1885, https://doi.org/10.1007/978-1-4939-8889-1_14,

sequencing) but may not provide a rapid final genotype nor facilitate the processing of many samples simultaneously ("high through-put"). This can be a disadvantage with respect to identifying the parental mutations if the disease-associated gene has a wide spectrum of potential mutations. The application of real-time PCR offers a means for rapid and potentially high throughput assays, without compromising accuracy, making it an ideal approach for genotyping parental and fetal DNA samples in the context of prenatal diagnosis.

1.1 An Introduction to Real-Time PCR for Genotyping Applications

Real-time PCR integrates microvolume rapid-cycle PCR with fluorometry, allowing real-time fluorescent monitoring of the amplification reaction for quantitative PCR and/or qualitative characterization of PCR products. The latter application provides a means for rapid genotyping, precluding any post-PCR sample manipulation. Several real-time PCR instruments are available on the market, and in addition there are a number of detection chemistries, some of which can be used on any instrument and others which are instrument-specific. Real-time PCR machines can be classified as either "flexible" or high throughput. The "flexible" instruments, usually faster and with a wider choice of running parameters, are more suitable for smaller batches of samples, whereas the high throughput instruments are more appropriate for running large batches of samples requiring a smaller repertoire of assays. Flexible instruments are probably more appropriate for PND applications since the processing of samples in small batches precludes potential errors, e.g., through the occurrence of a tube-switch. However, high throughput instruments may be advantageous when screening parental samples to characterize mutations before performing the prenatal diagnosis.

There are a number of detection chemistries suitable for genotyping but those more commonly described for use in genotyping monogenic diseases include hybridization probes, Taqman probes and molecular beacons [1].

The protocol that we describe in this chapter employs the use of a flexible instrument (the LightCycler™ 1.0, LightCycler™ 1.5, or LightCycler™ 480 II, Roche Molecular Biochemicals) with "hybridization probes."

Hybridization probes [2] involve a dual probe system. The two fluorescently labeled probes hybridize to adjacent sequences within the amplified target DNA, one of which covers the region expected to contain the mutation(s). Close proximity of annealed probes facilitates fluorescence resonance energy transfer (FRET) between them, and a fluorescent signal is only generated when both of the probes are hybridized to the target amplicon (Fig. 1a). The two probes of the pair are designed to have different melting temperatures (Tm), whereby the probe with the lower Tm lies over the mutation site. Monitoring the emitted fluorescent signal under conditions of increasing temperature will detect a loss of

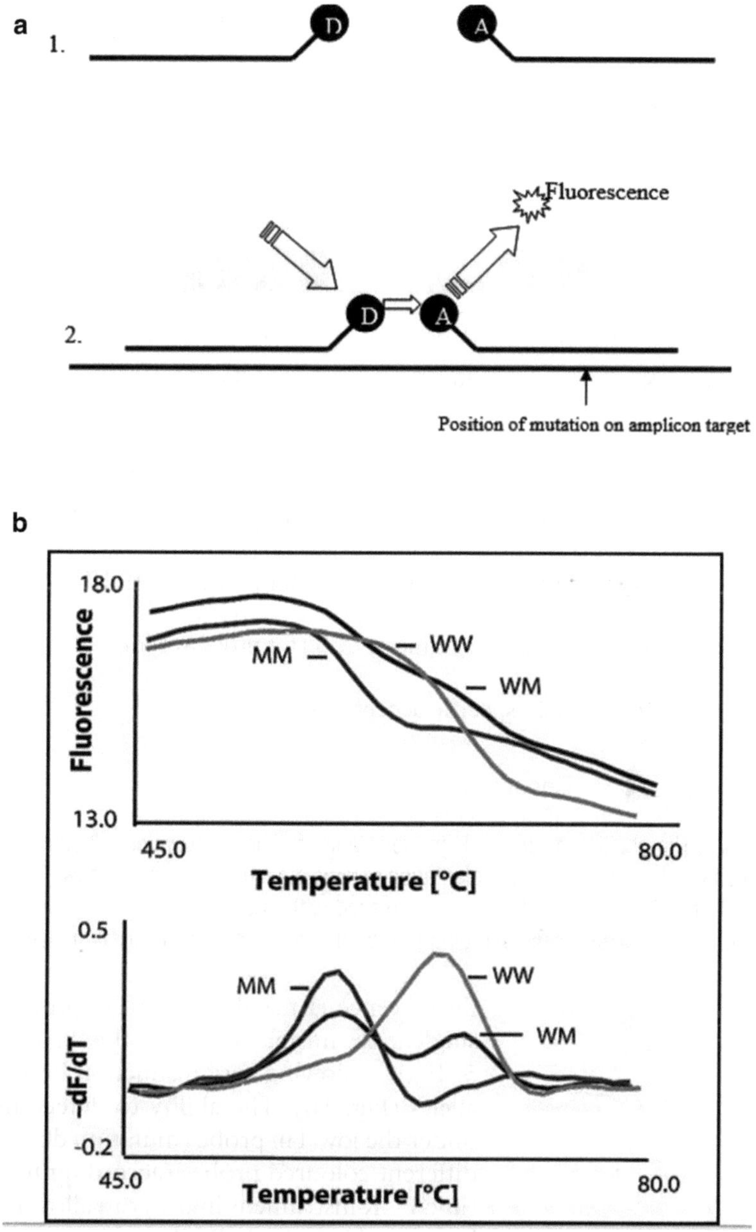

Fig. 1 (**a**) Principle of hybridization probes for allele discrimination. (1) One probe is labeled with a donor fluorophor (D) and the other with an acceptor fluorophore (A). The probe with the acceptor fluorophore is complimentary to the region including the expected mutation(s). (2) Close proximity of annealed probes facilitates fluorescence resonance energy transfer (FRET) and the emission of a fluorescent signal. (**b**) Plots of fluorescence versus temperature from melting curve analysis using hybridization probes. Top plot shows the raw melting peak data with fluorescence (F) versus temperature (T); Bottom plot shows the melting peaks displayed when the computer software automatically converts and displays the first negative derivative of fluorescence to temperature vs. temperature (-dF/dT vs. T). The latter facilitates easy discrimination between wild type and mutant alleles

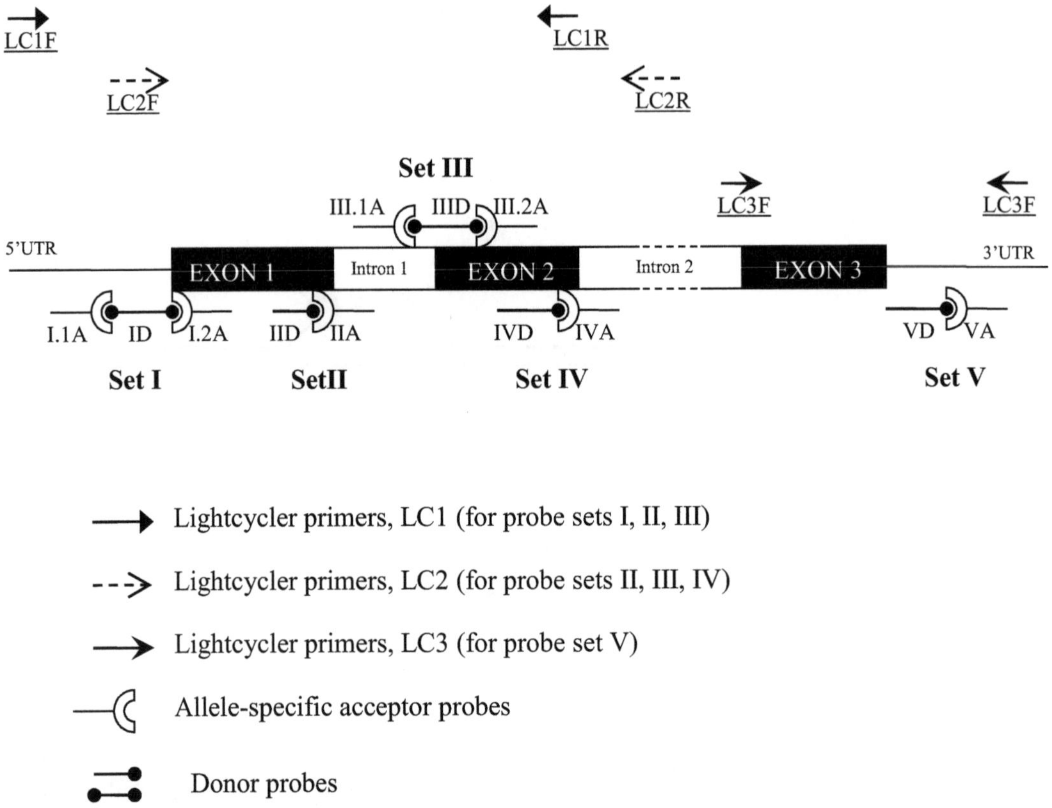

Fig. 2 The position of the β-globin gene primers and LightCycler™ hybridization probe sets appropriate for prenatal diagnosis and preimplantation genetic diagnosis protocols. Three PCR primer sets can be used (either LC1 or LC2, which can both be multiplexed with LC3 if required). F = forward primer; R = reverse primer. Probe sets I-V are used according to the mutations under investigation (see Table 1)

fluorescence (F) as the lower Tm probe melts off the template. A single base mismatch under this probe results in a Tm shift of 5–10 °C, allowing easy distinction between wild type and mutant alleles (Fig. 1b). The ability to detect any nucleotide mismatches under the low Tm probe (mutation detection probe) and the use of different coloured probes (according to the properties of the real-time PCR instrument in use) can allow more than one mutation to be assayed in a single PCR reaction (Fig. 2).

1.2 Molecular Basis of the β-Hemoglobinopathies and Design of Real-Time PCR Mutation Detection Assays

The β-globin gene (*HBB:* OMIM 141900) is a relatively small gene (<2000 bp) located in the short arm of chromosome 11. (11p15.5, GenBank: NM_000518). Although more than 200 causative mutations have been identified for β-thalassemia syndromes (HbVar http://globin.bx.psu.edu/hbvar/menu.html), the spectrum of mutations and their frequency in most populations usually includes a limited number of common mutations (e.g., up to approximately six) plus a slightly larger number of rare mutations (e.g., around 10). In most populations worldwide the majority of the most common mutations tend to cluster within small distances within *HBB*. The probes sets described in this chapter were designed based on those mutations most commonly found in the Mediterranean populations, although they are also suitable for detecting several of the common mutations found in other world populations (e.g., Asian Indian, SE Asian, and Chinese) [3, 4]. Overall they facilitate mutation detection with the use of a small number of probe sets within a minimal number of amplicons.

All the allele-specific (mutation-detection) probes described in this chapter were designed to be complementary to the wild-type sequence of *HBB*, rather than complementary to each specific mutation. This potentially allows the distinction of normal alleles from any allele with a nucleotide variation under the length of the probe, minimizing the number of assays that need to be performed, and potentially reducing costs and time required to identify the mutations in parental samples, and subsequently perform the PND. Although most mutations have a distinct melting profile and can be implicated by comparison with controls, the definitive characterization of each mutation should be achieved by a second method such as an ARMS-PCR assay [5, 6]. This is recommended for best-practice, and any laboratory performing DNA diagnostics and PND should have more than one available mutation detection method [7, 8].

The LightCycler™ PCR primers (sets LC1, LC2 and LC3) were designed with the aid of computer software (Amplify version 2.0, Bill Engels, 1992–1995). LC1 and LC2 amplify two overlapping regions of *HBB* surrounding the majority of the most common β-thalassemia mutations in all world populations, along with the HbS mutation, and when multiplexing mutation detection they should be selected according to the mutations under investigation (Table 1 and Fig. 2). LC3 amplifies a 3′ region of *HBB* which contains some rare β-thalassemia mutations and if necessary can be multiplexed with either set LC1 or LC2.

Design of LightCycler™ mutation detection probe sets took into account secondary structure properties (e.g., hairpin-loops) and potential primer-dimer formation between the probes themselves and the PCR primers, evaluated by computation prior to synthesis (TIB MOLBIOL, Berlin, Germany). In addition, design of mutation detection probes avoided the regions of *HBB* known to contain common polymorphic point mutations such as codon 2 (CAC > CAT). The LightCyclerTM systems 1.0 and 1.5 can detect 2 fluorescent labels (LightCyclerTM Red 640 [LC Red 640] and LightCyclerTM Red 705 [LC Red 705]), as well as SYBR® green. The choice of fluorescent label used, for each probe will depend upon the relative frequency of mutations in the population under study and the potential requirement for multiplexed assays when more than one mutation is investigated within a single sample. For example in the Greek population, HBB:c.93-21G>A

Table 1
Lightcycler mutation detection probe sets for the most common β-thalassemias mutations worldwide (and HbS mutation)

Probe set	Acceptor probe name and sequence	Donor probe name and sequence	Beta-gene mutation (s) detected	HGVS*** nomenclature
Set I	I.1A:	ID:	CAP +20 (C>T) *	HBB:c.−31C>T
	5′-ttc tga cac aac tgt gtt cac tag ca-3′ **LC Red****	**FITC** 5′-cct caa aca gac acc atg gtg cac c-3′ **FITC**	CAP+22 (G>A)	HBB:c.−29G>A
	I.2A:		HbS (Cd 6 A>T)	HBB:c.20A>T
	LC Red** 5′-gac tcc tga gga gaa gtc tgc-3′ **P**		Cd5 (−CT)	HBB:c.17_18delCT
			Cd6 (−A)	HBB:c.20delA
			Cd8 (−AA)	HBB:c.25_26delAA
			Cd 8/9 (+G)	HBB:c.27_28insG
Set II	IIA:	IID:	IVSI-1 (G>A)	HBB:c.92+1G>A
	LC Red** 5′-tgt aac ctt gat acc aac ctg ccc a-3′ **P**	5′-tgc cca gtt tct att ggt ctc ctt aaa cct gtc-3′ **FITC**	IVSI-1 (G>T)	HBB:c.92+1G>T
			IVSI-2 (T>G)	HBB:c.92+2T>G
			IVSI-2 (T>C)	HBB:c.92+2T>C
			IVSI-2 (T>A)	HBB:c.92+2T>A
			IVSI-5 (G>A)	HBB:c.92+5G>A
			IVSI-5 (G>C)	HBB:c.92+5G>C
			IVSI-5 (G>T)	HBB:c.92+5G>T
			IVSI-6 (T>C)	HBB:c.92+6T>C
Set III	III.1A:	IIID:	IVSI-110 (G>A)	HBB:c.93−21G>A
	5′-tct gcc tat tgg tct att ttc cc-3′ **LC Red****	**FITC** 5′-ccc tta ggc tgc tgg tgg tc-3′ **FITC**	IVSI-116 (T>G)	HBB:c.93−15T>G
	III.2A:		Cd39 (C>T)	HBB:c.118C>T
	LC Red** 5′-acc ctt gga ccc aga ggt tct t-3′ **P**		Cd37 (TGG>TGA)	HBB:c.114G>A
			Cd41/42 (delTTCT)	HBB: c.126_129delCTTT

Set IV	<u>IVA</u>: **LC Red**** 5′-tct cag gat cca cgt gca gct tg-3′**P**	<u>VID:</u> 5′-gtc cca tag act cac cct gaa g-3′ **FITC**.	IVSII-1(G>A)	HBB:c.315+1G>A
SetV	<u>VA:</u> **LC Red**** 5′gct caa ggc cct ttc ata ata tcc cc	<u>VD:</u> 5′ ttt ttc att agg cag aat cca ga-3′ **FITC.**	polyA signal mutation AATAAA>AACAAA AATAAA>AATGAA AATAAA>AATAGA AATAAA>AATAAG AATAAA>AA- - AA AATAAA>A- - - - -	HBB:c.*110T>C HBB:c.*111A>G HBB:c.*112A>G HBB:c.*113A>G HBB:c. [*109_*110delAT or *110_*111delTA] HBB:c. *108_*112delAATAA

The β-globin gene specific PCR primers include (see Fig. 2):
For probes sets I, II, III: **LC1F**: 5′-GCT GTC ATC ACT TAG ACC TCA-3′; **LC1R** 5′-CAC AGT GCA GCT CAC TCA G-3′;
For probes sets II, III,IV: **LC2F** 5′-CAA CTG TGT TCA CTA GCA AC-3′; **LC2R** 5′-AAA CGA TCC TGA GAC TTC CA-3′;
For probe set V: **LC3F** 5′-ATT TCT GAG TCC AAG CTG GGC -3′; **LC3R** 5′-AAA TGC ACT GAC CTC CCA-3′
FITC: Fluorescein; P = Phosphorylated
* = Polymorphism linked with the IVSII-745 (C>G) mutation ** LC Red: The fluorescent label used for each probe will depend upon the relative frequency of mutations in the population under study and the potential requirement of multiplexed assays. ***HGVS = Human Genome Variation Society

(IVSI-110 G>A) is the most common mutation, so the probes for most other mutations encountered in Greece are labeled with the opposite fluorescent marker to that used for HBB:c.93-21G>A. More specifically, two of the probe combinations (named set I and set III) include 2 acceptor (mutation detection) probes with one central donor probe, (Fig. 2), foreseeing the use of one or both acceptor probes of the set according to the needs of any genotyping assay. Each of the acceptor probes in sets I and III are labeled with different acceptor fluorophores and the central donor probe, designed to span the distance between the two acceptor probes, is labeled with a fluorescein (F) molecule at both 5′ and 3′ ends. Sets II and V were designed to screen for several neighboring mutations with use of a single mutation detection (acceptor) probe. Set IV was designed to detect a single mutation each and involved a donor probe which was labeled with fluorescein only at the end adjacent to the acceptor probe (Table 1, Fig. 2). In all sets the mutation-screening (acceptor) probes were designed to have a lower Tm relative to the donor probes, thereby ensuring that the fluorescent signal generated during the melting curve is determined only by the specificity of mutation-screening probe.

2 Materials

2.1 Equipment

The method described was set up using a LightCycler™ system instrument version 1.0 or 1.5 (Roche Diagnostics Corporation, Indianapolis, IN, USA) (*see* Subheading 4.1 **Notes 1** and **2**).

1. Aluminum cooling block, which holds 32 LightCycler™ Centrifuge Adapters (Roche Diagnostics Corporation, Indianapolis, IN, USA), in which the real-time PCR reactions are set up.
2. LightCycler™ glass capillary tubes (20 μl) (Roche Diagnostics Corporation, Indianapolis, IN, USA), in which the real-time PCR reactions are run in the LightCycler™ instrument.
3. A bench centrifuge with a well-depth of approximately 4.5 cm, for centrifugation (maximum 3000 × *g*) to pull the reaction volume (20 μl) to the base of the glass capillary, prior to loading in the LightCycler™ instrument.

2.2 Reagents

1. QIAMP DNA mini kit (Qiagen, Hilden, Germany) for extracting DNA from chorionic villi samples or amniocytes.
2. Pair(s)of PCR primers selected according to mutations under study (either LC1F/LC1R or LC2F/LC2R, if necessary with LC3F/LC3R, as shown in Table 1 and Fig. 2).
3. Fluorescently labeled mutation detection probe sets, appropriate for mutations under study (see Table 1 and Fig. 2).

4. LightCycler™ DNA Master Hybridization probes Kit (Roche Diagnostics Corporation, Indianapolis, IN, USA), which also includes $MgCl_2$ (25 mM) and PCR-grade water.

2.3 Handling and Storage of PCR Reagents

1. All PCR primers to be used on the LightCycler™ are diluted as stock solutions of 100 μM, divided into aliquots of convenient volume (e.g., 25 μl) and stored at −20 °C. For primer working solutions the stock solutions are diluted to 10 μM and can be subsequently stored at 4 °C for up to 3 months.
2. The LightCycler™ hybridization probes are diluted to 3 μM and stored in aliquots of relatively small volume (e.g., 20 μl) at −20 °C. A thawed aliquot should not be refrozen, but can be used up to 1 month when stored at 4 °C.
3. The "Master Mix" from the LightCycler™ -DNA Master Hybridization probes Kit should not be refrozen once thawed but can be used for up to 1 month when stored at 4 °C.

3 Methods

3.1 DNA Extraction from Chorionic Villi Samples or Amniocytes

The real-time PCR genotyping method described below assumes that assays are performed on good quality genomic DNA samples (parental or fetal) with a concentration of 30–50 ng/μl. Extract DNA using the QIAMP DNA mini kit according to the "Blood and Body Fluid Spin Protocol" outlined in the manual supplied with the kit.

3.2 Real-Time PCR Reaction Setup for the Lightcycler^{tm} 1.0 and 1.5 (See Subheading 4.2 Notes 1 and 2)

1. In an eppendorf tube make a premix for the amplification reactions for a total reaction volume of 20 μl (or 10 μl) per sample. Each reaction should contain the ready-to-use reaction mix provided by the manufacturer (LightCycler™ DNA Master Hybridization Probes) plus $MgCl_2$, a β-globin gene PCR primer pair (i.e., LC1, LC2, LCR3) and LightCycler™ fluorescent probe sets for the relevant mutations. A typical PCR reaction for single color detection for one sample is shown in Table 2.
2. When calculating the premix volume, make premix enough for the number of samples being genotyped, a PCR premix blank plus controls for the mutation(s) under investigation. The controls should include a homozygous wild-type sample (N/N), a sample heterozygous for the mutation (M/N) and a sample homozygous for the mutation (M/M).
3. Place the appropriate number of LightCyclerTM glass capillary tubes in the centrifuge adapters in an aluminum-cooling block.
4. Distribute accurately 18 μl (or 9 μl) of premix in all the capillaries.

Table 2
A typical PCR reaction for single color detection for one sample

	Stock Conc[a]	Final Conc[a]	[b]μl/sample
H_2O (PCR grade)			9.6 μl
$MgCl_2$	25 mM	4 mM	2.4 μl
Beta globin forward primer			
LC1(F) or LC2(F) or LC3(F)	10 μM	0.5 μM	1 μl
Beta globin reverse primer			
LC1(R) or LC2(R) or LC3(R)	10 μM	0.5 μM	1 μl
LC Red allele-specific			
probe (640 or 705)	3 μM	0.15 μM	1 μl
FITC donor	3 μM	0.15 μM	1 μl
Master Mix			2 μl
Premix volume			**18 μl**
DNA sample volume			**2 μl**
Total reaction volume			**20 μl[b]**

The volume of water is always adjusted to give final reaction volume of 20 μl/sample even when more than one primer or probe set is included in the reaction. For example a PCR reaction with dual color detection using 2 allele-specific LC probes (one labeled with Red 640 and the other with Red 705) and a common (central) doubly labeled FITC probe, or even two sets of LC donor-acceptor probes (i.e., 4 probes)

[a]Conc = concentration

[b]All volumes in the reaction may be halved without compromising the result

5. Add 2 μl (or 1 μl) genomic DNA (approximately 50 ng) per sample and controls, and finally add the same volume of double-distilled water to the PCR blank.
6. Once the PCR reactions have been set up in the capillaries at 4 °C place the caps carefully on each capillary without pressing down completely yet.
7. Remove the aluminum centrifuge adaptors containing the capillaries from the cooling block and place in a bench centrifuge with wells deep enough to hold the aluminum centrifuge adaptors (approximately 4.5 cm).
8. Spin at a maximum speed of 3000 × *g* for 10 s to pull the reaction volume to the base of the glass capillary.
9. Place each glass capillary carefully into the LightCycler™ carousel by letting it simply "slip" in place. Then gently press the cap completely in to the capillary and simultaneously the glass capillary fully down into position in the LightCycler™ carousel.

10. Put the loaded carousel in to the LightCycler™ and initiate the PCR cycles and melting curve protocols using the LightCycler software version 3.5.1, according to the manufacturer's specifications.

3.3 Amplification and Melting Curve Analysis

1. Preprogram the LightCycler™ software (according to the instrument model and the manufacturer's guidelines) for the following amplification steps: a first denaturation step of 30 s at 95 °C followed by 40 cycles of 95 °C for 3 s, 58 °C for 5 s and 72 °C for 20 s with a temperature ramp of 20 °C/s. During the PCR, emitted fluorescence can be measured at the end of the annealing step of each amplification cycle to monitor progression of amplification.
2. Immediately after the amplification step, the LightCycler™ is programmed to perform melting curve analysis to determine the genotypes. This involves a momentary rise of temperature to 95 °C, cooling to 45 °C for 2 min to achieve maximum probe hybridization, and then heating to 85 °C with a rate of 0.4 °C/s during which time the melting curve is recorded.
3. Emitted fluorescence is measured continuously (by both channels F2 (640 nm) and F3 (705 nm) if necessary) to monitor the dissociation of the fluorophore-labeled detection probes from the complementary single-stranded DNA (F/T) (*F*: Fluorescence emitted, *T*: Temperature). The computer software automatically converts and displays the first negative derivative of fluorescence to temperature versus temperature (-dF/dT vs. T) and the resulting melting peaks allow easy discrimination between wild type and mutant alleles (Fig. 1b).

4 Notes

4.1 LightCycler

1. The assay reactions described have also been used on a LightCyclerTM 480 II instrument without any modifications.
2. The Real-time PCR reaction set up for the LightCyclerTM 480 II is done in 96-well plates, sealed with Lightcycler 480 Sealing Foil, which precludes the use of adaptors, capillaries and caps as described in Subheading 3.2.

4.2 Melting Curves

1. Trouble with melting curve analysis usually occurs when a relatively high number of samples are included in a single run. Under these circumstances wide melting peaks are observed with only minor differences in the central Tm peak of the melting curve for all genotypes, e.g., M/M, N/N, and M/N; furthermore heterozygous DNAs will not give a double peak following melting curve analysis but a single peak which lies between that of the N/N and M/M controls/ samples.

2. The LightCyclerTM (system 1.0 and 1.5, software version 3.5) is designed to run a maximum of 32 samples in a single run, but our experience indicates that analysis of more than approximately 20 samples produces wide and "flattened" melting curves. The problem is probably due to the way that the LightcyclerTM performs the melting curve analysis. During the LightCyclerTM melting curve analysis the temperature increases from 45 °C to 90 °C, which takes about 150 s when using the "continuous acquisition" mode and a temperature increment of 0.3 °C/s. In "continuous acquisition" mode the temperature increases continuously, and does not take in to account that the measurement of fluorescence between one capillary and the next takes a certain time. If a small number of samples are analyzed, the fluorescence of each will be read more often during the 150 s of melting curve data acquisition, compared to a run with more samples. In the latter situation there are too few measurement points to calculate a detailed melting curve. There are three possible solutions to this problem:
   (a) For high sample numbers it is recommended that the temperature increment used for the melting curve is decreased, e.g., to 0.1 °C/s when using "continuous acquisition" mode, or to 0.4 °C/s when using "stepwise acquisition" mode.
   (b) If the melting curve still fails to give a satisfactory result, we have found that additional melting curves can be performed using other temperature increments, although it must be noted that the quality of the melting curves is reduced each time an analysis is performed (and this is not recommended by the manufacturer).
   (c) In cases when the melting curve still fails to give satisfactory result when analyzing more than about 20 samples, pause the LightCycler™ program following the amplification step and perform melting curve analyses in batches (including the appropriate controls with each melting curve analysis).

References

1. Wilhelm J, Pingoud A (2003) Real-time polymerase chain reaction. Chembiochem 4 (11):1120–1128. https://doi.org/10.1002/cbic.200300662
2. Lyon E (2001) Mutation detection using fluorescent hybridization probes and melting curve analysis. Expert Rev Mol Diagn 1(1):92–101. https://doi.org/10.1586/14737159.1.1.92
3. Vrettou C, Traeger-Synodinos J, Tzetis M, Malamis G, Kanavakis E (2003) Rapid screening of multiple beta-globin gene mutations by real-time PCR on the LightCycler: application to carrier screening and prenatal diagnosis of thalassemia syndromes. Clin Chem 49(5):769–776
4. Vrettou C, Traeger-Synodinos J, Tzetis M, Palmer G, Sofocleous C, Kanavakis E (2004) Real-time PCR for single-cell genotyping in sickle cell and thalassemia syndromes as a rapid, accurate, reliable, and widely applicable protocol for preimplantation genetic diagnosis. Hum

Mutat 23(5):513–521. https://doi.org/10.1002/humu.20022

5. Old JM, Varawalla NY, Weatherall DJ (1990) Rapid detection and prenatal diagnosis of beta-thalassaemia: studies in Indian and Cypriot populations in the UK. Lancet 336 (8719):834–837
6. Kanavakis E, Traeger-Synodinos J, Vrettou C, Maragoudaki E, Tzetis M, Kattamis C (1997) Prenatal diagnosis of the thalassaemia syndromes by rapid DNA analytical methods. Mol Hum Reprod 3(6):523–528
7. Old J, Petrou M, Varnavides L, Layton M, Modell B (2000) Accuracy of prenatal diagnosis for haemoglobin disorders in the UK: 25 years' experience. Prenat Diagn 20(12):986–991
8. Traeger-Synodinos J, Harteveld CL, Old JM, Petrou M, Galanello R, Giordano P, Angastioniotis M, De la Salle B, Henderson S, May A, Ehbp m (2015) EMQN Best Practice Guidelines for molecular and haematology methods for carrier identification and prenatal diagnosis of the haemoglobinopathies. Eur J Hum Genet 23(4):426–437. https://doi.org/10.1038/ejhg.2014.131

Chapter 15

Prenatal Diagnosis of Cystic Fibrosis

Anastasia M. Fedick, Jinglan Zhang, Lisa Edelmann, and Ruth Kornreich

Abstract

Cystic fibrosis (CF) is an inherited disease characterized by the accumulation of thick, sticky mucus which damages epithelia in organs such as the lungs, pancreas, liver, intestines, and other parts of the body. The most common symptoms are sinopulmonary disease and chronic gastrointestinal tract problems resulting from decreased mucociliary clearance and inflammation. CF is the most common life-limiting autosomal recessive disorder in people of northern European ancestry and it affects other populations with different prevalence. CF can be diagnosed by many methods including testing for blood immunoreactive trypsin, sweat chloride, transepithelial nasal potential difference, and molecular genetic testing.

Key words Cystic fibrosis, Recessive, Mutation, Chronic pulmonary disease, Congenital bilateral absence or atrophy of the vas deferens

1 Introduction

Cystic fibrosis (CF) is a severe autosomal recessive disease with its highest prevalence found in Caucasian populations at an estimated one in 2000–3000 births. The major clinical symptoms of CF include chronic pulmonary disease leading to progressive lung failure, pancreatic exocrine insufficiency, and male infertility due to congenital bilateral absence or atrophy of the vas deferens (CBAVD) or obstructive azoospermia. Respiratory failure is responsible for 80–95% of CF mortalities, which usually occur around the age of 37. Symptoms of CF usually present in early childhood, however there are rare instances of adult diagnoses. Although multidisciplinary care for CF is available, its morbidity and mortality often results from airway obstruction and pulmonary defense system impairment associated with chronic infection and neutrophil inflammation of the small and large airways. Persistent infections, especially with Pseudomonas aeruginosa and *Staphylococcus aureus*, cause chronic sputum production, and eventually bronchiectasis and lung destruction.

Brynn Levy (ed.), *Prenatal Diagnosis*, Methods in Molecular Biology, vol. 1885, https://doi.org/10.1007/978-1-4939-8889-1_15,

1.1 Molecular Genetics of Cystic Fibrosis

CF is a monogenic disorder caused by mutations in the *CFTR* gene. The CF disease gene, cystic fibrosis transmembrane conductance regulator (*CFTR*), was identified in 1989 [1, 2]. *CFTR* is a transmembrane protein that consists of five domains: two membrane-spanning segments each consisting of six regions (TM1-TM12) that form the chloride channel pore, two ATP-binding domains (NBF1 and NBF2) that control channel activity by interacting with cytosolic nucleotides, and a regulatory domain that also controls channel activity via phosphorylation [3]. The *CFTR* gene is ~215 kb in size and located on chromosome 7q31.2 with 26 introns and 27 exons. Over 1980 mutations have been reported to date in the Cystic Fibrosis Mutation Database (www.genet.sickkids.on.ca/cftr/app) including missense, nonsense, frameshift, splicing, and small and large insertions or deletions, located in both the promoter region and throughout the entire gene. Mutations in CF patients are usually inherited from both of their carrier parents although de novo *CFTR* mutations occur very rarely. Uniparental disomy (UPD) of chromosome 7 resulting in homozygosity of a *CFTR* mutation has also rarely been causative of CF [4–6], as well as mosaicism for UPD7 [7].

CFTR mutations can be categorized into five different groups based on the impact that they have on gene function. Class I mutations cause defective protein production due to premature stop codons, Class II mutations block protein processing due to mislocalization, Class III mutations effect the nucleotide binding domains causing errors in regulation and non-functional chloride channels, Class IV mutations effect the membrane spanning domains and impact conductance and/or gating properties, and Class V mutations include those that reduce the synthesis of the *CFTR* protein [3, 8]. While phenotype-genotype correlations have not been established using the above categorization for most CF phenotypes, there has been a correlation observed for most category I, II, and III mutations with severe pancreatic-insufficiency [3, 8].

The three base pair deletion of phenylalanine at position 508 (c.1521_1523delCTT, p.Phe508del) is the most common CF mutation, accounting for approximately two-thirds of all cases [9]. While CF is pan-ethnic, various ethnic populations have different risks of being carriers for the disease [10]. CF is most common in Ashkenazi Jews (carrier frequency of 1 in 25) and Caucasians (carrier frequency of 1 in 26) and least common in Asians (carrier frequency of 1 in 94). Certain mutations are also more prevalent in specific ethnic populations due to founder effects, such as the c.3846G>A, p.Trp1282X mutation in the Ashkenazi Jewish population which accounts for around 60% of all mutations [11] and the c.3302T>A, p.Met1101Lys mutation in the Hutterites of South Dakota which accounts for around 69% of all mutations [12].

When conducting molecular genetic tests, especially targeted genotyping assays, false positive results can occur if there is a variant at or near the same location of a known mutation. For example, three variants: c.1516A>G, p.Ile506Val; c.1519A>G, p.Ile507Val; and c.1523T>G, p.Phe508Cys have been known to cause erroneous results when testing for the c.1519_1521delATC, p.Ile507del or c.1521_1523delCTT deletions. Depending on the method used, it may be necessary to test for the additional variants whenever a c.1521_1523delCTT mutation is identified. It is particularly evident when an individual who is a carrier for the deletion appears to be homozygous because he or she is also a carrier for one of the above non-pathogenic variants. In such instances where the patient does not show any symptoms of CF, follow-up tests should be done for those specific variants to ensure that the results are accurate [13].

1.2 Genetic Testing for Cystic Fibrosis: Carrier and Diagnosis

The American College of Obstetricians and Gynecologists (ACOG) and The American College of Medical Genetics (ACMG) both published guidelines for prenatal and preconception carrier screening for CF in 2001. Both committees originally recommended conducting carrier screening for 25 common mutations that caused classic CF and had mutant allele frequencies of 0.1% or greater in the general United States population. The ACMG then updated their recommendation in 2004 and removed two mutations: c.948delT, p.Phe316LeufsX12 due to an observed frequency of less than 0.1% and c.443T>C, p.Ile148Thr because it is not a true pathogenic variant (it can occur in cis with the severe CF mutation c.3067_3072delATAGTG, p.Ile1023_Val1024del), reducing the recommended panel to 23 mutations. By screening for the 23 mutations, it is estimated that the approximate carrier risk after a negative test drops from 1:24 to 1:380 for Ashkenazi Jews, 1:25 to 1:200 for non-Hispanic whites, 1:58 to 1:200 for Hispanic whites, 1:61 to 1:170 for African Americans, and 1:94 to 1:180 for Asian Americans [14]. Genetic counseling is recommended both pre- and post-testing so that patients understand their remaining residual risk of having an affected child, especially based on ethnic background and test detection rates [15].

Since the publication of the guidelines in 2001, it has been routine for most pregnant women to have CF testing. When undergoing carrier screening, couples can choose to either be tested at the same time or in tiers, where one partner is screened first and the second is only screened if the first is found to be a carrier. In the event that one partner is determined to be a carrier of a common mutation, the second partner may want to be screened for more than just the mutations recommended by ACMG or ACOG due to the high heterogeneity of *CFTR*. For targeted mutations, low throughput genotyping methods were originally used to diagnose individuals, which included: the classic dot blot involving target

DNA immobilized on a membrane and then hybridized to a labeled probe, the reverse dot blot which had an unlabeled probe immobilized on a membrane and then hybridized to a labeled PCR product, and gel-based restriction enzyme analysis which involved DNA being cut at specific restriction sites and then run on gels to genotype based on band sizes and patterns. Now with the advent of high throughput genotyping, new methods involving fluorescent-based or molecular weight-based allelic discrimination are utilized which has allowed for many commercial laboratories to offer targeted mutation panels that extend beyond those specifically recommended by ACOG or ACMG. Sequencing can also be used for diagnostic purposes or even for screening [16], which would involve either Sanger or next generation sequencing, or a combination of both methods.

The ACMG has also recommended that reflex testing be done if carrier screening indicates that an individual has the c.350G>A, p.Arg117His mutation. Different phenotypes have been associated with the c.350G>A mutation depending on whether it is found in cis or trans with the 5T/7T/9T variant. If the 5T variant is found in trans with c.350G>A, then the CBAVD phenotype occurs without any other symptoms of CF, while if it is found in cis, classical CF is expressed. Since the frequency of the 5T variant alone is high in the general population, however, it is only recommended to screen for this variant if the c.350G>A mutation is detected first [17].

While the diagnosis of CF is typically performed by molecular genetic testing, confirmation is usually done via a sweat test which measures the amount of salt in a patient's sweat, with high salt levels confirming the diagnosis. Once a diagnosis of CF has been made, additional tests can include chest X-rays as well as lung function tests to monitor the pulmonary phenotype, a sinus X-ray to look for sinusitis, which can be a complication of CF, and sputum cultures to look for pulmonary infection with *Pseudomonas aeruginosa*, which is a bacteria that indicates advanced CF [18].

Currently, preconception carrier screening for couples is only recommended, however newborn screening for CF is required in all states in the United States. Testing can involve a two-tier system where immunoreactive trypsinogen (IRT) analysis is done first on dried neonatal blood spots, followed by DNA analysis for either the common delta c.1521_1523delCTT mutation or other CF mutations if the IRT levels are high [19].

1.3 Prenatal Testing and Counseling

Preconception screening is very important for couples so that they can make informed decisions about their reproductive options. If a couple is found to be at an increased-risk of having an affected child due to both parents carrying a mutation, the couple can consider preimplantation genetic diagnosis (PGD) on embryos at a fertility clinic so that only embryos known not to have CF will be candidates for implantation. Couples can also choose to conceive naturally but then undergo prenatal testing with the option of elective abortion if the fetus is found to be affected. Using donor sperm or eggs is another option, especially when the fathers are affected with CF since these men have high rates of infertility, as well as adoption.

Prenatal testing for CF should be offered in instances of increased risk either through direct or cultured chorionic villus sampling (CVS) at 10–12 weeks or amniocentesis at 15–18 weeks. Since CF screening is recommended for all pregnant women followed by partner screening in the case of carrier status, targeted mutation analysis can be done on the prenatal sample for the mutation(s) known to be present in the parents. In addition to known carrier status of the parents or a family history of CF, fetal intestinal obstruction, congenital viral infection, and intra-amniotic bleeding are other prenatal symptoms that can be associated with CF and indicate that molecular testing should be performed. Meconium ileus, which is a bowel obstruction that occurs when a newborn's stool is thicker and sticker than normal, is observed in 10–20% of newborns that have CF, and since it can be seen in second-trimester ultrasounds as an echogenic bowel, it can also be used as a prenatal predictor of CF [20]. In instances of ultrasound indications, molecular testing of the parents to identify the known mutation(s) is preferred, followed by testing the fetus in the same laboratory. If only one mutation is found in the fetus, its risk of being affected with CF can range from 13 to 43% based on the prior empirical risk, while the detection of two mutations would be diagnostic and the detection of no mutations decreases the risk to less than 1 in 645 for Caucasian fetuses [21].

Whenever prenatal testing is being performed, it is always important to test both the maternal blood sample and the fetal sample to ensure that there is no maternal cell contamination (MCC). Cytogenetic data has indicated that MCC can occur in 0.6–1.0% of cultured amniocytes, 0.1–0.9% of direct CVS, and 1.8–12.6% of cultured CVS [22]. Testing for MCC can be done by comparing the maternal and fetal samples using microsatellite or other polymorphic markers.

2 Materials

2.1 DNA Extraction

1. PureGene™ Genomic DNA purification kit (Qiagen, Germantown, MD, USA).

2.2 DNA-Based Molecular Diagnosis: Sanger Sequencing

CFTR PCR primers must span all exons and at least 20 nt of intronic sequences must be M13 tagged (for standardization of assays—not necessary for all laboratories) and synthesized by an established facility.

1. Primer working solutions: Prepare a 10 μM primer working solution.

Table 1
Sequences for *CFTR* coding exon gene specific primers

	Primer Sequence (5′ → 3′)		
Exon	Forward	Reverse	Product Length (bp)
1	CCCAGAGTAGTAGGTCTTTGGC	AAACCCAACCCATACACACG	204
2	GTGCATAATTTTCCATATGCC	ttagccaccatacttggctC	341
3	GGGTTAATCTCCTTGGATATAC TTG	TTCACCAGATTTCGTAGTC TTTTC	305
4	TCTTGTGTTGAAATTCTCAGGG	AAAACTACAACAGAGGCAG TTTACAG	525
5	GAACCTGAGAAGATAGTAAGC TAGATG	GAAAACTCCGCCTTTCCAG	321
6	TGATCATATAAGCTCCTTTTAC TTGC	TCCTGGTTTTACTAAAGTGGGC	343
7	TGCCCATCTGTTGAATAAAAG	CAAACATCAAATATGAGG TGGAAG	340
8	cttccattccaAGATCCCTG	TGAACATTCCTAGTATTAGC TGGC	476
9	TGCTTGGCAAATTAAC TTTAGAAC	gcACCTGGCCATTCCTCTAC	440
10	CAGTGTAATGGATCATGGGC	TGGAGAAGAGGATGACCACTG	853
11	cccttgtatcttttgtgcatagc	AACCGATTGAATATGGAGCC	465
12	GGAAGATGTGCCTTTCAAATTC	CCCACTAGCCATAAAACCCC	301
13	TGCATGTAGTGAACTG TTTAAGG	TGCAATCTATGATGGGACAG	255
14a	AAATGCTAAAATACGAGACATA TTGC	TCTTCGATGCCATTCATTTG	485
14b	GAAGGAGATGCTCCTGTCTCC	CTACTCAATTGCATTCTGTGGG	529
15	ACAATGGTGGCATGAAACTG	TGAGCTTTCGAATCTCTTAACC	547
16	AATTTAGATGTGGGCATGGG	GGATTACAATACATACAAACA TAGTGG	201
17	GGTTAAGGGTGCATGCTCTTC	AAAGCCAGCACTGCCATTAG	473
18	GAGAAATTGGTCGTTACTTGAA TC	GCAATAGACAGGACTTCAACCC	457
19	GACTAGGAATAGAA TGGGGAGAGTA	CATTTGGGAACCCAGAGAAA	1055
20	TCTATTCAAAGAATGGCACCAG	CAATGGAAATTCAAAGAAA TCAC	549

(continued)

Table 1
(continued)

	Primer Sequence (5′ → 3′)		
Exon	**Forward**	**Reverse**	**Product Length (bp)**
21	TGGTTGAATACTTACTATA TGCAGAGC	TGACAGATACACAGTGACCCTC	449
22	AGCAAGTGTTGCATTTTACAAG	GCTAACACATTGCTTCAGGC	428
23	GGTGACAGGATAAAATATTCCAA TG	TTGCAGAGTAATATGAATTTC TTGAG	362
24	TGATGGTAAGTACATGGGTG TTTC	TTGTGCACACACATACATGC	334
25	TCAAATGGTGGCAGGTAGTG	GTGTCACCATGAAGCAGGC	385
26	CTACCCCATGGTTGAAAAGC	TGAGTAAAGCTGGATGGCTG	421
27	CAAAATGCAAGGCTCTGGAC	TCCTCAATTCCCCTTACCAA	494

CFTR PCR primers were M13 tagged (not shown on the above table)

2. Molecular biology grade water.
3. dNTPs.
4. Platinum Taq DNA Polymerase.
5. 10× PCR Buffer.
6. 50 mM $MgCl_2$.
7. Shrimp Alkaline Phosphatase.
8. Exonuclease (USB, Thermo Fisher Scientific, Waltham, MA, USA).
9. Primer sequences are described in Table 1.

2.3 DNA-Based Molecular Diagnosis: CF60 Luminex

1. xTAG Cystic Fibrosis 60 kit v2 (Luminex Corporation, Austin, TX, USA).

3 Methods

3.1 CFTR Gene Sequence Analysis by Sanger Sequencing

3.1.1 DNA Preparation, PCR, and Sequencing

1. Extract DNA from prenatal cells using the PureGene™ Genomic DNA purification kit (*see* **Note 1**).
2. Dilute purified DNAs to a concentration of 50 ng/μL.
3. Prepare PCR master mix for the number of samples to be tested including a reagent blank and two extra for pipetting.
4. Distribute a 1.0 μL aliquot of the prepared DNAs (50 ng/μL) to thin-walled PCR (0.2 mL) tubes with 1.2 μL of exon F/R

primer mix (10 μM working solution), 15.4 μL distilled water, 2.5 μL 10× PCR buffer, 0.75 mM $MgCl_2$, 4.0 μL 0.2 μM dNTP, and 0.2 μL Platinum Taq (5 U/μL).

5. Run the following PCR profile: 95 °C for 5 min (95 °C for 30 s, 60 °C for 30 s, 72 °C for 30 s) × 35, 72 °C for 7 min and 4 °C hold.
6. Perform Exo/SAP treatment to clean up the PCR products (2.5 μL Shrimp Alkaline Phosphatase and 1 μL Exonuclease). Process the reactions in a thermal cycler programmed as follows: 37 °C for 30 min, 99 °C for 15 min, 4 °C hold.
7. Perform bi-directional DNA sequencing for *CFTR* exon (s) with 8–20 ng of the purified PCR product using procedures recommended by the manufacturer.

3.1.2 Sanger Sequencing Analysis

1. Separate PCR products by electrophoresis in agarose gels to ensure proper amplification, which should demonstrate a single strong band with the expected size for each exon to be analyzed. The blank must not contain any amplification products. If there is contamination in blank, all PCR reagents should be discarded and new amplification reactions should be set up.
2. The chromatograms containing the sequencing data should have unique, nonoverlapping peaks for homozygous samples. A heterozygous missense or nonsense mutation will produce an overlapped peak at the mutant position and deletion or insertion in one strand will produce overlapped peaks at all positions after the change. Sequencing results must show the variation in both the forward and reverse directions.

3.2 CFTR Targeted Mutation Analysis by Luminex Beads-Based Genotyping

3.2.1 CF60: DNA Preparation, PCR and ASPE

1. Extract DNAs for *CFTR* genotyping from blood samples or direct or cultured prenatal cells using the PureGene™ Genomic DNA Purification Kit (*see* **Note 2**).
2. For multiplex PCR, add the following into each specimen tube: 9.75 μL DNase and RNase Free Distilled Water, 5.0 μL 5× Platinum Tfi Reaction Buffer, 1.75 μL Tfi 50 mM $MgCl_2$, 2.5 μL xTAG CFTR PCR Primer Mix V2, 1 μL Platinum Tfi exo(−) DNA Polymerase and 5.0 μL of appropriate DNA sample.
3. Run the following PCR profile: 94 °C for 2 min, (94 °C for 15 s, 58 °C for 30 s, 72 °C for 30 s) × 30, 72 °C for 5′ and 4 °C hold. Set the thermal cycler temperature as BLOCK Temperature with the heated lid enabled.
4. Prepare Enzyme Mix as follows: 2.5 μL Shrimp Alkaline Phosphatase and 1.0 μL Exonuclease I. Add 3.7 μL of the Enzyme Mix into each of the PCR tubes. Incubate the tubes in a thermal cycler programmed as follows: 37 °C for 30 min and 99 °C for 5 min and 4 °C hold.

5. For multiplex ASPE, there will be two different ASPE Master Mixes (A and B). Add the reagents in the order listed below to prepare the ASPE A Master Mix: 6.8 μL DNase and RNase Free Distilled Water, 4.0 μL 5× Platinum Tfi Reaction Buffer, 1.2 μL Tfi 50 mM $MgCl_2$, 2.0 μL xTAG ASPE Primer A Mix v2, and 1.0 μL Platinum Tfi exo(−) DNA Polymerase. For the ASPE B Master Mix, repeat the above steps, but instead use xTAG ASPE Primer B Mix v2. Add 5.0 μL of the same treated PCR product to both ASPE Master Mixes. Cap each tube immediately after addition of sample.
6. Place tubes in thermal cycler and cycle under the following conditions: 94 °C for 2 min, (94 °C for 15 s, 56 °C for 30 s, 74 °C for 30 s) × 30, 99 °C for 5 min and 4 °C hold. Set the thermal cycler temperature as BLOCK temperature with the heated lid enabled.
7. Thaw and bring both the xTAG CFTR Bead Mix A v2 and the xTAG CFTR Bead Mix B v2to room temperature, limiting its exposure to light.
8. Vortex the A and B Bead Mixes for 10 s and then sonicate for 10 s to disperse the beads. Repeat this step.
9. Vortex for several seconds and aliquot 22.5 μL of the A Bead Mix into one set of eight labeled tubes, and aliquot 22.5 μL of the B Bead Mix into a different set of eight labeled tubes.
10. Aliquot 2.5 μL of the A ASPE product into the A Bead Mix tube and aliquot 2.5 μL of the B ASPE product into the B Bead Mix tube.
11. Place tubes in a thermocycler programmed as follows: 96 °C for 2 min, 37 °C for 30 min, and 37 °C hold.
12. Before proceeding to the next step (about 5 min before completion of the half hour incubation) prepare the Reporter Solution. Vortex the tube of Streptavidin, R-Phycoerythrin (SA-PE) conjugate for 2–5 s. For one sample, add 1.25 μL of SA-PE to 123.75 μL of xTAG 1× Wash Buffer.
13. Add 100 μL reporter (made from above step) to each well, briefly pipette up and down and transfer into Costar plate. There will be both an "A" plate or column and a "B" plate or column.
14. Incubate the plate(s) at room temperature for 15 min. Run samples on Luminex machine according to manufacturer's instructions.

3.2.2 CF60: Results Analysis for CFTR Genotyping Using Luminex Bead Technology

1. Data interpretation is accomplished using the TDAS CFTR Analysis Software.
2. Select both the "A" and "B" output data files that you want to analyze and analyze them using the xTAG Cystic Fibrosis v2 assay with 60 variations detected.

3. A negative control (blank) must be included in every run. Identify your negative control in the software.
4. In the Mask Editor dialog box, click on both checkboxes next to the ACMG Panel column header and the Full Panel column header.
5. Positive control samples are rotated on each run. If the signals obtained for the blank are too high, the run is invalid and must be repeated. Samples with insufficient signals or low bead counts are repeated.

4 Notes

1. Any equivalent DNA extraction method may be used.
2. The QIASymphony DNA extraction Technology or any equivalent DNA extraction method may be used.

References

1. Riordan JR, Rommens JM, Kerem B, Alon N, Rozmahel R, Grzelczak Z, Zielenski J, Lok S, Plavsic N, Chou JL et al (1989) Identification of the cystic fibrosis gene: cloning and characterization of complementary DNA. Science 245(4922):1066–1073
2. Rommens JM, Iannuzzi MC, Kerem B, Drumm ML, Melmer G, Dean M, Rozmahel R, Cole JL, Kennedy D, Hidaka N et al (1989) Identification of the cystic fibrosis gene: chromosome walking and jumping. Science 245(4922):1059–1065
3. Welsh MJ, Smith AE (1993) Molecular mechanisms of CFTR chloride channel dysfunction in cystic fibrosis. Cell 73 (7):1251–1254
4. Spence JE, Perciaccante RG, Greig GM, Willard HF, Ledbetter DH, Hejtmancik JF, Pollack MS, O'Brien WE, Beaudet AL (1988) Uniparental disomy as a mechanism for human genetic disease. Am J Hum Genet 42 (2):217–226
5. Voss R, Ben-Simon E, Avital A, Godfrey S, Zlotogora J, Dagan J, Tikochinski Y, Hillel J (1989) Isodisomy of chromosome 7 in a patient with cystic fibrosis: could uniparental disomy be common in humans? Am J Hum Genet 45(3):373–380
6. Le Caignec C, Isidor B, de Pontbriand U, David V, Audrezet MP, Ferec C, David A (2007) Third case of paternal isodisomy for chromosome 7 with cystic fibrosis: a new patient presenting with normal growth. Am J Med Genet A 143A(22):2696–2699. https://doi.org/10.1002/ajmg.a.31999
7. Reboul MP, Tandonnet O, Biteau N, Belet-de Putter C, Rebouissoux L, Moradkhani K, Vu PY, Saura R, Arveiler B, Lacombe D, Taine L, Iron A (2006) Mosaic maternal uniparental isodisomy for chromosome 7q21-qter. Clin Genet 70(3):207–213. https://doi.org/10.1111/j.1399-0004.2006.00664.x
8. Zielenski J, Tsui LC (1995) Cystic fibrosis: genotypic and phenotypic variations. Annu Rev Genet 29:777–807. https://doi.org/10.1146/annurev.ge.29.120195.004021
9. Kerem B, Rommens JM, Buchanan JA, Markiewicz D, Cox TK, Chakravarti A, Buchwald M, Tsui LC (1989) Identification of the cystic fibrosis gene: genetic analysis. Science 245(4922):1073–1080
10. Bobadilla JL, Macek M Jr, Fine JP, Farrell PM (2002) Cystic fibrosis: a worldwide analysis of CFTR mutations—correlation with incidence data and application to screening. Hum Mutat 19(6):575–606. https://doi.org/10.1002/humu.10041
11. Shoshani T, Augarten A, Gazit E, Bashan N, Yahav Y, Rivlin Y, Tal A, Seret H, Yaar L, Kerem E et al (1992) Association of a nonsense mutation (W1282X), the most common mutation in the Ashkenazi Jewish cystic fibrosis patients in Israel, with presentation of severe disease. Am J Hum Genet 50(1):222–228
12. Zielenski J, Fujiwara TM, Markiewicz D, Paradis AJ, Anacleto AI, Richards B, Schwartz RH,

Klinger KW, Tsui LC, Morgan K (1993) Identification of the M1101K mutation in the cystic fibrosis transmembrane conductance regulator (CFTR) gene and complete detection of cystic fibrosis mutations in the Hutterite population. Am J Hum Genet 52(3):609–615

13. Grody WW, Cutting GR, Klinger KW, Richards CS, Watson MS, Desnick RJ, Subcommittee on Cystic Fibrosis Screening AoGSCAACoMG (2001) Laboratory standards and guidelines for population-based cystic fibrosis carrier screening. Genet Med 3(2):149–154. doi:10.109700125817-200103000-00010
14. American College of O, Gynecologists Committee on G (2011) ACOG Committee Opinion No. 486: update on carrier screening for cystic fibrosis. Obstet Gynecol 117 (4):1028–1031. https://doi.org/10.1097/AOG.0b013e31821922c2
15. Culling B, Ogle R (2010) Genetic counselling issues in cystic fibrosis. Paediatr Respir Rev 11 (2):75–79. https://doi.org/10.1016/j.prrv.2010.01.001
16. Umbarger MA, Kennedy CJ, Saunders P, Breton B, Chennagiri N, Emhoff J, Greger V, Hallam S, Maganzini D, Micale C, Nizzari MM, Towne CF, Church GM, Porreca GJ (2014) Next-generation carrier screening. Genet Med 16(2):132–140. https://doi.org/10.1038/gim.2013.83
17. Watson MS, Cutting GR, Desnick RJ, Driscoll DA, Klinger K, Mennuti M, Palomaki GE, Popovich BW, Pratt VM, Rohlfs EM, Strom CM, Richards CS, Witt DR, Grody WW (2004) Cystic fibrosis population carrier screening: 2004 revision of American College of Medical Genetics mutation panel. Genet Med 6(5):387–391. doi:10.109701.GIM.0000139506.11694.7C
18. Dogru D, Pekcan S, Yalcin E, Ozcelik U, Kiper N, Gurcan N, Sener B (2013) The role of serum Pseudomonas aeruginosa antibodies in the diagnosis and follow-up of cystic fibrosis. Turk J Pediatr 55(1):50–57
19. Crossley JR, Elliott RB, Smith PA (1979) Dried-blood spot screening for cystic fibrosis in the newborn. Lancet 1(8114):472–474
20. Goetzinger KR, Cahill AG (2010) An update on cystic fibrosis screening. Clin Lab Med 30 (3):533–543. https://doi.org/10.1016/j.cll.2010.04.005
21. Richards CS, Bradley LA, Amos J, Allitto B, Grody WW, Maddalena A, McGinnis MJ, Prior TW, Popovich BW, Watson MS, Palomaki GE (2002) Standards and guidelines for CFTR mutation testing. Genet Med 4(5):379–391. doi:10.109700125817-200209000-00010
22. Richards CS, Grody WW (2004) Prenatal screening for cystic fibrosis: past, present and future. Expert Rev Mol Diagn 4(1):49–62. https://doi.org/10.1586/14737159.4.1.49

Chapter 16

Prenatal Diagnosis of Tay-Sachs Disease

Jinglan Zhang, Hongjie Chen, Ruth Kornreich, and Chunli Yu

Abstract

Tay-Sachs disease (TSD) is an autosomal recessive lysosomal storage disorder caused by mutations of the *HEXA* gene resulting in the deficiency of hexosaminidase A (Hex A) and subsequent neuronal accumulation of G_{M2} gangliosides. Infantile TSD is a devastating and fetal neurodegenerative disease with death before the age of 3–5 years. A small proportion of TSD patients carry milder mutations and may present juvenile or adult onset milder disease. TSD is more prevalent among Ashkenazi Jewish (AJ) individuals and some other genetically isolated populations with carrier frequencies of approximately ~1:27 which is much higher than that of 1:300 in the general population. Carrier screening and prenatal testing for TSD are effective in preventing the birth of affected fetuses greatly diminishing the incidence of TSD. Testing of targeted *HEXA* mutations by genotyping or sequencing can detect 98% of carriers in AJ individuals; however, the detection rate is much lower for most other ethnic groups. When combined with enzyme analysis, above 98% of carriers can be reliably identified regardless of ethnic background. Multiplex PCR followed by allele-specific primer extension is one method to test for known and common mutations. Sanger sequencing or other sequencing methods are useful to identify private mutations. For prenatal testing, only predefined parental mutations need to be tested. In the event of unknown mutational status or the presence of variants of unknown significance (VUS), enzyme analysis must be performed in conjunction with DNA-based assays to enhance the diagnostic accuracy. Enzymatic assays involve the use of synthetic substrates 4-methylumbelliferyl-N-acetyl-β-glucosamine (4-MUG) and 4-methylumbelliferyl-6-sulfo-2-acetamido-2-deoxy-β-D-glucopyranoside (4-MUGS) to measure the percentage Hex A activity (Hex A%) and specific Hex A activity respectively. These biochemical and molecular tests can be performed in both direct specimens and cultured cells from chorionic villi sampling or amniocentesis.

Key words Tay-Sachs disease, Hexosaminidase A (Hex A) deficiency, *HEXA* gene, Targeted mutation, *HEXA* sequencing, 4-methylumbelliferyl-N-acetyl-β-glucosamine (4-MUG), 4-methylumbelliferyl-6-sulfo-2-acetamido-2-deoxy-β-D-glucopyranoside (4-MUGS), Percentage Hex A activity (Hex A%), Specific Hex A activity, Prenatal diagnosis

1 Introduction

The G_{M2} gangliosidoses are a group of related lysosomal storage disorders with a deficiency of either β-hexosaminidase or an activator protein causing the inability to break down the gangliosides G_{M2}. As a result, the G_{M2} gangliosides and related substrates are accumulated in the lysosomes of neuronal cells and lead to neuronal

Brynn Levy (ed.), *Prenatal Diagnosis*, Methods in Molecular Biology, vol. 1885, https://doi.org/10.1007/978-1-4939-8889-1_16,

swelling and neurological degeneration [1–4]. Infantile Tay-Sachs disease (TSD) is the prototype G_{M2} gangliosidoses which is characterized by hypotonia, loss of motor skills, decreased attentiveness, and increased startle response with onset from 3 to 6 months of age followed by progressive neurological deterioration including blindness, dementia, seizures, and subsequent death before the age of 3–5 years. Juvenile (subacute), chronic and adult-onset variants of TSD have later onset, milder and variable neurological findings with slower progression [2–4]. The other two G_{M2} gangliosidoses, Sandhoff disease and G_{M2} activator deficiency, have clinical presentations indistinguishable from TSD, except that there are also other symptoms involved in Sandhoff disease such as organomegaly, skeletal abnormalities, and oligosacchariduria [3].

Two lysosomal β hexosaminidase isoenzymes (Hex A and Hex B) are critical for the degradation of gangliosides G_{M2} in the central nervous system and other substrates such as glycolipids and glycoproteins throughout the body. The enzymatic functions are specific toward the substrates' terminal nonreducing sugars *N*-acetylglucosamine (GlcNAc) or *N*-acetylgalactosamine (GalNAc) in β-linkage [2, 5]. Hex A (αβ) and Hex B (ββ) enzymes consist of α- and β-subunits, which are encoded by the *HEXA* and *HEXB* genes, respectively [6]. Neutral water soluble substrate such as artificial 4-methylumbelliferyl-N-acetyl-β-glucosamine (4-MUG) is specific for the β-subunit and therefore can be hydrolyzed by both Hex A and Hex B. The negatively charged hydrophobic gangliosides GM2 can only be hydrolyzed by the α-subunit and hence Hex A in the presence of GM2 activator protein which binds the membrane bound GM2 gangliosides to form soluble complex for Hex A cleavage [5]. The synthetic 4-methylumbelliferyl-6-sulfo-2-acetamido-2-deoxy-β-D-glucopyranoside (4-MUGS) is also specific toward the α-subunit of hexosaminidase and is used to measure the specific Hex A activity in vitro without the requirement of the activator protein [7]. Three forms of GM2 gangliosidoses are autosomal recessive disorders with deficiencies of Hex A enzyme. TSD is caused by mutations of the *HEXA* gene and profound deficiency of Hex A, while Sandhoff disease is caused by mutations of the *HEXB* gene and deficiencies of both Hex A and Hex B. GM2 activator protein deficiency results from mutations of the *G2MA* gene leading to nonfunctional Hex A activity in vivo [2–4]. Due to the severe clinical outcome and lack of effective therapy, carrier screening and prenatal testing for at risk pregnancies are important to prevent the birth of affected fetuses. The prenatal testing strategy and biochemical and molecular methods used for carrier and prenatal testing for TSD are the focus of this chapter.

1.1 Molecular Genetics of TSD

TSD is an autosomal recessive disease caused by mutations in the *HEXA* gene. The *HEXA* gene is 35 kb in size and located on chromosome 15q23-24 with 13 introns and 14 exons. Before population-based carrier screening programs started in the 1970s, TSD was most commonly found in the Ashkenazi Jewish (AJ) population with an incidence of 1:3600 births and a carrier frequency of ~1:28 [8, 9]. In some genetically isolated populations such as French Canadians in Quebec, Cajuns from Louisiana and the Old Order Amish in Pennsylvanian, TSD carrier frequency is also increased and similar to that of AJ individuals due to the founder effects. Overall, TSD incidence is 100 times lower in the general population with a carrier frequency of approximately 1:300 [2, 4]. Three mutations c.1274_1277dupTATC (1278+TATC), c.1421+1G>C (IVS12+1G>C), and c.805G>A (p.G269S) account for more than 98% disease alleles in AJ individuals [9, 10]. Founder mutations c.1073+1G>A (IVS9+1G>A) in the Irish [11] and g.2644_10588del (del7.6 kb) in French Canadians have also been identified [12]. More than 170 mutations in the *HEXA* gene have been reported to date in Human Gene Mutation Database (http://www.hgmd.cf.ac.uk/). Most of the mutations are associated with infantile TSD. The genotype and phenotype correlation has been well studied for TSD. The residual Hex A activity correlates inversely with the severity of the disease. Individuals with acute infantile TSD usually have two null alleles and no Hex A enzymatic activity (e.g., c.1274_1277dupTATC, c.1421+1G>C, c.1073+1G>A, and g.2644_10588del). Individuals with juvenile or chronic and adult onset TSD are usually compound heterozygotes for a null allele and an allele that results in low residual Hex A activity, or compound heterozygotes of two alleles that result in low residual Hex A activity [2, 4, 13]. Missense mutations at two codons (178 and 258), c.532C>T (p.R178C), c.533G>A (p. R178H), c.533G>T (p.R178L), and c.772G>C (p.D258H), are associated with B1 variant of TSD, accounting for a small proportion of TSD patients [14]. The B1 variants have normal enzyme activities toward the 4-MUG substrate; however are inactive toward natural substrates in vivo or the Hex A-specific 4-MUGS substrate [15]. For this reason, some B1 variant carriers might be falsely negative by the routine heat inactivation assay with the 4-MUG substrate. Individuals with a null allele and a B1 variant present with juvenile TSD. Individuals with two B1 alleles usually have chronic and adult onset disease [2, 14]. False positive carrier screening results for TSD by enzyme analysis are caused by the presence of one of two known non-pathogenic pseudo-deficiency alleles, c.739C>T (p.R247W) or c.745C>T (p.R249W). These two variants are not associated with the disease, but result in the production of a Hex A enzyme with decreased activity toward the 4-MUG substrate used in enzyme assays [16]. It has been reported about 35% of non-Jewish and 2% of Jewish individuals who are carriers by enzyme analysis are carriers for one of these two pseudo-deficiency alleles [16].

1.2 Biochemical Enzyme Assays

The biochemical diagnosis of TSD is established when Hex A activity is absent or extremely low with normal or even elevated Hex B activity. Enzyme analysis has also been the primary method for carrier testing of TSD in non-Jewish populations. The natural substrate G_{M2} gangliosides is most specific for testing Hex A activity but it is expensive, and assays using it are time-consuming and difficult to perform in clinical laboratories. Synthetic artificial substrates have been widely used for enzyme testing for TSD [17]. The enzyme assay can be performed using serum (or plasma), white blood cells, chorionic villi, amniotic fluid, and other tissues. In women who are either pregnant [18] or using birth control medication [19], interfering Hex P in serum (or plasma) may impact the percentage Hex A activity (Hex A%) and cause false positive results; therefore, the enzyme assay for these individuals should not be performed in serum or plasma. 4-MUG is the most sensitive and commonly used artificial substrate in TSD biochemical carrier screening tests. The Hex A and Hex B isoenzymes are both reactive toward 4-MUG with similar kinetics; however they have different thermal stabilities. At pH 4.4, Hex B is stable up to 55 °C, whereas Hex A is inactivated under heat. The half-life of Hex A is approximately 10 min at 50 °C and 3 min at 55 °C. The differential thermal stabilities of Hex A and Hex B are the basis for the routinely used heat-inactivation hexosaminidase activity assay. The total hexosaminidase activities (Hex A and Hex B) are measured with 4-MUG before and after the denaturation of the Hex A at 50–55 °C for 2–3 hour. The Hex A% is calculated from the difference and divided by the total activity to reflect the proportion of Hex A from total hexosaminidase [2]. Both total hexosaminidase activity and Hex A % are routinely reported for the 4-MUG-based enzyme assay; however, only Hex A% is used for the clinical diagnosis of TSD and TSD carriers. TSD is characterized by a very low Hex A% (<10%) and normal total activity (Hex B). Carriers of TSD have an intermediate Hex A% (20–50%) that can be discriminated from non-carriers (60–65% ±5%). When testing for Tay-Sachs carriers with a 4-MUG-based enzyme assay, Sandhoff carriers can also be revealed by a characteristic high Hex A% activity (≥75–80%) and relatively low total activity. In the individuals affected with Sandhoff disease, the total activity is absent or extremely low with an extremely high Hex A% (>80–90%). Another commonly used synthetic sulfated substrate 4-MUGS is used to measure the specific Hex A activity as it is almost exclusively hydrolyzed by Hex A. 4-MUGS substrate has been used in the diagnosis of TSD, and particularly the B1 variant [15]. TSD and Sandhoff disease patients demonstrate absent or extremely low specific Hex A activity (0–15 nmol/hour/mg protein) compared to normal individuals (>200 nmol/hour/mg protein). The B1 variant could be falsely normal or intermediate when tested with 4-MUG substrate, therefore should be tested with 4-MUGS substrate. The 4-MUGS substrate is not appropriate for carrier testing of TSD.

1.3 Molecular Genetic Testing

Molecular testing for TSD includes targeted DNA assays for founder mutations in various populations at higher risk for TSD. Five *HEXA* mutations c.1274_1277dupTATC, c.1421+1G>C, c.805G>A, c.1073+1G>A, and g.2644_10588del are included in many DNA-based TSD carrier screening programs together with two non-pathogenic pseudo-deficiency alleles c.739C>T and c.745C>T [9]. One commonly used genotyping technology to test these *HEXA* mutations is based on allele specific primer extension (ASPE) and is deployed on many different platforms. ASPE usually involves an enzymatic reaction to determine the target genotype by specific nucleotide incorporation followed by a platform-specific detection step to quantify the allele-specific nucleotide incorporation. However, the detection rate of this five-mutation panel is much lower in the general population and thus makes targeted mutation testing less effective. Therefore, it is recommended to always perform the enzymatic test with targeted mutation analysis and reflex to full gene sequencing to screen for the pathogenic mutation when the enzyme test results are positive or inconclusive. Generally, only targeted genotyping or sequencing of the predefined pathogenic mutations identified in parents should be performed for TSD prenatal testing. When a fetus is negative for at least one of parental pathogenic alleles, the likelihood this fetus is affected by TSD is greatly diminished. Maternal cell contamination studies (e.g., testing maternal and fetal microsatellite DNA sequences) should always be performed to ensure that negative results such as a heterozygote call in the fetus are not caused by the presence of maternal DNA. Microsatellites (short tandem repeats, STRs) are small arrays of tandem repeats (1–4 bp) interspersed throughout the genome occurring on average once every 50 Kb. Because of the highly variable number of repeats, microsatellites are widely used in linkage studies and paternity tests. Microsatellite markers can be used to determine the status of maternal cell contamination in prenatal samples. Usually, the fluorescently labeled PCR products are run by capillary electrophoresis on a genetic analyzer.

1.4 Prenatal Testing and Counseling

Prenatal testing for TSD should be offered for at-risk pregnancies. Chorionic villus sampling (CVS) at 10–12 weeks or amniocentesis at 15–18 weeks can be performed to obtain fetal cells. DNA-based testing can be performed with either direct or cultured CVS cells or amniocytes. Enzyme analysis can be performed using direct or cultured CVS and cultured amniocytes. In addition, enzyme analysis can also be performed with cell-free amniotic fluid specimens. If both parental disease-causing alleles are identified, DNA-based assays for the parental mutations in the fetus are sufficient and accurate. If the risk for TSD of a pregnancy is determined solely by parental enzyme analysis and the underlying *HEXA* mutation(s) are unknown, enzyme testing in combination with specific mutation analysis can be pursued with formal genetic counseling. With the increasing trend of pan-ethnic carrier screening and utilization of sequencing-based DNA assays in clinical testing, identifications of novel mutations and variants of unknown significance (VUS) have increased. It is important that both enzyme and DNA-based assay are performed concurrently in these situations. Both 4-MUG and 4-MUGS assays should be performed to increase test sensitivity as well as testing a reference enzyme β-galactosidase to ensure sample integrity. Normal and positive controls of the appropriate specimen type are always tested with the fetal specimen. Maternal cell contamination should be excluded by molecular marker studies.

2 Materials

2.1 Enzymatic Assays

1. 0.9% saline (normal saline).
2. 0.05% trypsin-EDTA solution.
3. Serum Buffer: 12 mM citrate-20 mM Na_2HPO_4, pH 4.4.

   Dissolve 461 mg citric acid (MW = 192.1) and 568 mg Na_2HPO_4 (MW = 142.0) in 150 mL deionized water. Adjust pH to 4.4, and then bring volume to 200 mL. Store at −20 °C for up to 2 years.
4. WBC buffer: 6 mM citrate–10 mM Na_2HPO_4, pH 4.4/ 0.6% HAS.

   Dilute 50 mL serum buffer to a final volume of 100 mL with deionized water. Add 0.6 g of Human Serum Albumin (HSA). Store at −20 °C for up to 2 years.
5. Citrate–Na_2HPO_4 Buffer: 0.1 M citrate–0.2 M Na_2HPO_4 (0.1/0.2 M C–P), pH 4.2.

   0.2 M citrate: dissolve 19.21 g of citric acid in 500 mL deionized water.

   0.4 M Na_2HPO_4: dissolve 28.4 g of Na_2HPO_4 in 500 mL deionized water.

   Mix 58.8 mL of 0.2 M citrate with 41.2 mL of 0.4 M Na_2HPO_4, adjust pH to 4.2 by adding either 0.2 M citrate or 0.4 M Na_2HPO_4. Bring volume to 200 mL with deionized water. Discard after making the 4-MUGS substrate.
6. Sodium acetate Buffer: 100 mM sodium acetate/sodium chloride, pH 4.0.

   Dissolve 1.64 g sodium acetate (MW = 82.04) and 1.17 g sodium chloride (MW = 58.44) in 180 mL deionized water, adjust pH to 4.0 with acetic acid, and bring the volume to 200 mL. Discard after making the β-Galactosidase substrate.
7. 4-MUG substrate: 3.0 mM 4-MUG.

   Dissolve 16 mg of 4-MUG (MW = 379.36) in 14 mL of either serum or WBC buffer for a batch of 20 samples. This substrate is freshly made for use before the enzyme reaction.

8. 4-MUGS substrate: 3.0 mM 4-MUGS.

   Dissolve 14.9 mg 4-MUGS potassium salt (MW = 497.5) in 10 mL of 0.1/0.2 M C-P buffer, pH 4.2. Store at −20 °C for 2 years.

9. β-Galactosidase substrate: 0.5 mM β-Galactosidase.

   Dissolve 1.7 mg 4-methylumbelliferyl-β-D-galactopyranoside (MW = 338.3) in 10 mL 100 mM sodium acetate/sodium chloride buffer, pH 4.0. Store at −20 °C for 2 years.

10. Stop solution (for stopping enzyme reaction): 0.1 M ethylene diamine.

    Dilute 6.75 mL anhydrous ethylene diamine (MW = 60.1, density = 0.899 g/mL) with deionized water to a final volume of 1000 mL. Store at room temperature in amber glass dispense bottle for up to 1 year.

11. 4-MU stock solution: 25 mM 4-MU.

    Dissolve 44 mg of 4-MU (MW = 176.2) in 10 mL DMSO.

12. 4-MU intermediate stock solution: 100 μM 4-MU.

    Dilute 50 μL of the 25 mM 4-MU stock solution with DMSO to a final volume of 12.50 mL.

13. 4-MU working solution: 10 μM 4-MU.

    Dilute 0.5 mL of the 100 μM 4-MU intermediate stock solution with DMSO to a final volume of 5 mL.

2.2 DNA Extraction

1. PureGeneTM Genomic DNA purification kit (Qiagen, Germantown, MD, USA).

2.3 DNA-Based Molecular Diagnosis: Sanger Sequencing

HEXA PCR primers must span all exons and at least 20 nt of intronic sequences must be M13 tagged (for standardization of assays—not necessary for all laboratories) and synthesized by an established facility. 10 μM working solutions of the primers are prepared.

1. Primer working solutions: Prepare a 10 μM primer working solution.
2. DNase and RNase-free molecular biology grade distilled water.
3. dNTPs.
4. Platinum Taq DNA Polymerase.
5. 10× PCR Buffer.
6. 50 mM $MgCl_2$ (Invitrogen, Carlsbad, CA, USA).
7. Shrimp Alkaline Phosphatase.
8. Exonuclease (USB, Thermo Fisher Scientific, Waltham, MA, USA).
9. Primer sequences are described in Table 1.

Table 1
Sequences for *HEXA* coding exon gene-specific primers

Exon	Primer sequence (5′→3′) Forward	Reverse	Product length (bp)
1	CCAGGCCGGAAGTGAAAG	CTCCTGATTGAACCGTAGTCCTA	638
2	TAGGGTCTTGGTTTTGCCTG	AGGCCATCCAGAGTTACAGC	267
3	GTCCAGTGATTTATATAGAATATCTGGTC	AACACCAACCTTCCCACATC	249
4	TGCTCTGCTACATTGAGAACC	CAATATTGGGATCCAACCCC	230
5	TTGTCTTCATCTCCCTGTGC	GGAACTTGGTCTGTCCGTTG	292
6	CCAACATCGCAAGTTTGAGG	GCCACAGCCAGATTCAGAC	268
7	TGTGGGCATTTTGAGTATCTTC	AGCCAGTGCCCTGAAGC	315
8	TTACGTGTAGGACTGTGCGTG	CCTCGGGTGCTAACTTCTATTC	357
9–10	TAATCCCCAGGCATTAGGC	TCTGTAGAGGCAGGGAGGAG	629
11–12	GACATACTTTGCTGCTGGGG	CTTCAGAAGGCTCGTTGCAC	782
13	GGTAGCAGCCTGTGGATGTC	CTCTCTAAGGGGTTCCCCAG	286
14	GTGTGAAAAGTGTTGCTGGG	TGCCACATTACTCTTTATTGAATG	345

HEXA PCR primers were M13 tagged (not shown on the above table)

2.4 DNA-Based Molecular Diagnosis: Luminex

1. Primer sequences provided by Luminex (Luminex Corporation Austin, TX, USA).
2. 10× PCR Primer Mix (Luminex Corporation Austin, TX, USA).
3. ASPE Primer Mix (Luminex Corporation Austin, TX, USA).
4. Bead Mix (Luminex Corporation Austin, TX, USA).
5. DNase and RNase-free molecular biology grade distilled water.
6. dNTPs.
7. HotStarTaq® DNA Polymerase (Qiagen, Germantown, MD, USA).
8. 10× Qiagen HotStar® PCR Buffer (Qiagen, Germantown, MD, USA).
9. 25 mM $MgCl_2$ (Qiagen, Germantown, MD, USA).
10. Shrimp Alkaline Phosphatase.

Table 2
Sequences for microsatellite marker primers used in maternal cell contamination studies

Maker	Primer sequence (5′→3′) Forward	Reverse	Product length (bp)
D7S1817	[6-FAM]CAAATTAATGGCAAAAACTGC	CCCCCCATTGAGG TTATTAC	122
D2S406	[5-HEX]GTGATGGTAAATAATTTCTGAGACC	GACAACTGAC TTTCCCAGGA	184
DxS981	[6-FAM]TCAGAGGAAAAGAAGTAGACATACT	TTCTCTCCAC TTTTCAGAGTCA	187
D7S821	[5-HEX]ACAAAACCCCAAGTACGTGA	TATGACAGGCATC TGGGAGT	248
D11S1392	[6-FAM]GCAGGTATATTGCATCCATACG	AGAAGGCC TTGAGACATCCA	196
CSF1PO	[6-FAM]AACCTGAGTCTGCCAAGGACTAGC	TTCCACACACCAC TGGCCATCTTC	319
TPOX	[5-HEX]GCACAGAACAGGCACTTAGG	CGCTCAAACG TGAGGTTG	270
VWA	[5-HEX]GCCCTAGTGGATGATAAGAATAATC AGTATGTG	GGACAGATGA TAAATACA TAGGATGGATGG	151
D7S820	[6-FAM]ATGTTGGTCAGGCTGACTATG	GATTCCACATTTA TCCTCATTGAC	243

Fluorescent dyes were conjugated to the 5′-end of forward PCR primers

11. Exonuclease (USB, Thermo Fisher Scientific, Waltham, MA, USA).
12. 10× Wash Buffer (Luminex Corporation Austin, TX, USA).
13. Streptavidin, R-Phycoerythrin conjugate (Invitrogen, Carlsbad, CA, USA).

2.5 DNA-Based Marker Studies for Maternal Cell Contamination Analysis

1. PCR primers for microsatellite markers are diluted to a working concentration of 20 μM.
2. Primer sequences are described in Table 2.

3 Methods

3.1 Methods for Enzymatic Assays

3.1.1 Quality Control

Normal and affected controls must be performed with the prenatal specimen. Affected controls are aliquots of previously diagnosed affected samples kept at −80 °C. Concurrent normal controls are provided from the prenatal sampling facilities or tissue culture facilities.

3.1.2 Blanks and Standards

For 4-MUG assays, the WBC buffer is used as blank for direct and cultured CVS and cultured amniocytes; and serum buffer is used as blank for cell-free amniotic fluid. For 4-MUGS and β-galactosidase assays, water is used as blank for all specimen types. In addition, a self-blank is used for 4-MUGS assay in amniotic fluid, where the stopping solution is added before the substrate. One point 4-MU calibration containing 1 nmol 4-MU standard (100 μL of 10 μM 4-MU standard) is used in every prenatal assay for calculation of enzyme activities. Full range 4-MU calibration is performed every 6 months.

3.1.3 Preparation of Direct CVS Sample

1. Clean and wash the direct CVS samples with normal saline (performed by a cell culture laboratory).
2. Add 300–1000 μL of normal saline to the freshly prepared or frozen CVS sample according to the size of the sample.
3. Freeze and thaw the CVS sample in a dry ice/ethanol bath and a 37 °C water batch for five times to lyse the cells.
4. Centrifuge at 4600 × *g* for 1 min.
5. Use the supernatant for enzyme assay or store at −20 °C until assay.

3.1.4 Preparation of Cultured CVS Cells or Amniocytes

1. Decant the culture media and wash with 10 mL normal saline.
2. Add 0.75 mL 0.05% trypsin-EDTA to T25 flask and incubate at 37 °C incubator for 5 min. Check under a microscope to make sure the cells are detached then add 0.75 mL saline.
3. Transfer the cell suspension into a 1.5 mL Eppendorf microfuge tube and centrifuge at 4600 × *g* for 3 min.
4. Discard the supernatant and wash the cell pellet with 1.5 mL normal saline twice.
5. Remove the normal saline by inverting the tube over a paper towel.
6. Add 300–1000 μL of chilled water depending on the size of the pellet. Vortex to resuspend the pellet.
7. Sonicate the sample for 10 s using Fisher F60 sonic dismembrator with output power setting of 4.
8. Centrifuge at 4600 × *g* for 1 min and the resultant supernatant is ready for enzyme assay or store at −20 °C until analysis.

3.1.5 Total Hexosaminidase and Hex A% Activity with 4-MUG Substrate

The general procedures described below apply to all prenatal specimen types with minor differences in buffers, dilution factor, and reaction times.

1. Dilute cell lysates from direct CVS, cultured CVS, and cultured amniocytes with WBC buffer and a 1:20 dilution, e.g., 570 μL WBC buffer +30 μL lysates. Dilute amniotic fluid sample with serum buffer and a 1:10 dilution, e.g., 540 μL serum buffer +60 μL of amniotic fluid sample.
2. Label four sets of 12 × 75 mm glass tubes for blank, normal control (NC), affected control (AC), and prenatal sample in duplicates (set-0, 1h, 2h, and 3h).
3. Place 50 μL of diluted controls and patient sample in each tube and cover with parafilm to avoid evaporation of the samples during heat inactivation. 50 μL WBC buffer is used as blank for lysates. 50 μL serum buffer is used as blank for amniotic fluid sample.
4. Place "0" set of tubes in ice-water bath for non-heat or total hexosaminidase.
5. Place the other rack containing 1h, 2h, and 3h sets in 50 °C water bath for heat-inactivation.
6. Take out sample tubes labeled 1h, 2h, and 3h after 1 hour, 2 hour, and 3 hour heat-inactivation respectively. Place on ice-water bath immediately.
7. Add 100 μL of the freshly prepared 3.0 mM 4-MUG substrate in WBC buffer to all samples. 3.0 mM 4-MUG substrate in serum buffer is used for amniotic fluid samples.
8. Incubate in 37 °C water bath for 15 min (30 min for amniotic fluid sample).
9. Add 2.35 mL of stop solution to each tube to stop enzyme reaction.
10. Read fluorescence at 360 nm excitation and 450 nm emission.
11. Determine protein concentration in mg/mL by method of preference (e.g., Lowry or Bradford methods).
12. Total β-hexosaminidase (Hex) activity (nmol/hour/mg protein or nmol/hour/mL) is expressed as nmol of 4-MU produced per hour per mg of protein in the cell lysates or per mL of amniotic fluid, where 4-MU turnover is calculated from comparing fluorescence intensity of sample to the 1 nmol 4-MU standard.
13. The Hex A% or [Hex A/(Hex A + Hex B)]% is calculated from the fluorescence difference of the non-heated and heated samples divided by the fluorescence of the non-heated samples and multiplied by 100 (*see* **Note 1**). Hex A% of 1h is reported.

3.1.6 Specific Hex A Activity with 4-MUGS Substrate

1. Label 12 × 75 mm glass test tubes in duplicate for blank, normal control, affected control, and sample.
2. Place 20 μL of lysates for 4-MUGS assay. Add 30 μL of water to controls and sample. Pipette 50 μL of water for blank.
3. Add 50 μL of 4-MUGS substrate to each sample. Quickly vortex or shake all the samples for 10 s and incubate in 37 °C water bath for 30 min.
4. After incubation, remove tubes from the water bath and immediately place in ice-water bath.
5. Add 2.4 mL of stop solution to all tubes to stop enzyme reaction.
6. Read the fluorescence density at 365 nm excitation and 450 nm emission.
7. The specific Hex A activity is expressed as nmol of 4-MU produced per hour per mg of protein in the cell lysates or per mL of amniotic fluid.

3.1.7 Reference Enzyme β-Galactosidase Activity

1. Label 12 × 75 mm glass test tubes for blank, normal control, affected control, and sample.
2. Place 10 μL of lysates for β-galactosidase activity assay. Add 40 μL of water to controls and patient samples. Pipette 50 μL of water for the blank.
3. Add 50 μL of 3.0 mM β-galactosidase substrate to each sample. Quickly vortex or shake all the samples for 10 s and incubate in 37 °C water bath for 30 min.
4. After incubation, remove tubes from the water bath and immediately place in ice-water bath.
5. Add 2.4 mL of stop solution to all tubes to stop enzyme reaction.
6. Read the fluorescence density at 365 nm excitation and 450 nm emission.
7. The β-galactosidase activity is expressed as nmol of 4-MU produced per hour per mg of protein.

3.1.8 Result Interpretation

The Hex A% after 1 hour heat-inactivation and specific Hex A activity are reported for the prenatal sample along with the normal and affected controls. It is important for the prenatal testing laboratory to establish normal and affected ranges for Hex A% and specific Hex A activity in different specimen types. The affected ranges of Hex A% in all specimen types are <5–10%. The affected ranges of specific Hex A activity are less than 5–10% of the normal mean of tested specimen type. The enzyme results are not valid if there are significant maternal cell contaminations or sample integrity is questionable reflected by low reference enzyme activity.

3.2 Methods for HEXA Gene Sequence Analysis by Sanger Sequencing

3.2.1 DNA Preparation, PCR, and Sequencing

1. Extract DNA from prenatal cells using the PureGene™ Genomic DNA purification kit (*see* **Note 2**).
2. Dilute purified DNA to a concentration of 50 ng/μL.
3. Prepare PCR master mix for the number of samples to be tested including a reagent blank and two extra for pipetting loss.

   Distribute a 1.0 μL aliquot of the prepared DNA (50 ng/μL) to thin-walled PCR (0.2 mL) tubes with 1.2 μL of exon F/R primer mix (10 μM working solution), 15.4 μL distilled water, 2.5 μL 10× PCR buffer, 0.75 mM $MgCl_2$, 4.0 μL 0.2 μM dNTP, and 0.2 μL Platinum Taq (5 U/μL).
4. Run the following PCR profile:
   (a) One cycle: 95 °C for 5 min.
   (b) Thirty-five cycles: 95 °C for 30 s, 60 °C for 30 s, 72 °C for 30 s.
   (c) One cycle: 72 °C for 7 min.
   (d) 4 °C hold.
5. Perform Exo/SAP treatment to clean up the PCR products (2.5 μL Shrimp Alkaline Phosphatase and 1 μL Exonuclease). Process the reactions in a thermal cycler programmed as follows:
   (a) One cycle: 37 °C for 30 min.
   (b) One cycle: 99 °C for 15 min.
   (c) 4 °C hold.
6. Perform bi-directional DNA sequencing for *HEXA* exon (s) with 8–20 ng of the purified PCR product using procedures recommended by the manufacturer.

3.2.2 Sanger Sequencing Analysis

1. Separate PCR products by electrophoresis in agarose gels to ensure proper amplification, which should demonstrate a single strong band with the expected size for each exon to be analyzed. The blank must not contain any amplification products. If there is contamination in blank, all PCR reagents should be discarded and new amplification reactions should be set up.
2. The chromatograms containing the sequencing data should have unique, non-overlapping peaks for homozygous samples. A heterozygous missense or nonsense mutation will produce an overlapped peak at the mutant position and deletion or insertion in one strand will produce overlapped peaks at all positions after the change. Sequencing results must show the variation in both the forward and reverse directions.

3.3 HEXA Targeted Mutation Analysis by Luminex Beads-Based Genotyping

3.3.1 DNA Preparation, PCR, and ASPE

1. Extract DNA for *HEXA* genotyping from blood samples or direct or cultured prenatal cells using the PureGene™ Genomic DNA Purification Kit (*see* **Note 3**).
2. For multiplex PCR, add the following into each specimen tube: 4.0 μL DNase and RNase Free Distilled Water, 1.9 μL 10× Qiagen HotStar® PCR Buffer, 1.0 μL Qiagen 25 mM $MgCl_2$, 2.5 μL PCR Primer Mix (with dNTPs), 0.6 μL HotStarTaq® DNA Polymerase and 2.5 μL of appropriate DNA sample.
3. Set the thermal cycler temperature as BLOCK Temperature with the heated lid enabled and run the following PCR profile:
   (a) One cycle: 95 °C for 15 min.
   (b) Thirty-three cycles: 95 °C for 30 s, 58 °C for 30 s, 72 °C for 2 min.
   (c) One cycle: 72 °C for 5 min.
   (d) 4 °C hold.
4. Prepare Enzyme Mix as follows: 1.3 μL Shrimp Alkaline Phosphatase and 0.5 μL Exonuclease I. Add 1.8 μL of the Enzyme Mix into each of the PCR tubes. Incubate the tubes in a thermal cycler programmed as follows:
   (a) One cycle: 37 °C for 30 min.
   (b) One cycle: 99 °C for 5 min.
   (c) 4 °C hold.
5. For multiplex ASPE, add the reagents in the order listed below to prepare the ASPE Master Mix. 10.5 μL DNase and RNase Free Distilled Water, 3.0 μL 10× Qiagen HotStar® PCR Buffer, 1.6 μL Qiagen 25 mM $MgCl_2$, 2.0 μL ASPE Primer Mix (with dNTPs), 0.4 μL HotStarTaq® DNA Polymerase. Add 2.5 μL of treated PCR product to the appropriately labeled ASPE tube. Cap each tube immediately after addition of sample.
6. Set the thermal cycler temperature as BLOCK Temperature with the heated lid enabled and place tubes in thermal cycler. Run the following program:
   (a) One cycle: 95 °C for 15 min.
   (b) Forty cycles: 95 °C for 30 s, 56 °C for 30 s, 72 °C for 1 min.
   (c) One cycle: 99 °C for 15 min.
   (d) 4 °C hold.
7. Thaw and bring the 2× Beads Mix to room temperature, limiting its exposure to light, and prepare a 1.1× Wash Buffer solution from the 10× Wash Buffer stock.

8. Vortex the 2× Bead Mix tube for 10 s and then sonicate for 10 s to disperse the beads. Repeat this step.
9. Use black tube (1.5 mL or 5 mL) to dilute 2× beads mix with 1.1× wash buffer at 1:1 volume ratio. The final concentration for beads mix should be 1×.
10. Vortex for several seconds and aliquot 45 μL of the Bead Mix into the eight labeled tubes.
11. Aliquot 5 μL of the ASPE reaction into the corresponding labeled tube or well.
12. Place tubes in a thermal cycler programmed as follows:
    (a) One cycle: 96 °C for 2 min.
    (b) One cycle: 37 °C for 60 min.
    (c) 37 °C hold.
13. Add 100 μL 1× wash buffer to each well, then place the strips/plate on the Magnetic Particle Concentrator (The concentrator has 13 columns, which enables the 96-well plate to shift its position). Hold 10 s and shift strips/plate position by one column. Hold another 10 s and then shift the strips/plate back by one column. Hold at least 1 min for beads precipitation. Brown palates should be seen along one side of the well inner wall.
14. Add 120 μL 1× wash buffer to each well and repeat the shifting and pouring procedures once.
15. Before proceeding to the next step (about 5 min before completion of the 1 hour incubation) prepare the Reporter Solution. Vortex the tube of Streptavidin, R-Phycoerythrin (SA-PE) conjugate for 2–5 s. For eight samples, add 6 μL of SA-PE (1 mg/mL) to 2 mL of 1× Wash Buffer (Tm Bioscience) in a 15 mL sterile centrifuge tube.
16. Add 100 μL reporter (made from above step) to each well, briefly pipette up and down, and transfer into Costar plate.
17. Incubate the plate at room temperature for 15 min. Run samples on Luminex machine according to the manufacturer's instructions.

3.3.2 Results Analysis for HEXA Genotyping Using Luminex Bead Technology

1. Data interpretation is accomplished by obtaining the raw data as a comma delimited file (csv file) which subtracts the background from each variation in each sample, calculates the allelic ratio for each variation, and ultimately defines a "SNP Call" for each sample and variation.
2. The calls are made using a combination of thresholds that require each signal to be significantly higher than the background and that the allelic ratios fall within empirically derived ranges. The following QC cutoff is used to accept a genotyping

result: minimum MFI of 300, minimum bead count of 100. Genotype is called based on allelic ratios: if $\geq$0.85: homozygous mutation; if >0.7 and <0.85 or >0.15 and <0.3: No Call; if $\geq$0.3 and $\leq$0.7: heterozygous; if $\geq$0.0 and $\leq$0.15: wild type.

3. A negative control (blank) must be included in every run. Positive control samples are rotated on each run. If the signals obtained for the blank are too high, the run is invalid and must be repeated. Samples with insufficient signals or low bead counts are repeated.

3.4 Maternal Cell Contamination Study

3.4.1 Method for Marker Studies Using PCR and Capillary Electrophoresis

1. Extract DNA from maternal blood and prenatal samples.
2. PCR Amplification. Add the reagents in the order listed below to prepare the PCR Master Mixes. 9.8 μL DNase and RNase Free Distilled Water, 2.6 μL 10× Qiagen HotStar® PCR Buffer, 1.5 μL Qiagen 25 mM $MgCl_2$, 4.0 μL 1.25 mM dNTP and 2.5 μL R/F primers, 1 U platinum Taq polymerase, and 2.5 μL of appropriate DNA sample into each specimen tube.
3. Run the following PCR profile:
   (a) One cycle: 94 °C for 3 min.
   (b) Twenty-five cycles: 94 °C for 15 s, 58 °C for 20 s, 72 °C for 20 s.
   (c) One cycle: 72 °C for 5 min.
   (d) 4 °C hold.
4. After thermal cycling, store the fluorescent PCR products in the dark at 4 °C until ready to proceed, and store at −20 °C for longer-term storage.
5. Prepare the samples for loading in the Genetic Analyzer by denaturing the samples at 95 °C for 3 min and then placing the plate on ice for 3 min.
6. Run the samples on the Genetic Analyzer according to the manufacturer's instructions.
7. Analyze the data according to the Genemapper instructions.

3.4.2 Analysis for the Marker Study

1. Most samples will be heterozygous and show two major bands due to the high heterozygosity of the markers. Homozygous samples will show one major band.
2. The stutter bands and nonspecific bands should be minimal and distinguishable from real products. The maternal and fetal patterns are compared.
3. At least one band should be in common between the maternal and fetal samples. A marker is considered informative if the patterns are different between the maternal and fetal samples.

4. If none of the initial five markers tested are informative, additional markers are tested.
5. If maternal cell contamination is not present, there will be a band present in the maternal sample that is not observed in the fetal sample.

4 Notes

1. Multiple heat-inactivation time points are the experience of this testing laboratory.
2. Any equivalent DNA extraction method may be used.
3. The QIASymphony DNA extraction Technology or any equivalent DNA extraction method may be used.

References

1. Moriwaki S, Takashima S, Yoshida H, Kawano N, Goto M (1977) Histological observation of the brain of Tay-Sachs disease with seizure and chronic DPH intoxication—report of an autopsy case. Acta Pathol Jpn 27 (3):387–407
2. Gravel RA, Clarke JTR, Kaback MM, Mahuran D, Sandhoff K, Suzuki K (1995) The GM2 gangliosidoses. In: Scriver CR, Beaudet AL, Sly WS et al (eds) The metabolic and molecular basis of inherited disease, 7th edn. McGraw-Hill, New York, pp 2839–2879
3. Sandhoff K, Harzer K (2013) Gangliosides and gangliosidoses: principles of molecular and metabolic pathogenesis. J Neurosci 33 (25):10195–10208. https://doi.org/10.1523/JNEUROSCI.0822-13.2013
4. Kaback MM, Desnick RJ (1993) Hexosaminidase A deficiency. In: Pagon RA, Adam MP, Ardinger HH et al (eds) GeneReviews(R). University of Washington, Seattle, Seattle, WA
5. Zwierz K, Zalewska A, Zoch-Zwierz A (1999) Isoenzymes of N-acetyl-beta-hexosaminidase. Acta Biochim Pol 46(3):739–751
6. Mahuran DJ, Tsui F, Gravel RA, Lowden JA (1982) Evidence for two dissimilar polypeptide chains in the beta 2 subunit of hexosaminidase. Proc Natl Acad Sci U S A 79(5):1602–1605
7. Bayleran J, Hechtman P, Saray W (1984) Synthesis of 4-methylumbelliferyl-beta-D-N-acetylglucosamine-6-sulfate and its use in classification of GM2 gangliosidosis genotypes. Clin Chim Acta 143(2):73–89
8. Kronn D, Jansen V, Ostrer H (1998) Carrier screening for cystic fibrosis, Gaucher disease, and Tay-Sachs disease in the Ashkenazi Jewish population: the first 1000 cases at New York University Medical Center, New York, NY. Arch Intern Med 158(7):777–781
9. Scott SA, Edelmann L, Liu L, Luo M, Desnick RJ, Kornreich R (2010) Experience with carrier screening and prenatal diagnosis for 16 Ashkenazi Jewish genetic diseases. Hum Mutat 31(11):1240–1250. https://doi.org/10.1002/humu.21327
10. Fernandes MJ, Kaplan F, Clow CL, Hechtman P, Scriver CR (1992) Specificity and sensitivity of hexosaminidase assays and DNA analysis for the detection of Tay-Sachs disease gene carriers among Ashkenazic Jews. Genet Epidemiol 9(3):169–175. https://doi.org/10.1002/gepi.1370090303
11. van Bael M, Natowicz MR, Tomczak J, Grebner EE, Prence EM (1996) Heterozygosity for Tay-Sachs disease in non-Jewish Americans with ancestry from Ireland or Great Britain. J Med Genet 33(10):829–832
12. De Braekeleer M, Hechtman P, Andermann E, Kaplan F (1992) The French Canadian Tay-Sachs disease deletion mutation: identification of probable founders. Hum Genet 89 (1):83–87
13. Maegawa GH, Stockley T, Tropak M, Banwell B, Blaser S, Kok F, Giugliani R, Mahuran D, Clarke JT (2006) The natural history of juvenile or subacute GM2 gangliosidosis: 21 new cases and literature review of 134 previously reported. Pediatrics 118(5): e1550–e1562. https://doi.org/10.1542/peds.2006-0588
14. Mahuran DJ (1999) Biochemical consequences of mutations causing the GM2

gangliosidoses. Biochim Biophys Acta 1455 (2–3):105–138

15. Peleg L, Meltzer F, Karpati M, Goldman B (1995) GM2 gangliosidosis B1 variant: biochemical and molecular characterization of hexosaminidase A. Biochem Mol Med 54 (2):126–132
16. Cao Z, Natowicz MR, Kaback MM, Lim-Steele JS, Prence EM, Brown D, Chabot T, Triggs-Raine BL (1993) A second mutation associated with apparent beta-hexosaminidase A pseudodeficiency: identification and frequency estimation. Am J Hum Genet 53(6):1198–1205
17. Lowden JA, Zuker S, Wilensky AJ, Skomorowski MA (1974) Screening for carriers of Tay-Sachs disease: a community project. Can Med Assoc J 111(3):229–233
18. Navon R, Mark Z, Mashiah S, Padeh B (1973) Determination of Tay-Sachs genotypes in pregnant women. Clin Genet 4(3):286–287
19. Nitowsky HM, Davis J, Nakagawa S, Fox D (1979) Human hexosaminidase isozymes. IV. Effects of oral contraceptive steroids on serum hexosaminidase activity. Am J Obstet Gynecol 134(6):642–647

Chapter 17

Next Generation Sequencing of Prenatal Structural Chromosomal Rearrangements Using Large-Insert Libraries

Benjamin B. Currall, Caroline W. Antolik, Ryan L. Collins, and Michael E. Talkowski

Abstract

Precise tests for genomic structural variation (SV) are essential for accurate diagnosis of prenatal genome abnormalities. The two most ubiquitous traditional methods for prenatal SV assessment, karyotyping and chromosomal microarrays, do not provide sufficient resolution for some clinically actionable SVs. Standard whole-genome sequencing (WGS) overcomes shortcomings of traditional techniques by providing base-pair resolution of the entire accessible genome. However, while sequencing costs have continued to decline in recent years, conventional WGS costs remain high for most routine clinical applications. Here, we describe a specialized WGS technique using large inserts (liWGS; also known as "jumping libraries") to resolve large (>5000–10,000 nucleotides) SVs at kilobase-resolution in prenatal samples, and at a fraction of the cost of standard WGS. We explicate the protocols for generating liWGS libraries and supplement with an overview for processing and analyzing liWGS data.

Key words Jumping libraries, Whole-genome sequencing, Prenatal diagnosis, Structural variation, Chromosomal abnormalities, Copy-number variation

1 Introduction

Structural variation (SV), including copy-number variations (CNVs; deletions and duplications) and balanced chromosomal abnormalities (BCAs; SV absent gross gain or loss of DNA, such as translocations or inversions), represents a highly penetrant class of deleterious genetic mutations that can arise sporadically in offspring and perturb genes essential in human development. Traditional cytogenetic techniques revolutionized genetic analysis of large genomic structural variation (SV) and are a cornerstone of prenatal diagnosis for many genetic disorders; however, these mainstay techniques have substantial limitations [1–3]. Conventional G-banded karyotyping, while sensitive to all forms of extremely large SV, cannot provide breakpoint resolution below the size of individual chromosome banding patterns (~3–10 million

Brynn Levy (ed.), *Prenatal Diagnosis*, Methods in Molecular Biology, vol. 1885, https://doi.org/10.1007/978-1-4939-8889-1_17,

nucleotides) [4–7]. Fluorescence in situ hybridization (FISH) provides improved resolution over karyotyping, but requires prior knowledge of the approximate genomic location of an SV, and thus is only a tenable approach when specific SV are already suspected [8]. Array-based comparative genomic hybridization (aCGH) has far higher resolution, but is only sensitive to CNVs and therefore blind to all BCAs.

Whole-genome sequencing (WGS) represents a major advance beyond traditional methods by providing comprehensive data about the accessible genome in its entirety, thus in theory permitting delineation of all forms and sizes of SV to base-pair resolution [9, 10]. Standard WGS preparation involves acoustic or enzymatic fragmentation of genomic DNA, attaching adapters that are compatible with the selected sequencing technology, and identifying indices to isolate these fragments [11]. The resulting DNA "libraries" are often further amplified by polymerase chain reaction (PCR) before high throughput sequencing. At present, Illumina sequencing instruments are the most widely used, such as the HiSeq 2000/2500 and MiSeq, and employ Solexa "sequencing-by-synthesis" chemistry. Other approaches are also viable, and each offers technical advantages and disadvantages. High throughput sequencing yields an abundance of short (generally ~150 nucleotide) reads from the original genomic DNA. These reads are computationally mapped back against a reference genome, and unexpected read mappings can be used to flag sites of divergence versus the reference genome (e.g., sites of genetic variation in the sequenced sample). Standard WGS approaches, however, can be clinically cumbersome due to high sequencing costs and requirements of computational infrastructure and expert knowledge [12].

An alternative WGS method, known as long-insert WGS (liWGS; also known as "jumping libraries"), can provide a cost-effective alternative to conventional WGS while still capturing nearly all large SV in the genome [13–16]. Importantly, the resolution of liWGS is roughly four orders of magnitude (1000-fold) higher than karyotyping and one order of magnitude (tenfold) higher than most clinical aCGH platforms. In contrast to standard WGS, liWGS involves an initial fragmentation of genomic DNA to a target size of typically 3–5 thousand nucleotides. These fragments are circularized in a manner that allows specific retention of the junction sites following fragmentation of the circle. DNA libraries are prepared from the smaller junction fragments, which contain the ends of the initial, larger fragments. Paired sequencing reads from such libraries effectively span the sample genome in "jumps" proportional to the initial fragment size, permitting liWGS to infer ~10-fold more covered genomic bases per sequenced fragment as compared to standard WGS. The resultant sequencing data can be processed and analyzed analogously to standard WGS. At current sequencing costs, this liWGS approach results in an approximate eightfold cost reduction to achieve comparable nucleotide coverage of the genome by conventional short-insert WGS compared to the physical coverage of the inserts produced by liWGS. However, this improved efficiency comes at a significant tradeoff in the genomic information that can be obtained. Given the low nucleotide coverage achieved by liWGS, only relatively large SVs are accessible, and the lower size threshold is directly proportional to the size of the insert. The method cannot detect small SVs ($\leq$~5000 nucleotides) nor single nucleotide variants (SNVs) and small insertion/deletions (1–49 nucleotides). The demonstrated value of liWGS has been in the delineation of large SVs with high confidence and the genomic features that they disrupt, providing clinically relevant information that is otherwise inaccessible to conventional technologies such as karyotyping and aCGH [17, 18].

Herein, we describe a liWGS preparation method we developed in our laboratory for detecting chromosomal abnormalities in prenatal samples, which we have applied to samples received within our hospital and collaborating hospitals [19]. Notably, the method is also applicable to pediatric and adult populations, as has been demonstrated in numerous research studies [13, 18, 20–25].

2 Materials

2.1 Fragmentation of Human Genomic DNA

1. miniTUBE Red 5.0 kb (Covaris, Woburn, MA).
2. 1× Tris-EDTA buffer.
3. Covaris focused ultrasonicator such as E220*evolution* (Covaris, Woburn, MA).

2.2 End-Repair of Sheared DNA

1. End-It DNA End-Repair Kit (Epicentre, Madison, WI).
2. QIAquick PCR Purification Kit (Qiagen, Germany).

2.3 EcoP15I Cap Adapter Ligation

1. Cap Adapter 1: /5Phos/ACAGCAG (Integrated DNA Technologies, Coralville, IA).
2. Cap Adapter 2: /5Phos/CTGCTGTAC (Integrated DNA Technologies, Coralville, IA).
3. Nuclease-Free Duplex Buffer (Integrated DNA Technologies, Coralville, IA).
4. Quick Ligation Kit (New England Biolabs, Inc., Ipswich, MA).
5. QIAquick PCR Purification Kit (Qiagen, Germany).

2.4 Gel Size Selection

1. 1 Kb Plus DNA Ladder (Thermo Fisher Scientific, Cambridge, MA).
2. QIAquick Gel Extraction Kit (Qiagen, Germany).

2.5 T4 Circularization

1. Internal adapter 1: /5Phos/CGTTC/iBiodT/CCGT (Integrated DNA Technologies, Coralville, IA).
2. Internal adapter 2: /5Phos/GGAGAACGGT (Integrated DNA Technologies, Coralville, IA).
3. Nuclease-Free Duplex Buffer (Integrated DNA Technologies, Coralville, IA).
4. T4 DNA Ligase (New England Biolabs, Inc., Ipswich, MA).
5. QIAquick PCR Purification Kit (Qiagen, Germany).

2.6 DNase Treatment

1. Plasmid-Safe ATP-Dependent DNase (Epicentre, Madison, WI).
2. QIAquick PCR Purification Kit (Qiagen, Germany).

2.7 EcoP15I Digestion

1. EcoP15I (New England Biolabs, Inc., Ipswich, MA).
2. InSolution sinefungin (EMD Millipore, Billerica, MA). Make up solution for protocol at 10 mM.

2.8 End-Repair of Digested DNA

1. DNA Polymerase I, Large (Klenow) Fragment (New England Biolabs, Inc., Ipswich, MA).
2. dNTPs, 25 mM.

2.9 Bead Binding

1. 1× wash buffer:
   (a) 60 μL Tris–HCl, 1 M pH 7.5.
   (b) 2.4 mL NaCl, 5 M.
   (c) 12 μL EDTA, 0.5 M.
   (d) 0.5 μL Tween 20.
   (e) QS to 12 mL with sterile water.
2. 2× binding buffer:
   (a) 60 μL Tris–HCl, 1 M pH 7.5.
   (b) 2.4 mL NaCl, 5 M.
   (c) 12 μL EDTA, 0.5 M.
   (d) QS to 6 mL with sterile water.
3. Dynabeads MyOne Streptavidin C1 (Thermo Fisher Scientific, Waltham, MA).
4. Magnetic rack.

2.10 dA-Tailing

1. NEBNext dA-Tailing Module (New England Biolabs, Inc., Ipswich, MA).

2.11 Adapter Ligation

1. Universal adapter: ACACTCTTTCCCTACAC-GACGCTCTTCCGATC*T (Integrated DNA Technologies, Coralville, IA).

2. Indexed adapter: /5Phos/GATCGGAAGAGCACACGTCT-GAACTCCAGTCAC(6BPindex) (Integrated DNA Technologies, Coralville, IA).
3. Quick Ligation Kit (New England Biolabs, Inc., Ipswich, MA).

2.12 PCR on Beads

1. Universal forward primer: AATGATACGGCGACCACCGA-GATCTACACTCTTTCCCTACACGACGCTCTTCC-GATC*T (Integrated DNA Technologies, Coralville, IA).
2. Custom reverse indexed primer: CAAGCAGAAGACGGCA-TACGAGAT(+6BPprimerindex)GTGACTGGAGTTC (reverse primer index is the reverse complement of the barcode adapter index) (Integrated DNA Technologies, Coralville, IA).
3. Phusion High-Fidelity PCR Master Mix with HF Buffer (New England Biolabs, Inc., Ipswich, MA).
4. QIAquick PCR Purification Kit (Qiagen, Germany).

2.13 Final Gel Selection

1. 1 Kb Plus DNA Ladder (Thermo Fisher Scientific, Cambridge, MA).
2. QIAquick Gel Extraction Kit (Qiagen, Germany).

3 Methods

3.1 Fragmentation of Human Genomic DNA

1. Load 5–10 μg of DNA into a red miniTUBE and combine with 1× TE for a total volume of 200 μL (*see* **Note 1**).
2. Shear DNA to a target size of 3 kb using a Covaris focused-ultrasonicator with red miniTUBEs and the 5k shear protocol as specified by the manufacturer.
3. Transfer fragmented DNA (200 μL) to clean 1.5 mL tube.
4. Use the QIAquick PCR Purification Kit to purify sample as specified by the manufacturer's protocol, eluting in 35 μL Buffer EB.

3.2 End-Repair of Sheared DNA

1. Use the End-It End-Repair Kit to end-repair fragmented DNA: to the fragmented and purified DNA, add 5 μL End-It Buffer (10×), 5 μL End-It dNTPs (2.5 nM), 5 μL End-It ATP (10 nM), and 1 μL enzyme mix (*see* **Note 2**).
2. Mix sample, spin down, and incubate at room temperature for 30–40 min.
3. Purify end-repaired DNA using QIAquick PCR Purification Kit, eluting in 52 μL Buffer EB.

3.3 EcoP15I Cap Adapter Ligation

3.3.1 Prepare Cap Adapters

1. Resuspend cap adapters 1 and 2 together in Nuclease-Free Duplex Buffer to a final concentration of 50 μM.
2. Incubate at 94 °C for 2 min, then allow to cool on ice.

3.3.2 Ligate Cap Adapters

1. Determine concentration of DNA and calculate the volume of duplexed cap adapters required for an adapter:fragment ratio of 10:1 (*see* **Notes 3** and **4**).
2. To each sample, add: the volume of cap adapters calculated for that sample, 55 μL Quick Ligase Buffer (2×), and 2 μL Quick Ligase (2,000,000 U/mL).
3. Mix sample, spin down, and incubate at room temperature for 15 min.
4. Purify samples using QIAquick PCR Purification Kit, eluting in 30 μL Buffer EB.

3.4 Gel Size Selection

3.4.1 Run Agarose Gel and Select Band from Gel

1. Prepare a 1% agarose gel with ~0.17 μg of ethidium bromide per milliliter.
2. Add an appropriate loading dye to DNA ladder and samples, mix, and load ladder and samples on gel. Load 1 Kb Plus Ladder each in the right- and leftmost lanes of each row of gel; load samples so that empty wells are left between the ladder and sample lanes, as well as between lanes containing different samples, to reduce the risk of contamination.
3. Run gel at 100 V for approximately 1 h, until a bromophenol dye indicator has migrated about 2 cm (*see* **Note 5**).
4. Use a razor blade or scalpel to select a DNA band in the 3–5 kb range from each sample on the gel (*see* **Notes 6** and **7**).

3.4.2 Extract DNA Using Qiagen's QIAquick Gel Extraction Kit

1. Weigh gel slice and add 3 volumes of Buffer QG (*see* **Note 8**).
2. Let it sit at room temperature until gel is completely dissolved.
3. Use columns to purify sample as directed in the manufacturer's protocol, but wash sample two times with 600 μL Buffer PE during the wash step.
4. Elute in 100 μL Buffer EB (*see* **Note 9**).

3.5 T4 DNA Circularization

3.5.1 Prepare Internal Adapters

1. Resuspend internal adapters 1 and 2 together to a final concentration of 2 μM in Nuclease-Free Duplex Buffer.
2. Incubate at 94 °C for 2 min, then allow to cool on ice.

3.5.2 Circularize DNA

1. Determine concentration of DNA using Nanodrop instrument and calculate the volume of duplexed internal adapters to add for an adapter:fragment ratio of 3:1 (*see* **Note 10**).

2. To each sample, add 78 μL water, 20 μL T4 Ligation Buffer (10×), the calculated amount of internal adapters, and 2 μL T4 DNA Ligase (*see* **Note 11**).
3. Mix sample, spin down, and incubate at room temperature for at least 3 h.
4. Purify with QIAquick PCR Purification Kit, eluting in 60 μL Buffer EB.

3.6 DNase Treatment

1. Using the Plasmid-Safe DNase Kit, add the following to each sample: 24.5 μL water, 10 μL Plasmid-Safe Buffer (10×), 5 μL ATP (25 mM), 2 μL Plasmid-Safe DNase (100 U/μL) (*see* **Note 12**).
2. Mix, spin down, and incubate at 37 °C for 40 min.
3. Purify with QIAquick PCR Purification Kit, eluting in 63 μL Buffer EB (*see* **Note 13**).

3.7 EcoP15I Digest

1. Add the following to each sample: 10 μL NEB Buffer 3.1 (10×), 20 μL ATP (10×), 1 μL sinefungin (10 mM), and 6 μL EcoP15I enzyme (10,000 U/mL).
2. Mix samples by pipetting and digest at 37 °C overnight.
3. After digestion is complete, inactivate enzyme by heating for 20 min at 65 °C; cool on ice for 5 min after heat inactivation.

3.8 End Repair of Digested DNA

1. Add 1.5 μL dNTPs (25 mM) and 1.5 μL of DNA Polymerase I, Large (Klenow) Fragment (5000 U/mL) to each sample. Mix samples by pipetting and incubate at room temperature for 30 min.
2. Inactivate by heating for 20 min at 65 °C, then cool on ice for 5 min.

3.9 Streptavidin Bead Binding

1. Aliquot 30 μL beads (10 mg/mL) per sample into a 1.5 mL tube (*see* **Note 14**). Separate beads from solution on magnetic rack and discard supernatant.
2. Add 500 μL 1× wash buffer to sample, remove from magnet, and gently mix. Separate beads from solution on magnet and discard supernatant.
3. Repeat **step 3** twice for a total of three washes.
4. Add 500 μL 1× binding buffer, remove from magnet, and gently mix. Separate beads from solution on magnet and discard supernatant (*see* **Note 15**).
5. Resuspend beads in the original volume using 1× binding buffer.
6. Add 105 μL 2× binding buffer and 30 μL beads to each sample and mix by pipetting (*see* **Note 16**).

7. Bind for 30 min at room temperature, mixing by pipetting every 10 min.
8. Separate beads from solution on magnet and discard supernatant.
9. Wash beads four times with 200 μL wash buffer (*see* **Note 17**).

3.10 dA-Tailing

1. Using the NEBNext dA-Tailing Module, add 42 μL water, 5 μL dA-Tailing Buffer (10×), and 3 μL Klenow (exo-) fragment (5000 U/mL) to each sample. Mix by pipetting and incubate for 30 min at 37 °C.
2. Separate beads from solution on magnet and discard supernatant.
3. Wash beads four times with 200 μL wash buffer, then wash once with ~50 μL Quick Ligase Buffer (1×) (*see* **Note 18**).

3.11 Adapter Ligation

3.11.1 Prepare Adapters

1. Resuspend universal adapter with individual barcoded adapters in Nuclease-Free Duplex Buffer to a final concentration of 15 μM.
2. Incubate for 2 min at 94 °C, then allow to cool on ice.

3.11.2 Ligate Adapters to Samples

1. Using the Quick Ligation Kit, add 24.5 μL water, 25 μL Quick Ligase Buffer (2×), 1 μL duplexed adapter (15 μM), and 1.3 μL Quick Ligase (2,000,000 U/mL) to each sample, using a different barcoded adapter for each sample.
2. Incubate at room temperature for 45 min.
3. Separate beads from solution on magnet and discard supernatant.
4. Wash beads four times with 200 μL wash buffer, then wash once with 200 μL Buffer EB.
5. Resuspend beads in 30 μL Buffer EB.

3.12 Amplify Samples on Beads to Add Illumina Adapters Using Phusion HF PCR Master Mix with HF Buffer

1. Add 1 μL universal forward primer (25 μM), 1 μL sample-specific reverse indexed primer (25 μM), and 75 μL Phusion Master Mix (2×) to each sample (*see* **Note 19**).
2. Mix samples by pipetting and split individual samples into three reactions of 50 μL each for PCR.
3. PCR amplify using the following conditions (*see* **Note 20**):
   (a) One cycle: 98 °C for 30 s.
   (b) Eleven cycles: 98 °C for 10 s, 65 °C for 30 s, 72 °C for 30 s.
   (c) One cycle: 72 °C for 5 min.
   (d) 10 °C hold.

4. After PCR is complete, combine replicates for each sample into single 1.5 mL tube.
5. Separate beads from solution on magnet and transfer supernatant to a new 1.5 mL tube.
6. Purify with QIAquick PCR Purification Kit, eluting in 30 μL Buffer EB.

3.13 Gel Purification of Final Product

1. Prepare a 1.5–2% agarose gel with ~0.17 μg of ethidium bromide per mL.
2. Add an appropriate loading dye to DNA ladder and samples, mix, and load 1 Kb Plus Ladder (1 μg/μL) and samples on gel. Load one ladder each in the right- and leftmost lanes of each row of gel, then load samples onto gel, leaving an empty well between ladder and sample.
3. Run gel at 100 V for approximately one and a half hours.
4. Use a razor blade or scalpel cut the band ~200 bp from the gel for each sample (*see* **Notes 21** and **22**).
5. Extract sample using QIAquick Gel Extraction kit as described in Subheading 3.4.2, but elute in 20 μL EB.

3.14 Quantify and Pool Libraries

1. Quantify using Agilent Bioanalyzer, Agilent Tapestation, or qPCR.
2. Pool libraries in desired ratio for Illumina sequencing (*see* **Note 23**).

3.15 Sequencing and Data Processing

1. Sequence libraries with paired 25 bp read chemistry and a 6 bp barcode read on an Illumina sequencing platform.
2. Demultiplex reads corresponding to the sample-specific 6 bp barcode index attached to the prepared library, in accordance with Illumina's standard recommended protocols.
3. Reverse-complement the raw reads; this can be done with tools such as *fastx* or *seqtk* (https://github.com/lh3/seqtk) [26].
4. Align reads using a pairwise-aware aligner appropriate for short (25 bp) reads, such as *BWA-backtrack* (*see* **Note 24**), against a human genome reference assembly (*see* **Note 25**) [27].
5. Mark duplicate sequenced fragments; this can be done with tools such as *Picard MarkDuplicates* (http://broadinstitute.github.io/picard/) or *SAMBLASTER* [28].
6. Sort aligned reads by numerical coordinate ordering; this can be done with tools such as *samtools* or *sambamba* [29, 30].
7. Evaluate alignment metrics of the processed library; this can be done with *PicardTools* (recommended; http://broadinstitute.github.io/picard/), *sambamba/samtools flagstat*, *bamtools stats*, and numerous other programs (*see* **Note 26** and Table 1) [29–31].

Table 1
liWGS library alignment metrics on nine multiethnic samples sequenced to deep coverage as part of the 1000 Genomes Project: Human Genome Structural Variation Consortium

Sample	Raw read pairs	Alignment rate Read	Alignment rate Pair	Proper pair rate	Duplication rate Read	Duplication rate Pair	Chimeric pair rate	Median insert size	Haploid physical coverage
HG00512	183,274,642	97.2%	95.1%	88.0%	12.4%	10.3%	7.4%	3401	161.4
HG00513	195,273,608	96.8%	94.4%	88.1%	11.9%	10.2%	6.6%	3315	166.9
HG00514	178,875,771	96.0%	93.5%	86.9%	14.1%	11.6%	7.0%	3325	147.5
HG00731	187,721,771	95.8%	93.2%	88.0%	15.5%	12.6%	5.5%	3439	159.9
HG00732	180,471,734	95.4%	92.9%	85.0%	18.4%	16.5%	8.4%	3525	144.6
HG00733	211,630,514	96.9%	94.6%	80.8%	8.1%	7.0%	14.4%	3736	193.8
GM19238	198,430,973	96.2%	93.6%	79.1%	12.9%	10.7%	15.4%	3493	158.1
GM19239	182,791,861	97.0%	94.7%	87.2%	13.0%	11.2%	7.8%	3420	158.3
GM19240	208,381,715	97.2%	95.2%	85.3%	11.9%	9.8%	10.3%	3497	184.1
Mean	191,872,510	96.5%	94.1%	85.4%	13.1%	11.1%	9.2%	3461	163.9

8. Perform visual quality assurance on the distribution of insert sizes as determined by *Picard CollectInsertSizeMetrics* (*see* Fig. 1, Table 1, and **Note 27**; http://broadinstitute.github.io/picard/).

3.16 Data Analysis

1. Isolate anomalous read-pairs using *samtools* or *sambamba* [29, 30].
2. Search across anomalous read-pairs for unexpected aggregations of anomalous pairs in close proximity (<5 kb) with high alignment and read qualities.

4 Notes

1. 3 μg of DNA is recommended as a minimum starting input, but the protocol can also be done with less DNA input if optimized.
2. Aliquot ATP from kit into smaller, single use tubes to reduce freeze-thaw cycles. Always keep ATP-containing solutions on ice during reaction preparation.
3. The amount of DNA used in this step and the subsequent gel purification can affect the percentage of chimeras present in the final sequencing reads. To greatly reduce the amount of chimeras, limit the DNA used in this step to no more than 4 μg

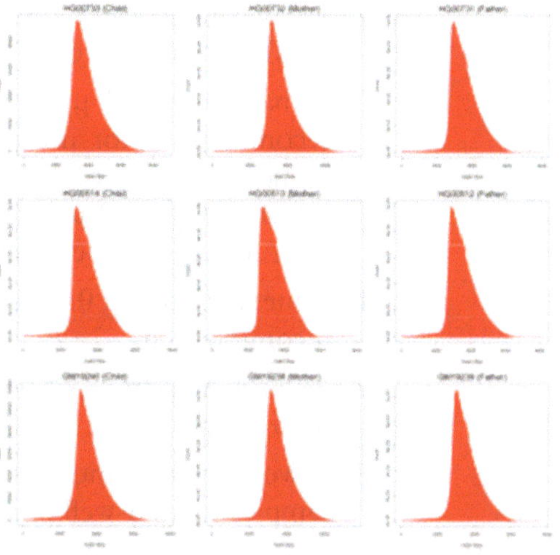

Fig. 1 Example insert size distributions of sequenced fragments from nine libraries generated by the Talkowski Laboratory with this protocol for the Human Genome Structural Variation project. Given an original input of 5 μg genomic DNA and a targeted insert size of 3.5 kb, the below distribution of proper sequenced fragments were obtained when sequenced to a yield of 180 M individual fragments with 25 bp reads on an Illumina HiSeq 2500. Reads were processed as described in Subheading 3.14 and the below distribution was generated from aligned BAM files by *PicardTools* (http:/broadinstitute.github.io/picard/). These data are available freely through the 1000 Genomcs Project ftp server, accessible here: http:/www.1000genomes.org/human-genome-structural-variation-consortium/. Notably, for detection of known structural variation, coverage can be greatly reduced as desired; 30–50× physical coverage is typically sufficient for confirmation of known rearrangements

(80 ng/μL in 50 μL volume), though reactions can be split into multiple samples if more complex libraries are desired.

4. The volume of cap adapter added to a sample should not exceed 4 μL; samples that require higher volumes should be diluted and total sample should be reduced.

5. Exceeding the recommended gel run time will likely require multiple Qiagen columns for purification to retain the desired size range.

6. Capturing pre- and post-size selection images of the gel is recommended.

7. A straight edge is recommended to ensure accurate and uniform size selection of bands, and selection should be below the 6 kb threshold to minimize chimera rates (expected size of concatemerization of two 3 kb fragments).

8. The gel slice should weigh ~0.4 g. If exceeded, two spin columns may be required.

9. To maximize yield during extraction, two elution steps of 50 μL each (total vol = 100 μL) should be used.
10. A maximum of 1 μg DNA (10 ng/μL in 100 μL volume) is recommended for use in this step. If DNA concentration is higher, increase volume of total reaction or split into multiple tubes to obtain ~1 μg of DNA per reaction. Higher amounts of DNA can increase chimera rates.
11. Generally, adding 0.6–0.7 μL of internal adapters per sample is recommended.
12. Aliquot ATP from kit into smaller, single-use tubes to reduce freeze-thaw cycles.
13. If working with more than eight samples at once, transferring samples to a 96-well plate at this time is suggested.
14. Beads should be at room temperature prior to use; mix beads thoroughly before use to ensure solution is uniform.
15. A brief spin in a centrifuge is recommended at this stage to ensure complete removal of any residual wash buffer.
16. Mix samples slowly on beads to prevent excessive air bubble formation, which can interfere with wash buffer removal.
17. Take care to remove all wash buffer after this step before proceeding. Residual wash buffer can interfere with later reactions.
18. Washing with a small amount of Quick Ligase Buffer (1×) aids in removing any remaining traces of wash buffer.
19. For each sample, use the specific reverse primer that corresponds to the adapter added in the previous step.
20. The number of cycles can be adjusted based on anticipated library complexity and tolerance of duplications for a specific experiment. Increasing cycles will increase final yield but may increase duplication rates.
21. Product should be visible as a ~200 bp band on the gel. If the size is lower than ~200 bp, run the gel longer to avoid possible contamination with adapter/primer dimers during gel extraction.
22. Capturing pre- and post-size selection images of the gel is recommended.
23. It is recommended to save an aliquot of the final pool.
24. Many common aligners are not appropriate for 25 bp reads generated by this protocol. Ensure your choice of aligner is appropriate. BWA-Backtrack is the recommended aligner [27].
25. The most current human reference genome assembly is available directly from the NCBI Genome Reference Consortium (GRC; http://www.ncbi.nlm.nih.gov/projects/genome/assembly/grc/).

26. Given average read quality and sufficient sequencing depth for minimal analysis of a human whole-genome (>40 M sequenced read-pairs), desirable alignment quality metrics might be: pairwise alignment rate $\geq$90%; chimeric pair rate $\leq$10%; pairwise duplication rate $\leq$10%; median insert size = 3500 bp. An example of typical metrics for a high coverage library (~150× haploid coverage) such as those generated for the 1000 Genomes Project/Human Genome Structural Variation Consortium is provided in Table 1.
27. Desirable insert size distributions of sequenced libraries will feature a sharp left tail (right skew) leading to a peak at the approximate desired library insert size. The right tail can be elongated, but generally is not advised to extend significantly beyond ~8 kb for a 3.5 kb median insert library, at which point the distribution kurtosis will adversely impact read alignment algorithms. *See* Fig. 1 and Table 1 for an example of desirable insert size distributions and related alignment statistics.

References

1. Hillman SC, McMullan DJ, Williams D, Maher ER, Kilby MD (2012) Microarray comparative genomic hybridization in prenatal diagnosis: a review. Ultrasound Obstet Gynecol 40 (4):385–391. https://doi.org/10.1002/uog.11180
2. Lichtenbelt KD, Knoers NV, Schuring-Blom GH (2011) From karyotyping to array-CGH in prenatal diagnosis. Cytogenet Genome Res 135(3–4):241–250. https://doi.org/10.1159/000334065
3. Miller DT, Adam MP, Aradhya S, Biesecker LG, Brothman AR, Carter NP, Church DM, Crolla JA, Eichler EE, Epstein CJ, Faucett WA, Feuk L, Friedman JM, Hamosh A, Jackson L, Kaminsky EB, Kok K, Krantz ID, Kuhn RM, Lee C, Ostell JM, Rosenberg C, Scherer SW, Spinner NB, Stavropoulos DJ, Tepperberg JH, Thorland EC, Vermeesch JR, Waggoner DJ, Watson MS, Martin CL, Ledbetter DH (2010) Consensus statement: chromosomal microarray is a first-tier clinical diagnostic test for individuals with developmental disabilities or congenital anomalies. Am J Hum Genet 86 (5):749–764. https://doi.org/10.1016/j.ajhg.2010.04.006
4. Cheung VG, Nowak N, Jang W, Kirsch IR, Zhao S, Chen XN, Furey TS, Kim UJ, Kuo WL, Olivier M, Conroy J, Kasprzyk A, Massa H, Yonescu R, Sait S, Thoreen C, Snijders A, Lemyre E, Bailey JA, Bruzel A, Burrill WD, Clegg SM, Collins S, Dhami P, Friedman C, Han CS, Herrick S, Lee J, Ligon AH, Lowry S, Morley M, Narasimhan S, Osoegawa K, Peng Z, Plajzer-Frick I, Quade BJ, Scott D, Sirotkin K, Thorpe AA, Gray JW, Hudson J, Pinkel D, Ried T, Rowen L, Shen-Ong GL, Strausberg RL, Birney E, Callen DF, Cheng JF, Cox DR, Doggett NA, Carter NP, Eichler EE, Haussler D, Korenberg JR, Morton CC, Albertson D, Schuler G, de Jong PJ, Trask BJ (2001) Integration of cytogenetic landmarks into the draft sequence of the human genome. Nature 409(6822):953–958. https://doi.org/10.1038/35057192
5. Furey TS, Haussler D (2003) Integration of the cytogenetic map with the draft human genome sequence. Hum Mol Genet 12 (9):1037–1044
6. Smeets DF (2004) Historical prospective of human cytogenetics: from microscope to microarray. Clin Biochem 37(6):439–446. https://doi.org/10.1016/j.clinbiochem.2004.03.006
7. Warburton D (1991) De novo balanced chromosome rearrangements and extra marker chromosomes identified at prenatal diagnosis: clinical significance and distribution of breakpoints. Am J Hum Genet 49(5):995–1013
8. Shaffer LG, Bejjani BA (2006) Medical applications of array CGH and the transformation of clinical cytogenetics. Cytogenet Genome Res 115(3–4):303–309. https://doi.org/10.1159/000095928
9. Francescatto L, Katsanis N (2015) Newborn screening and the era of medical genomics.

Semin Perinatol 39(8):617–622. https://doi.org/10.1053/j.semperi.2015.09.010

10. Tattini L, D'Aurizio R, Magi A (2015) Detection of genomic structural variants from next-generation sequencing data. Front Bioeng Biotechnol 3:92. https://doi.org/10.3389/fbioe.2015.00092
11. Metzker ML (2010) Sequencing technologies—the next generation. Nat Rev Genet 11 (1):31–46. https://doi.org/10.1038/nrg2626
12. Zhang W, Cui H, Wong LJ (2014) Application of next generation sequencing to molecular diagnosis of inherited diseases. Top Curr Chem 336:19–45. https://doi.org/10.1007/128_2012_325
13. Talkowski ME, Ernst C, Heilbut A, Chiang C, Hanscom C, Lindgren A, Kirby A, Liu S, Muddukrishna B, Ohsumi TK, Shen Y, Borowsky M, Daly MJ, Morton CC, Gusella JF (2011) Next-generation sequencing strategies enable routine detection of balanced chromosome rearrangements for clinical diagnostics and genetic research. Am J Hum Genet 88(4):469–481. https://doi.org/10.1016/j.ajhg.2011.03.013
14. Korbel JO, Urban AE, Affourtit JP, Godwin B, Grubert F, Simons JF, Kim PM, Palejev D, Carriero NJ, Du L, Taillon BE, Chen Z, Tanzer A, Saunders AC, Chi J, Yang F, Carter NP, Hurles ME, Weissman SM, Harkins TT, Gerstein MB, Egholm M, Snyder M (2007) Paired-end mapping reveals extensive structural variation in the human genome. Science 318(5849):420–426. https://doi.org/10.1126/science.1149504
15. Collins FS, Weissman SM (1984) Directional cloning of DNA fragments at a large distance from an initial probe: a circularization method. Proc Natl Acad Sci U S A 81(21):6812–6816
16. Hanscom C, Talkowski M (2014) Design of large-insert jumping libraries for structural variant detection using illumina sequencing. Curr Protoc Hum Genet 80:7.22.1–7.2229. https://doi.org/10.1002/0471142905.hg0722s80
17. Talkowski ME, Ordulu Z, Pillalamarri V, Benson CB, Blumenthal I, Connolly S, Hanscom C, Hussain N, Pereira S, Picker J, Rosenfeld JA, Shaffer LG, Wilkins-Haug LE, Gusella JF, Morton CC (2012) Clinical diagnosis by whole-genome sequencing of a prenatal sample. N Engl J Med 367(23):2226–2232. https://doi.org/10.1056/NEJMoa1208594
18. Talkowski ME, Rosenfeld JA, Blumenthal I, Pillalamarri V, Chiang C, Heilbut A, Ernst C, Hanscom C, Rossin E, Lindgren AM, Pereira S, Ruderfer D, Kirby A, Ripke S, Harris DJ, Lee JH, Ha K, Kim HG, Solomon BD, Gropman AL, Lucente D, Sims K, Ohsumi TK, Borowsky ML, Loranger S, Quade B, Lage K, Miles J, Wu BL, Shen Y, Neale B, Shaffer LG, Daly MJ, Morton CC, Gusella JF (2012) Sequencing chromosomal abnormalities reveals neurodevelopmental loci that confer risk across diagnostic boundaries. Cell 149 (3):525–537. https://doi.org/10.1016/j.cell.2012.03.028
19. Wapner RJ, Martin CL, Levy B, Ballif BC, Eng CM, Zachary JM, Savage M, Platt LD, Saltzman D, Grobman WA, Klugman S, Scholl T, Simpson JL, McCall K, Aggarwal VS, Bunke B, Nahum O, Patel A, Lamb AN, Thom EA, Beaudet AL, Ledbetter DH, Shaffer LG, Jackson L (2012) Chromosomal microarray versus karyotyping for prenatal diagnosis. N Engl J Med 367(23):2175–2184. https://doi.org/10.1056/NEJMoa1203382
20. Brand H, Collins RL, Hanscom C, Rosenfeld JA, Pillalamarri V, Stone MR, Kelley F, Mason T, Margolin L, Eggert S, Mitchell E, Hodge JC, Gusella JF, Sanders SJ, Talkowski ME (2015) Paired-duplication signatures mark cryptic inversions and other complex structural variation. Am J Hum Genet 97(1):170–176. https://doi.org/10.1016/j.ajhg.2015.05.012
21. Brand H, Pillalamarri V, Collins RL, Eggert S, O'Dushlaine C, Braaten EB, Stone MR, Chambert K, Doty ND, Hanscom C, Rosenfeld JA, Ditmars H, Blais J, Mills R, Lee C, Gusella JF, McCarroll S, Smoller JW, Talkowski ME, Doyle AE (2014) Cryptic and complex chromosomal aberrations in early-onset neuropsychiatric disorders. Am J Hum Genet 95 (4):454–461. https://doi.org/10.1016/j.ajhg.2014.09.005
22. Talkowski ME, Mullegama SV, Rosenfeld JA, van Bon BW, Shen Y, Repnikova EA, Gastier-Foster J, Thrush DL, Kathiresan S, Ruderfer DM, Chiang C, Hanscom C, Ernst C, Lindgren AM, Morton CC, An Y, Astbury C, Brueton LA, Lichtenbelt KD, Ades LC, Fichera M, Romano C, Innis JW, Williams CA, Bartholomew D, Van Allen MI, Parikh A, Zhang L, Wu BL, Pyatt RE, Schwartz S, Shaffer LG, de Vries BB, Gusella JF, Elsea SH (2011) Assessment of 2q23.1 microdeletion syndrome implicates MBD5 as a single causal locus of intellectual disability, epilepsy, and autism spectrum disorder. Am J Hum Genet 89(4):551–563. https://doi.org/10.1016/j.ajhg.2011.09.011
23. Hodge JC, Mitchell E, Pillalamarri V, Toler TL, Bartel F, Kearney HM, Zou YS, Tan WH, Hanscom C, Kirmani S, Hanson RR, Skinner SA, Rogers RC, Everman DB, Boyd E, Tapp C,

Mullegama SV, Keelean-Fuller D, Powell CM, Elsea SH, Morton CC, Gusella JF, DuPont B, Chaubey A, Lin AE, Talkowski ME (2014) Disruption of MBD5 contributes to a spectrum of psychopathology and neurodevelopmental abnormalities. Mol Psychiatry 19 (3):368–379. https://doi.org/10.1038/mp.2013.42

24. Kloosterman WP, Guryev V, van Roosmalen M, Duran KJ, de Bruijn E, Bakker SC, Letteboer T, van Nesselrooij B, Hochstenbach R, Poot M, Cuppen E (2011) Chromothripsis as a mechanism driving complex de novo structural rearrangements in the germline. Hum Mol Genet 20 (10):1916–1924. https://doi.org/10.1093/hmg/ddr073

25. Kloosterman WP, Tavakoli-Yaraki M, van Roosmalen MJ, van Binsbergen E, Renkens I, Duran K, Ballarati L, Vergult S, Giardino D, Hansson K, Ruivenkamp CA, Jager M, van Haeringen A, Ippel EF, Haaf T, Passarge E, Hochstenbach R, Menten B, Larizza L, Guryev V, Poot M, Cuppen E (2012) Constitutional chromothripsis rearrangements involve clustered double-stranded DNA breaks and nonhomologous repair mechanisms. Cell Rep 1(6):648–655. https://doi.org/10.1016/j.celrep.2012.05.009

26. Blankenberg D, Gordon A, Von Kuster G, Coraor N, Taylor J, Nekrutenko A (2010) Manipulation of FASTQ data with Galaxy. Bioinformatics 26(14):1783–1785. https://doi.org/10.1093/bioinformatics/btq281

27. Li H, Durbin R (2009) Fast and accurate short read alignment with Burrows-Wheeler transform. Bioinformatics 25(14):1754–1760. https://doi.org/10.1093/bioinformatics/btp324

28. Faust GG, Hall IM (2014) SAMBLASTER: fast duplicate marking and structural variant read extraction. Bioinformatics 30 (17):2503–2505. https://doi.org/10.1093/bioinformatics/btu314

29. Tarasov A, Vilella AJ, Cuppen E, Nijman IJ, Prins P (2015) Sambamba: fast processing of NGS alignment formats. Bioinformatics. https://doi.org/10.1093/bioinformatics/btv098

30. Li H, Handsaker B, Wysoker A, Fennell T, Ruan J, Homer N, Marth G, Abecasis G, Durbin R (2009) The Sequence Alignment/Map format and SAMtools. Bioinformatics 25 (16):2078–2079. https://doi.org/10.1093/bioinformatics/btp352

31. Barnett DW, Garrison EK, Quinlan AR, Stromberg MP, Marth GT (2011) BamTools: a C++ API and toolkit for analyzing and managing BAM files. Bioinformatics 27 (12):1691–1692. https://doi.org/10.1093/bioinformatics/btr174

Chapter 18

Prenatal Diagnosis by Whole Exome Sequencing in Fetuses with Ultrasound Abnormalities

Vanessa Felice, Avinash Abhyankar, and Vaidehi Jobanputra

Abstract

Whole-exome sequencing (WES) has been used as a standard of care for postnatal diagnosis in the clinical setting in the past few years for children and adults with undiagnosed disease. Many rare disorders have been diagnosed through WES, which is less expensive than the traditional serial genetic testing where patients had previously spent years on an uninformative diagnostic odyssey. Seeking a diagnosis often entails enduring time consuming, and sometimes invasive procedures which may be associated with medical risks that are stressful for families and impose a heavy burden on the health-care system. However, the use of WES is considered impractical in the prenatal and neonatal testing period because of the technical and computational challenges of performing genomic sequencing from small amounts of genetic material, and the need for faster turnaround time (TAT) than the current 6–8 weeks TAT provided by most clinical labs offering postnatal testing. With the rapidly evolving methods of sequence analysis, there are clinical challenges such as the constantly increasing number of genes being identified which are not yet fully phenotypically characterized, especially when ascertained prenatally or neonatally before all the clinical features may be evident. Despite these challenges, there are many clinical benefits to acquiring genomic information in the prenatal and neonatal period. These include superior prognostic information which allows for prenatal planning of mode of delivery and hospital for delivery and optimized neonatal management. We have developed a clinical WES assay using small amounts of DNA with a TAT of 10 days for use in the prenatal or neonatal setting. This test is used to detect small nucleotide variants and indels in fetuses and neonates with structural abnormalities.

Key words Prenatal diagnosis, Whole-exome sequencing, Fetal anomalies

1 Introduction

The risk of major structural birth defects among live births in the United States is approximately 3% and is associated with inherited or de novo mutations as well as with maternal factors, such as advanced age and exposure to teratogens [1, 2]. With advances in imaging, the ability to detect birth defects prenatally and neonatally and subsequently use this information to optimize perinatal and neonatal management has increased tremendously. Simultaneously, molecular genetic diagnostics have improved the ability to more

Brynn Levy (ed.), *Prenatal Diagnosis*, Methods in Molecular Biology, vol. 1885, https://doi.org/10.1007/978-1-4939-8889-1_18,

precisely identify the underlying cause of these birth defects and provide additional prognostic information to improve prenatal and postnatal management. The first major improvement in genomic molecular prenatal diagnosis was chromosome microarray analysis (CMA) [3]. The introduction of prenatal CMA has provided an invaluable opportunity to evaluate the clinical value of new genomic technologies in prenatal care and to understand the challenges of interpretation of data in an evolving field.

Generally a combination of karyotype, Fluorescence *In Situ* Hybridization (FISH), and CMA are used to investigate the etiology of fetal anomaly identified by an ultrasound scan in the second trimester. Of cases that undergo diagnostic testing, a karyotype abnormality is found in 8% to 10% of cases, whereas a microdeletion/duplication is identified in another 6%, leaving most abnormal fetuses without a specific genetic diagnosis [3, 4]. Advances in throughput and decreased cost of next generation sequencing technology have enabled whole-exome sequencing (WES) which is ideal for diagnosing disorders that are genetically heterogeneous and for which gene discovery is incomplete. The use of clinical exome sequencing for the diagnosis of a wide range of indications including birth defects has been described in several studies [5–7]. The diagnostic yield of WES in pediatric patients with undiagnosed disease is approximately 25% [5], suggesting that it might complement genetic diagnosis in other settings. A case report [8] and a study of 30 fetuses and neonates with structural anomalies identified by ultrasound, illustrate the utility of identifying variants that potentially cause abnormal fetal development [9]. While these studies performed sequencing on prenatal specimens, the data were not produced within a timeframe that would have allowed the results to be used until after the birth of the baby. Since then, additional smaller studies show that prenatal WES, when the standard genetic testing is normal, can elucidate the pathogenic variants in approximately 10–50% of fetal structural anomalies [10–13].

There are many challenges to implementing genomic prenatal and neonatal testing. These include the technical and computational challenges of performing genomic sequencing from small amounts of genetic material, the need for faster turnaround time (TAT) than the current 6-8 weeks TAT in postnatal cases, and the rapidly evolving methods of sequence analysis. Clinical challenges include the constantly increasing number of genes being identified which are not yet fully phenotypically characterized, especially when ascertained prenatally or neonatally before all the clinical features may be evident. Despite these challenges, there are many clinical benefits with proper utilization of prenatally and neonatally acquired genomic information including increasingly precise prognostic information allowing prenatal planning of mode of delivery and hospital for delivery and optimized neonatal management. A few large studies are currently ongoing to determine the clinical utility of WES in prenatal setting.

At present, the American College of Medical Genetics and Genomics (ACMGG) and the Society for Maternal Fetal Medicine (SMFM) do not recommend routine use of WES for prenatal diagnosis outside of the context of clinical trials [14]. In select cases in which other approaches to diagnosis have been uninformative, it may be appropriate to offer WES. Examples of such cases include recurrent or multiple congenital anomalies, heterotaxy, and undiagnosed skeletal dysplasias. Prenatal WES also has a role in cases in which a fetus has structural abnormalities with reported consanguinity or homozygosity indicating relatedness on microarray [4]. We describe below our laboratory method for WES with rapid turnaround time which is emerging as a valuable tool for genetic diagnosis in the prenatal and neonatal setting.

2 Materials

2.1 DNA Library Preparation

1. SureSelectXT Library Prep Kit (Agilent Technologies, Santa Clara, CA, USA).
2. SureSelectXT Clinical Research Exome V2 (Agilent Technologies, Santa Clara, CA, USA).
3. Agencourt AMPure XP Kit (Beckman Coulter, Indianapolis, IN).
4. Dynabeads MyOne Streptavidin T1 (Thermo Fisher Scientific, Waltham, MA).
5. Ethanol, 200 proof for molecular biology.
6. Sterile, nuclease-free water.
7. DNA 1000 CHiP Kit (Agilent Technologies, Santa Clara, CA, USA).
8. Dynal DynaMag-2 magnetic stand (Thermo Fisher Scientific, Waltham, MA).
9. Covaris microTUBE plate (Covaris, Woburn, MA).
10. 96-Well Deep Well Plates.
11. 96-Well skirted PCR plates.

2.2 Illumina DNA Sequencing

1. HiSeq Paired End Flow Cell v4 (Illumina, Inc., San Diego, CA, USA).
2. HiSeq Paired End Cluster Kit v4 (Illumina, Inc., San Diego, CA, USA).
3. HiSeq Rapid Paired End Flow Cell v2 (Illumina, Inc., San Diego, CA, USA).
4. cBot Manifold (Illumina, Inc., San Diego, CA, USA).

5. 1.0 N Sodium Hydroxide, JT Baker 200 mM Tris–HCl, pH 8.0.
6. 200 mM Tris–HCl, pH 8.0.
7. Laboratory-grade water.

2.3 Laboratory Equipment

1. Thermo Mixer C 5382 (Eppendorf, Hauppauge, New York, USA).
2. Agilent Technologies 2100 Bioanalyzer (Agilent Technologies, Santa Clara, CA, USA).
3. PCR Thermal cycler.
4. Covaris LE-220 Sample Preparation System (Covaris, Woburn, MA).
5. Vacuum DNA concentrator.
6. Microsample Incubator.
7. High Speed Microplate Shaker.
8. HiSeq 2500 (Illumina, Inc., San Diego, CA, USA).
9. cBot (Illumina, Inc., San Diego, CA, USA).

3 Methods

The protocols described in this chapter require high molecular weight DNA of good quality. Any commercial DNA extraction kit may be utilized (*see* Chapter 7). In addition, maternal cell contamination studies should be performed (*see* Chapter 8) to ensure that WES results accurately reflect the genomic status of the fetus.

3.1 DNA Library Preparation

The library preparation process can be completed within 48 hours. This process includes shearing genomic DNA, repairing the ends of the fragments, adding an A-base to the 3′ ends, ligating Illumina adapters, and amplifying the DNA. The exome is then captured through a hybridization to RNA baits and enriched with PCR to prepare the samples for sequencing on Illumina next generation sequencing instruments.

3.1.1 DNA Shearing

The shearing process uses sonication to break up DNA into smaller fragments which will be selected out based on size in the subsequent steps.

1. Normalize 1500 ng of DNA in 130 μL of nuclease-free water and transfer to a Covaris plate.
2. Cover the plate with Covaris foil tape and spin down briefly (*see* **Note 1**).
3. Turn on the Covaris LE220 instrument.

4. Chill the water to 7 °C and degas the instrument for at least 45 min prior to starting fragmentation.
5. Select load Samples to bring the sample tray to the front of the instrument.
6. When the green "Open" button is illuminated, press the button and gently pull on the handle to open the instrument door.
7. Place the Covaris plate containing the samples to be sheared onto the sample platform.
8. Close the door and select the following conditions: Time = 380 s, Duty Cycle = 30%, PIP = 450, Cycles Per Burst = 200.
9. Ensure that the positions of the samples on the software setup page are correct and press Start to begin the fragmentation.
10. Once the fragmentation is complete, open the door and remove the plate.
11. Transfer the sheared samples from the Covaris plate to a new 96-well plate.
12. Be sure the AMPure beads have been removed from the refrigerator and have acclimated to room temperature for at least 30 min prior to proceeding.
13. Make 80% Ethanol just prior to starting this procedure.
14. Vortex the AMPure XP beads until they are well dispersed.
15. Add 180 μL of the AMPure XP beads to each well of the plate containing sample and pipette up and down 15 times.
16. Incubate the plate at room temperature for 10 min.
17. Place the plate on the appropriate magnetic stand and let it incubate at room temperature for an additional 5 min.
18. Remove and discard all the solution of the supernatant from each well.
19. With the plate still on the magnetic stand, add 200 μL of freshly prepared 80% ethanol to each well without disturbing the beads.
20. Incubate the plate at room temperature for 30 s, then remove and discard all the supernatant from each well.
21. Repeat **steps 19** and **20** once for a total of two ethanol washes.
22. Following the last ethanol wash, use a p10 to remove any residual ethanol from the bottom of the wells while keeping the plate on the magnetic stand.
23. Keep the plate on the magnetic stand for no more than 5 min to dry the beads (*see* **Note 2**).
24. Remove the plate from the magnet and add 52 μL of nuclease-free water to resuspend the beads by gently pipetting up and down ten times.

25. Incubate the plate with the resuspended samples for 2 min at room temperature.
26. Place the plate on the magnetic stand and let the plate incubate at room temperature for an additional 5 min.
27. With the plate still on the magnetic stand, transfer 48 μL of the supernatant to a new plate.

3.1.2 End Repair

Following shearing, the ends of the DNA are of varied lengths and have 3′ and 5′ overhangs. For adapter ligation to be efficient, the overhands must be repaired. The end repair step extends the overhangs to create blunt-ended DNA fragments.

1. Create an End repair master mix using the guidelines in Table 1.
2. Add 52 μL of End Repair/A-Tail Mix to each sample of the plate and pipette up and down to mix.
3. Seal the plate and spin down briefly.
4. Place the plate in the thermal cycler and run for 30 min at 20 °C.
5. Proceed immediately to the next step.

3.1.3 AMPure Bead Cleanup

1. Be sure the AMPure beads have been removed from the refrigerator and have been acclimated to room temperature for at least 30 min prior to proceeding.
2. Make 80% Ethanol just prior to starting this procedure, unless it was already prepared during the DNA shearing cleanup.
3. Vortex the AMPure XP beads until they are well dispersed.
4. Add 180 μL of the AMPure XP beads to each well of the plate containing sample and pipette up and down to mix.
5. Incubate the plate at room temperature for 10 min.

Table 1
End repair master mix setup

Reagent	Vol. for 1 library (μL)	Vol. for *N* library (μL)
Nuclease-free water	35.2	$(N+1) \times 35.2$
10× end repair buffer	10	$(N+1) \times 10$
dNTP mix	1.6	$(N+1) \times 1.6$
T4 DNA polymerase	1.0	$(N+1) \times 1.0$
Klenow DNA polymerase	2.0	$(N+1) \times 2.0$
T4 polynucleotide kinase	2.2	$(N+1) \times 2.2$
Total volume	52.0	$(N+1) \times 52.0$

6. Place the plate on the appropriate magnetic stand and let it incubate at room temperature for an additional 5 min.
7. Remove and discard all the solution of the supernatant from each well without disturbing the beads.
8. Use a p10 multichannel pipette to ensure that as much of the solution is removed as possible.
9. With the plate on the magnetic stand, add 200 μL of freshly prepared 80% ethanol to each well without disturbing the beads.
10. Incubate the plate at room temperature for 30 s, then remove and discard all the supernatant from each well.
11. Be careful not to disturb the beads.
12. Repeat **steps 10** and **11** once for a total of two ethanol washes.
13. Following the last ethanol wash, use a p10 to remove any residual ethanol from the bottom of the wells while keeping the wells on the magnetic stand.
14. Keep the plate on the magnetic stand for 5 min to dry.
15. Add 32 μL of nuclease-free water to each well and resuspend the beads by pipetting up and down.
16. Incubate the plate with the resuspended samples for 2 min at room temperature.
17. Place the plate on the magnetic stand and let the plate incubate at room temperature for an additional 5 min.
18. With the plate on the magnetic stand, transfer 30 μL of the supernatant from the plate to a new PCR plate and proceed to the next steps.

3.1.4 Adenylation of the 3′ Ends

The adapter ligation requires the presence of a 3′ A-base on the double stranded DNA fragments. The adenylation step uses dATPs and Exo(−) Klenow to adenylate the DNA fragments

1. Create an A-tail master mix using the guidelines in Table 2.
2. Obtain the post end repair plate from the thermocycler and add 20 μL of the master mix to each sample.
3. Incubate the plate for 30 min at 37 °C.
4. Proceed immediately to the next step.

3.1.5 AMPure Bead Cleanup

1. Vortex the AMPure XP beads until they are well dispersed.
2. Add 90 μL of the AMPure XP beads to each sample.
3. Incubate the plate at room temperature for 10 min.
4. Place the plate on the appropriate magnetic stand and let it incubate at room temperature for an additional 5 min.
5. Remove and discard all of the supernatant from each well.

Table 2
A-tail master mix setup

Reagent	Vol. for 1 library (μL)	Vol. for *N* libraries (μL)
Nuclease-free water	11.0	$(N+1) \times 11.0$
10× Klenow polymerase buffer	5.0	$(N+1) \times 5.0$
dATP	1.0	$(N+1) \times 1.0$
Exo(−) Klenow	3.0	$(N+1) \times 3.0$
Total volume	20.0	$(N+1) \times 20.0$

6. With the plate still on the magnetic stand, add 200 μL of freshly prepared 80% ethanol to each well without disturbing the beads.
7. Incubate the plate at room temperature for 30 s, then remove and discard all the supernatant from each well.
8. Repeat **steps 6** and 7 once for a total of two ethanol washes.
9. Following the last ethanol wash, use a p10 to remove any residual ethanol from the bottom of the wells while keeping the wells on the magnetic stand.
10. Keep the plate on the magnetic stand for not more than 5 min to dry the beads.
11. Add 15 μL of nuclease-free water to each well of the plate using a multichannel pipette. Resuspend the beads gently by pipetting 10 times.
12. Incubate the plate with the resuspended samples for 2 min at room temperature.
13. Place the plate on the magnetic stand and let the plate incubate at room temperature for an additional 5 min.
14. With the plate still on the magnetic stand, transfer 13 μL of the supernatant to a new PCR plate and proceed immediately to the next step.

3.1.6 Adapter Ligation

1. Create a master mix using the guidelines in Table 3.
2. Add 37 μL of Adapter Ligation Mix to each sample of the plate and pipette up and down to mix.
3. Seal the plate and spin down briefly.
4. Place the plate in the thermal cycler and run for 15 min at 20 °C.
5. Proceed immediately to the next step.

Table 3
Adapter ligation master mix setup

Reagent	Vol. for 1 library (μL)	Vol. for *N* libraries (μL)
Nuclease-free water	15.5	$(N+1) \times 15.5$
5× T4 DNA ligase	10.0	$(N+1) \times 10.0$
SureSelect adapter oligo mix	10.0	$(N+1) \times 10.0$
T4 DNA ligase	1.5	$(N+1) \times 1.5$
Total volume	37.0	$(N+1) \times 37.0$

3.1.7 AMPure Bead Cleanup

1. Vortex the AMPure XP beads until they are well dispersed.
2. Add 90 μL of the AMPure XP beads to each sample.
3. Incubate the plate at room temperature for 10 min.
4. Place the plate on the appropriate magnetic stand and let it incubate at room temperature for an additional 5 min.
5. Remove and discard all of the solution of the supernatant from each well.
6. With the plate still on the magnetic stand, add 200 μL of freshly prepared 80% ethanol to each well without disturbing the beads.
7. Incubate the plate at room temperature for 30 s, then remove and discard all the supernatant from each well.
8. Repeat **steps 6** and 7 once for a total of two ethanol washes.
9. Following the last ethanol wash, use a p10 to remove any residual ethanol from the bottom of the wells while keeping the wells on the magnetic stand.
10. Keep the plate on the magnetic stand for not more than 5 min to dry the beads.
11. Add 32 μL of nuclease-free water to each well of the plate using a multichannel pipette. Resuspend the beads gently by pipetting ten times.
12. Incubate the plate with the resuspended samples for 2 min at room temperature.
13. Place the plate on the magnetic stand and let the plate incubate at room temperature for an additional 5 min.
14. With the plate still on the magnetic stand, transfer 30 μL of the supernatant to a new PCR plate and proceed immediately to the next step.

Table 4
DNA enrichment master mix setup

Reagent	Vol. for 1 library (μL)	Vol. for *N* libraries (μL)
Nuclease-free water	21.0	$(N+1) \times 21.0$
SureSelect primer	1.25	$(N+1) \times 1.25$
ILM indexing PCR reverse primer	1.25	$(N+1) \times 1.25$
5× Herculase II reation buffer	10.0	$(N+1) \times 10.0$
100 nM dNTP	0.5	$(N+1) \times 0.5$
Herculase II fusion DNA polymerase	1.0	$(N+1) \times 1.0$
Total volume	35.0	$(N+1) \times 35.0$

3.1.8 PCR Enrichment

1. Create a PCR master mix for the samples using the guidelines in Table 4.
2. Pipette 35 μL of PCR master mix to the wells of a new PCR plate.
3. Add 15 μL of ligated DNA and mix by pipetting up and down at least ten times.
4. Seal the plate and spin down briefly.
5. Place the plate in the thermal cycler and run the Enrichment program as follows:
   (a) One cycle: 98 °C for 2 min.
   (b) Six cycles: 98 °C for 30 s, 65 °C for 30 s, 72 °C for 1 min.
   (c) One cycle: 72 °C for 10 min.
6. Proceed immediately to the next step.

3.1.9 AMPure Bead Cleanup

1. Vortex the AMPure XP beads until they are well dispersed.
2. Add 90 μL of the AMPure XP beads to each sample.
3. Incubate the plate at room temperature for 10 min.
4. Place the plate on the appropriate magnetic stand and let it incubate at room temperature for an additional 5 min.
5. Remove and discard all of the solution of the supernatant from each well.
6. With the plate still on the magnetic stand, add 200 μL of freshly prepared 80% ethanol to each well without disturbing the beads.
7. Incubate the plate at room temperature for 30 s, then remove and discard all the supernatant from each well.
8. Repeat **steps 6** and 7 once for a total of two ethanol washes.

9. Following the last ethanol wash, use a p10 to remove any residual ethanol from the bottom of the wells while keeping the wells on the magnetic stand.
10. Keep the plate on the magnetic stand for not more than 5 min to dry the beads.
11. Add 32 μL of nuclease-free water to each well of the plate using a multichannel pipette. Resuspend the beads gently by pipetting ten times.
12. Incubate the plate with the resuspended samples for 2 min at room temperature.
13. Place the plate on the magnetic stand and let the plate incubate at room temperature for an additional 5 min.
14. With the plate still on the magnetic stand, transfer 30 μL of the supernatant from the plate to a new PCR plate.
15. Run the whole genome libraries on the Agilent 2100 Bioanalyzer using the DNA 1000 chip.
16. Libraries that pass QC have a concentration >25 ng/μL and a library size >200 bp with and average peak >400 bp.

3.1.10 Capture Hybridization

1. Normalize 750 ng of library in 20 μL of nuclease-free water in a PCR plate.
2. Place the plate in a speed vacuum on medium heat until the samples have dried down completely.
3. While the samples are drying down, create three individual master mixes: Hybridization Mix, Capture Mix, and Block Mix.
4. Create a Capture master mix for the samples using the guidelines in Table 5 and keep the master mix on ice until ready to use.
5. Create a Hybridization master mix using the guidelines in Table 6 and keep at room temperature until ready touse.
6. Create a Blocking master mix using the guidelines in Table 7 and keep and keep on ice until ready to use.
7. After the samples have dried down, add 3.4 μL of nuclease-free water and resuspend the samples.
8. Add 5.6 μL of the Block master mix to each sample and mix by pipetting up and down.
9. Seal the plate and run the hybridization program as follows:
   (a) One cycle: 95 °C for 5 min.
   (b) 65 °C hold.
10. While the thermal cycler is cooling down to the 65 °C hold, prepare the capture/hybridization mix by combing the capture and hybridization master mixes as shown in Table 8.

Table 5
Capture master mix setup

Reagent	Vol. for 1 library (μL)	Vol. for *N* library (μL)
Nuclease-free water	1.5	$(N+1) \times 1.5$
SureSelect capture reagent	5	$(N+1) \times 5.0$
SureSelect RNAse block	0.5	$(N+1) \times 0.5$
Total volume	7.0	$(N+1) \times 7.0$

Table 6
Hybridization master mix setup

Reagent	Vol. for 1 library (μL)	Vol. for *N* library (μL)
SureSelect Hyb #1	6.63	$(N+1) \times 6.63$
SureSelect Hyb #2	0.27	$(N+1) \times 0.27$
SureSelect Hyb #3	2.65	$(N+1) \times 2.65$
SureSelect Hyb #4	3.45	$(N+1) \times 3.45$
Total volume	13.0	$(N+1) \times 13.0$

Table 7
Blocking master mix setup

Reagent	Vol. for 1 library (μL)	Vol. for *N* library (μL)
Indexing block #1	2.5	$(N+1) \times 2.5$
Block #2	2.5	$(N+1) \times 2.5$
Indexing block #3	0.6	$(N+1) \times 0.6$
Total volume	5.6	$(N+1) \times 5.6$

Table 8
Capture/hybridization master mix setup

Reagent	Vol. for 1 library (μL)	Vol. for *N* library (μL)
Capture mix	7	$(N+1) \times 7$
Hybridization mix	13	$(N+1) \times 13$
Total volume	20.0	$(N+1) \times 20.0$

11. Once the cycler has reached 65 °C, keep the plate on and remove the seal.
12. With the plate on the thermal cycler, quickly add 20 μL of the capture/hybridization mix to all the samples and pipette up and down several times.
13. Seal the plate and incubate at 65 °C for 18–24 h.

3.1.11 Preparation of Streptavidin T1 Magnetic Beads

1. Remove a vial of DynaBeads MyOne Streptavidin T1 beads from the 4 °C refrigerator and vortex vigorously to resuspend the beads in their storage buffer (*see* **Note 3**).
2. Obtain a new deep well plate and label it with "Wash Buffer 2."
3. Add 280 μL of SureSelect Wash Buffer 2 to six wells of the "Wash Buffer 2" plate for each sample being processed.
4. Seal the plate and place in the Hybex incubator set at 65 °C. Incubate at 65 °C until needed.
5. Aliquot 50 μL of Dynabeads to each well of a deep well plate that will contain sample.
6. Add 200 μL of SureSelect Binding Buffer to each well containing beads.
7. Mix the beads by pipetting up and down at least ten times.
8. Place the plate on a magnetic block and allow the beads to migrate to the magnet for at least 5 min.
9. Remove and discard the supernatant without disturbing the beads.
10. Repeat **steps 6–10** two times, for a total of three washes.
11. Add 200 μL of SureSelect Binding Buffer to each of the wells. Resuspend the beads by pipetting up and down.
12. The beads are now washed and ready to use.

3.1.12 Wash and Target Capture

1. With the thermal cycler still holding at 65 °C, open the lid and remove the seal.
2. Transfer the hybridization mixture to the associated wells in the deep well plate containing the washed beads.
3. Place the sealed plate on a plate shaker set on low speed for 30 min.
4. Following incubation, spin the plate briefly in a centrifuge.
5. Place the plate on a magnetic block and allow beads to migrate for 5 min.
6. Once the beads have bound to the magnet and the supernatant is clear, remove the supernatant and discard.
7. Remove the plate from the magnetic block and resuspend the beads in 500 μL of SureSelect Wash Buffer 1 by pipetting up and down.

8. Seal the plate and plate the place on a plate shaker.
9. Mix the samples on the plate shaker for 15 min at room temperature.
10. After the incubation, briefly spin the plate down.
11. Place the plate on a magnetic block for 5 min while the beads migrate to the magnet.
12. Once the beads have bound to the side of the well and the solution appears clear, remove the supernatant and discard.
13. Remove the plate from the magnetic block.
14. Resuspend the beads in 500 μL of the 65 °C pre-warmed SureSelect Wash Buffer 2.
15. Mix by pipetting up and down at least five times (*see* **Note 4**).
16. Seal the plate and incubate the samples for 10 min at 65 °C.
17. Following the incubation, briefly spin the plate down in a centrifuge.
18. Place the plate on the magnetic block and allow the beads to migrate for 5 min.
19. Once the beads have bound to the sides of the well, remove and discard the clear supernatant. Remove the plate from the magnetic block.
20. Repeat **steps 14–19** twice, for a total of three washes.
21. After the final wash has been completed, use a 10 μL pipette to make sure all the wash buffer has been removed.
22. Resuspend the beads in 30 μL of nuclease-free water.
23. The hybridized libraries are now bound to the Dynabeads.

3.1.13 DNA Fragment Enrichment

1. Create a PCR master mix for the samples using the guidelines in Table 9.
2. Pipette 35 μL of PCR master mix to the wells of a new PCR plate for each sample needed.
3. Add 14 μL of the library on bead to each well.
4. Add 1 μL of the index to each sample and mix by pipetting up and down (*see* **Note 5**).
5. Seal the plate and spin down briefly.
6. Place the plate in the thermal cycler and run the Enrichment program as follows:
   (a) One cycle: 98 °C for 2 min.
   (b) Ten cycles: 98 °C for 30 s, 57 °C for 30 s, 72 °C for 1 min.
   (c) One cycle: 72 °C for 1 min.
7. Proceed immediately to next step.

Table 9
DNA enrichment master mix setup

Reagent	Vol. for 1 library (μL)	Vol. for *N* libraries (μL)
Nuclease-free water	22.5	$(N+1) \times 22.5$
ILM post capture forward primer	1.0	$(N+1) \times 1.0$
5× Herculase II reation buffer	10.0	$(N+1) \times 10.0$
100 nM dNTP	0.5	$(N+1) \times 0.5$
Herculase II fusion DNA polymerase	1.0	$(N+1) \times 1.0$
Total volume	35.0	$(N+1) \times 35.0$

3.1.14 AMPure Bead Cleanup

1. Vortex the AMPure XP beads until they are well dispersed.
2. Add 90 μL of the AMPure XP beads to each sample.
3. Incubate the plate at room temperature for 10 min.
4. Place the plate on the appropriate magnetic stand and let it incubate at room temperature for an additional 5 min.
5. Remove and discard all of the solution of the supernatant from each well.
6. With the plate still on the magnetic stand, add 200 μL of freshly prepared 80% ethanol to each well without disturbing the beads.
7. Incubate the plate at room temperature for 30 s, then remove and discard all the supernatant from each well.
8. Repeat **steps 6** and 7 once for a total of two ethanol washes.
9. Following the last ethanol wash, use a p10 to remove any residual ethanol from the bottom of the wells while keeping the wells on the magnetic stand.
10. Keep the plate on the magnetic stand for not more than 5 min to dry the beads.
11. Add 32 μL of nuclease-free water to each well of the plate using a multichannel pipette. Resuspend the beads gently by pipetting ten times.
12. Incubate the plate with the resuspended samples for 2 min at room temperature.
13. Place the plate on the magnetic stand and let the plate incubate at room temperature for an additional 5 min.
14. With the plate still on the magnetic stand, transfer 30 μL of the supernatant from the plate to a new PCR plate.
15. Run the final libraries on the Agilent 2100 Bioanalyzer using the DNA 1000 chip.
16. Final libraries that pass QC have a concentration >2 ng/μL and a library size >200 bp with and average peak >400 bp.

3.2 DNA Sequencing on the Illumina HiSeq 2500

The final DNA library is diluted, denatured, and introduced into the lanes of the flow cell using the cBot according to the manufactures protocol. The libraries are loaded at a coverage of 100× for the proband sample and 60× for the parent samples. The DNA library templates are captured by the oligonucleotides that are affixed to the surface of the flow cell. Templates bound to the oligonucleotides on the flow cell are 3′ extended, producing covalently-attached discrete single molecules. The double-stranded molecule is denatured, and the original template is washed away. The free ends of the bound templates hybridize to the adjacent lawn primers to form U-shaped bridges. The DNA bridge is then copied from the primer to create a double-stranded DNA bridge. The resulting dsDNA is denatured, hybridized to lawn-primers to form new bridges and extended again. This process of iso-thermal bridge amplification is repeated 35 times to create a dense cluster of over 2000 molecules. The reverse strands in the cluster are removed by cleavage at the reverse strand-specific lawn primers, leaving a cluster with forward strands only. The free 3′-OH ends are blocked to prevent nonspecific priming. Sequencing primers are hybridized to the free ends of the DNA templates. The flow cell is now ready to be sequenced on the Illumina HiSeq 2500 and is loaded onto the sequencer according to the manufacturer's protocol (*see* **Note 6**).

3.3 Data Processing

1. Demultiplexing: Once the sequencing chemistry is complete the raw sequencing data is written in binary base call (BCL) format. Illumina's bcl2fastq software is used to demultiplex the raw sequencing data and convert it into standard FASTQ format for downstream analysis.
2. Alignment: Individual sequencing reads in the FASTQ files are mapped to reference human genome using Borrows-Wheeler Aligner (BWA) [15]. This process generates a BAM format file which is a compressed binary representation of aligned reads in Sequence Alignment Map (SAM) format [16].
3. Duplicate marking: Duplicate reads are defined as sequence reads originating from a single fragment of DNA. They can arise due to PCR-based library preparation or as a result of single amplification clusters on the flowcell being incorrectly detected as multiple clusters by the sequencing instrument optics. The BAM file generated in **step 2** is processed through Picard tools [http://broadinstitute.github.io/picard] which locates and tags duplicate reads.
4. Base Quality Score Recalibration (BQSR): Base quality scores are important quality indicators and are used by variant calling algorithms for accuracy. Multiple factors like library preparation and sequencing instrumentation can introduce biases in

the sequencer-assigned base qualities. To correct any systematic bias observed in the data, the duplicate marked BAM file is processed using BaseRecalibrator tool of the Genome Analysis Toolkit (GATK) [17]. At this stage the aligned BAM file is ready for variant discovery.

5. Variant discovery: Identifying short variants (Single Nucleotide Variants—SNVs and insertion/deletions—Indels) is typically a two-step process. GATK HaplotypeCaller tool is run on each sample separately in GVCF mode for scalable variant calling. This produces an intermediate file format called gVCF (for genomic VCF). GVCFs of multiple samples are then run through a joint genotyping step to produce a multi-sample VCF using GATK GenotypeGVCFs tool. Variant quality score recalibration (VQSR) using GATK VariantRecalibrator is then performed to filter low quality variants.
6. Variant annotation: To simplify and accelerate variant prioritization, the filtered VCF is processed through Ensembl Variant Effect Predictor (VEP) [18]. Relevant variant-level and gene-level annotations are added to each variant in this step. These annotations include, but are not limited to, variant consequence (missense, nonsense, frameshift, etc.), allele frequency in gnomAD database [http://gnomad.broadinstitute.org/about], in-silico damaging predictions from SIFT [19] and PolyPhen [20], association with human phenotypes from OMIM [https://omim.org] and previously reported variant clinical significance from ClinVar [21].
7. Variant prioritization: To identify candidate function-impacting variant(s) the annotations are used to perform step-wise variant filteration. The variants are first filtered based on the allele frequency in the population (gnomAD). Typically, for rare disorders any variant observed at a frequency of 1% or above is filtered out. It should be noted that this frequency cutoff should be determined based on the phenotype being investigated and ancestry of the case. When parental genotypes are available variants are further filtered based on the expected mode of inheritance. For example, if recessive mode of inheritance is being considered for a fully penetrant phenotype and the parents are unaffected, only homozygous variants in the proband are retained with both parents heterozygous for the variant allele. Similar filtration is done for other modes of inheritance. At this stage, retained variants and associated genes are manually evaluated for association with the phenotype being investigated using information from OMIM, ClinVar, and PubMed. Once variants possibly associated with the phenotype are identified, their clinical significance is assessed using ACMG standards and guidelines for interpretation of sequence variants [22]. According to the assessment the variants are

categorized into the following categories—Benign, Likely Benign, Uncertain Significance, Likely Pathogenic, and Pathogenic.

8. Pathogenic and likely pathogenic reportable variants may be confirmed by using standard Sanger sequencing.

4 Notes

1. Visually check each sample well to ensure that there are no air bubbles present prior to shearing and the metal rod is in the center of the Covaris tube. Air bubbles can cause variable shearing. If air bubbles are present, briefly centrifuge the plate and then check again.
2. Over drying the beads can lead to significant sample loss.
3. This step should be performed not more than 1 h prior to removal of the Hybridization plate from the thermal cycler. The Hybridization plate should remain incubating at 65 °C during this process.
4. When mixing the beads with the buffer incubated at 65 °C, this should be done as quickly as possible. If the temperature drops much below 65 °C, nonspecific binding can occur.
5. The list of Agilent adapters can be obtained at: https://www.agilent.com/cs/library/usermanuals/Public/G7530-90000.pdf
6. Introduction to Next Generation Sequencing technology can be found at: https://www.illumina.com/content/dam/illumina-marketing/documents/products/illumina_sequencing_introduction.pdf

References

1. Centers for Disease Control and Prevention, National Center on Birth Defects and Developmental Disabilities (2008) Update on overall prevalence of major birth defects—Atlanta, Georgia, 1978–2005. MMWR 57(1):1–5
2. Talkowski ME, Ordulu Z, Pillalamarri V et al (2012) Clinical diagnosis by whole-genome sequencing of a prenatal sample. N Engl J Med 367(23):2226–2232. https://doi.org/10.1056/NEJMoa1208594
3. Wapner RJ, Martin CL, Levy B et al (2012) Chromosomal microarray versus karyotyping for prenatal diagnosis. N Engl J Med 367(23):2175–2184. https://doi.org/10.1056/NEJMoa1203382
4. Jelin AC, Vora N (2018) Whole exome sequencing: applications in prenatal genetics. Obstet Gynecol Clin North Am 45(1):69–81. https://doi.org/10.1016/j.ogc.2017.10.003
5. Iglesias A, Anyane-Yeboa K, Wynn J et al (2014) The usefulness of whole-exome sequencing in routine clinical practice. Genet Med 16(12):922–931. https://doi.org/10.1038/gim.2014.58
6. Yang Y, Muzny DM, Reid JG et al (2013) Clinical whole-exome sequencing for the diagnosis of mendelian disorders. N Engl J Med 369(16):1502–1511. https://doi.org/10.1056/NEJMoa1306555
7. Yang Y, Muzny DM, Xia F et al (2014) Molecular findings among patients referred for clinical whole-exome sequencing. JAMA 312(18):1870–1879. https://doi.org/10.1001/jama.2014.14601

8. Macera MJ, Sobrino A, Levy B et al (2015) Prenatal diagnosis of chromothripsis, with nine breaks characterized by karyotyping, FISH, microarray and whole-genome sequencing. Prenat Diagn 35(3):299–301. https://doi.org/10.1002/pd.4456
9. Carss KJ, Hillman SC, Parthiban V et al (2014) Exome sequencing improves genetic diagnosis of structural fetal abnormalities revealed by ultrasound. Hum Mol Genet 23 (12):3269–3277. https://doi.org/10.1093/hmg/ddu038
10. Drury S, Williams H, Trump N et al (2015) Exome sequencing for prenatal diagnosis of fetuses with sonographic abnormalities. Prenat Diagn 35(10):1010–1017. https://doi.org/10.1002/pd.4675
11. Hillman SC, Willams D, Carss KJ et al (2015) Prenatal exome sequencing for fetuses with structural abnormalities: the next step. Ultrasound Obstet Gynecol 45(1):4–9. https://doi.org/10.1002/uog.14653
12. Vora NL, Powell B, Brandt A et al (2017) Prenatal exome sequencing in anomalous fetuses: new opportunities and challenges. Genet Med 19(11):1207–1216. https://doi.org/10.1038/gim.2017.33
13. Wapner RJ, Petrovski S, Brennan K et al (2017) Whole exome sequencing in the evaluation of fetal structural anomalies: a prospective study of sequential patients. Am J Obstet Gynecol 216(1 Supplement):S5–S6
14. Committee on Genetics and the Society for Maternal-Fetal Medicine (2016) Committee opinion no.682: microarrays and next-generation sequencing technology: the use of advanced genetic diagnostic tools in obstetrics and gynecology. Obstet Gynecol 128(6): e262–e268. https://doi.org/10.1097/AOG.0000000000001817
15. Li H, Durbin R (2009) Fast and accurate short read alignment with Burrows-Wheeler transform. Bioinformatics 25(14):1754–1760. https://doi.org/10.1093/bioinformatics/btp324
16. Li H, Handsaker B, Wysoker A et al (2009) The Sequence Alignment/Map format and SAMtools. Bioinformatics 25 (16):2078–2079. https://doi.org/10.1093/bioinformatics/btp352
17. McKenna A, Hanna M, Banks E et al (2010) The Genome Analysis Toolkit: a MapReduce framework for analyzing next-generation DNA sequencing data. Genome Res 20 (9):1297–1303. https://doi.org/10.1101/gr.107524.110
18. McLaren W, Gil L, Hunt SE et al (2016) The Ensembl variant effect predictor. Genome Biol 17(1):122. https://doi.org/10.1186/s13059-016-0974-4
19. Kumar P, Henikoff S, Ng PC (2009) Predicting the effects of coding non-synonymous variants on protein function using the SIFT algorithm. Nat Protoc 4(7):1073–1081. https://doi.org/10.1038/nprot.2009.86
20. Adzhubei I, Jordan DM, Sunyaev SR (2013) Predicting functional effect of human missense mutations using PolyPhen-2. Curr Protoc Hum Genet Chapter 7:Unit7.20. doi:https://doi.org/10.1002/0471142905.hg0720s76
21. Landrum MJ, Lee JM, Benson M et al (2018) ClinVar: improving access to variant interpretations and supporting evidence. Nucleic Acids Res 46(D1):D1062–D1067. https://doi.org/10.1093/nar/gkx1153
22. Richards S, Aziz N, Bale S et al (2015) Standards and guidelines for the interpretation of sequence variants: a joint consensus recommendation of the American College of Medical Genetics and Genomics and the Association for Molecular Pathology. Genet Med 17 (5):405–424. https://doi.org/10.1038/gim.2015.30

Chapter 19

Isolation and Characterization of Amniotic Fluid-Derived Extracellular Vesicles for Biomarker Discovery

Blake Ebert and Alex J. Rai

Abstract

Amniotic fluid, the fetal-protective liquid that fills the amniotic sac, represents a rich source of biomarkers. The diagnostic utility of amniotic fluid relies on the highly abundant maternal and fetal nucleic acid and proteomic content, which allows for the simultaneous determination of mother and fetal health status. Extracellular vesicles (ECVs) that are released by all cells and found in amniotic fluid could be harnessed to provide substantial clinically actionable data. ECVs are mediators of critical biological functions and reflect the health of the parent cell. Thus, ECVs released from cells in distress may provide important diagnostic information. Here, we describe a straightforward and optimized method for isolating ECVs from amniotic fluid. In addition, we validate our procedure through western blotting using antibodies targeting canonical ECV protein markers and via direct visualization using transmission electron microscopy.

Key words Amniotic fluid, Apoptotic vesicles, Exosomes, Extracellular vesicles, Microvesicles, Biomarkers

1 Introduction

Amniotic fluid (AF) is a dynamic and complex biological fluid comprised of fetal secretions from the respiratory and excretory systems, amniocytes, and maternal plasma [1]. AF changes in volume and composition throughout pregnancy in response to fetal development and is crucial for the healthy development of the fetus [1]. The embryo-containing amniotic sac forms 12 days after conception and is immediately filled with AF [2]. At this point, AF is composed primarily of water derived from the maternal plasma. By 12–14 weeks, fetal urine is the most abundant component. From 14–32 weeks, volume steadily increases to a maximum of approximately 1000 mL [2].

Changes in the AF cells, nucleic acids, proteins and extracellular vesicles may reflect fetal abnormalities [2]. In current clinical practice, AF status is assessed in vivo via ultrasound for detection of fetal malformations and is typically collected in the second trimester via

Brynn Levy (ed.), *Prenatal Diagnosis*, Methods in Molecular Biology, vol. 1885, https://doi.org/10.1007/978-1-4939-8889-1_19,

amniocentesis to assess certain pregnancy-related complications in high-risk mothers, including chromosomal abnormalities, fetal infection, and encephalopathies [3]. While the ultimate goal is to eliminate the need for amniocentesis by noninvasive fetal testing through maternal serum or urine, AF as a diagnostic resource has many benefits [4]. Namely, AF contains a higher abundance of cell-free fetal/maternal DNA, RNA, and proteins than maternal serum and urine [4]. In addition, AF reflects the health of both the mother and the fetus simultaneously [4]. Taken together, these findings suggest the utility of AF as a diagnostic tool for a wide spectrum of diseases and abnormalities.

In particular, AF-derived extracellular vesicles (ECVs) may represent a rich trove of biomarkers. Released from all cells and found ubiquitously in every biological fluid, ECVs carry genetic material and proteins throughout the body that reflect the original parent cell [5]. ECVs are primarily classified by size, although there are discrepancies in the literature with regard to size limits. In general, exosomes are the smallest, ranging from ~50–150 nm; microvesicles are larger, ranging up to 1000 nm, and apoptotic vesicles are the largest of the three, and can be up to 5000 nm. In recent years, evidence has accumulated suggesting that ECVs, and exosomes specifically, may be important regulators of key biological functions [5]. Thus, in an abnormal state, an assessment of vesicular contents may yield valuable clinically actionable information.

ECV-based biomarkers in amniotic fluid have the potential to significantly improve clinical risk assessment and maternal/fetal patient management [4]. Although AF is collected invasively through amniocentesis, the high concentration of cell-free fetal and maternal DNA, RNA, and proteins in AF relative to maternal circulation suggests its utility in discovery-based analysis. We report here an optimized methodology for isolating AF-derived ECVs and validate this procedure via western blotting and negative staining based transmission electron microscopy.

2 Materials

2.1 ECV Isolation

1. Centrifuge capable of 20,000 × *g* speed.
2. D-Dithiothreitol (DTT) (100 mg/mL in ddH_2O).

2.2 SDS-PAGE and Western Blotting

1. 2× LDS-reducing agent buffer.
   (a) 4× LDS Stock sample buffer (Thermo Fisher Scientific, Carlsbad, CA).
   (b) 10× stock sample reducing agent (Thermo Fisher Scientific, Carlsbad, CA).

   Prepare by adding 500 μL of 4× LDS Stock sample buffer, 200 μL 10× stock sample reducing agent, 300 μL ddH_2O.

2. 4–12% Bis-Tris 15 well gel (Thermo Fisher Scientific, Carlsbad, CA).
3. 1× MES SDS running buffer: Prepare by adding 50 mL 20× MES and 950 mL ddH_2O.
4. iBlot™ Transfer Stack, nitrocellulose, regular size (Thermo Fisher Scientific, Carlsbad, CA).
5. Ponceau S solution (Sigma Aldrich, St. Louis, MO). 0.1% in 5% acetic acid.
6. 1× PBS-Tween 20 (PBS-T): Prepare by adding 50 mL 20× PBS-T and 950 mL ddH_2O.
7. 5% milk in PBS-T: Prepare by dissolving 5 g nonfat dry milk in 100 mL PBS-T.
8. SuperSignal™ West Pico PLUS Chemiluminescent Substrate (Thermo Fisher Scientific, Carlsbad, CA): Contains SuperSignal west pico and luminol and peroxide chemiluminescence solutions.
9. XCell SureLock Mini-cell (Thermo Fisher Scientific, Carlsbad, CA).
10. 600 V Power Supply.
11. iBlot™ 2 Gel Transfer Device (Thermo Fisher Scientific, Carlsbad, CA).

2.3 Primary Antibodies

1. PDCD6IP Antibody—C-terminal region (ARP76945_P050) (Aviva Systems Biology, San Diego, CA).
2. CD81 Antibody—C-terminal region (ARP63231_P050) (Aviva Systems Biology, San Diego, CA).
3. CD9 antibody—N-terminal region (ARP61171_P050) (Aviva Systems Biology, San Diego, CA).
4. HSP90B1 antibody—C-terminal region (ARP40463_P050) (Aviva Systems Biology, San Diego, CA).
5. ACTN4 antibody—N-terminal region (ARP42202_T100) (Aviva Systems Biology, San Diego, CA).
6. Purified Mouse Anti-Flotillin-1 (Clone 18/Flotillin-1) (BD Biosciences, San Jose, CA).

2.4 Secondary Antibodies

1. Anti-rabbit IgG, HRP-linked antibody (Cell Signaling Technology, Danvers MA): 1:5000 in 5% milk
2. Anti-mouse IgG, HRP-linked antibody (Cell Signaling Technology, Danvers MA): 1:5000 in 5% milk.

2.5 Transmission Electron Microscopy, Negative Staining

1. 2% paraformaldehyde (PFA) in 0.1 M PBS.
2. Formvar-carbon-coated EM grids (Electron Microscopy Sciences, Hatfield, PA).

3. Uranyl-oxalate, pH 7 (prepare from stock solution of 4% uranyl acetate in ddH_2O and 0.15 M oxalic acid, brought to pH 7 by titrating with 25% NH_4OH).
4. JEM-1200 EXII transmission electron microscope (JEOL Ltd., Tokyo, Japan) (*see* **Note 1**).

3 Method

The method described herein is straightforward, inexpensive, and does not require complex equipment. These characteristics allow for its incorporation into a standard operating procedure and use in a CLIA-certified clinical laboratory setting. The first two steps involve low-speed centrifugation spins to remove dead cells and cellular debris. Successful isolation requires the addition of dithiothreitol (DTT), which removes high-abundance components and allows for the detection of lower-abundance proteins. See Fig. 1 for protocol details.

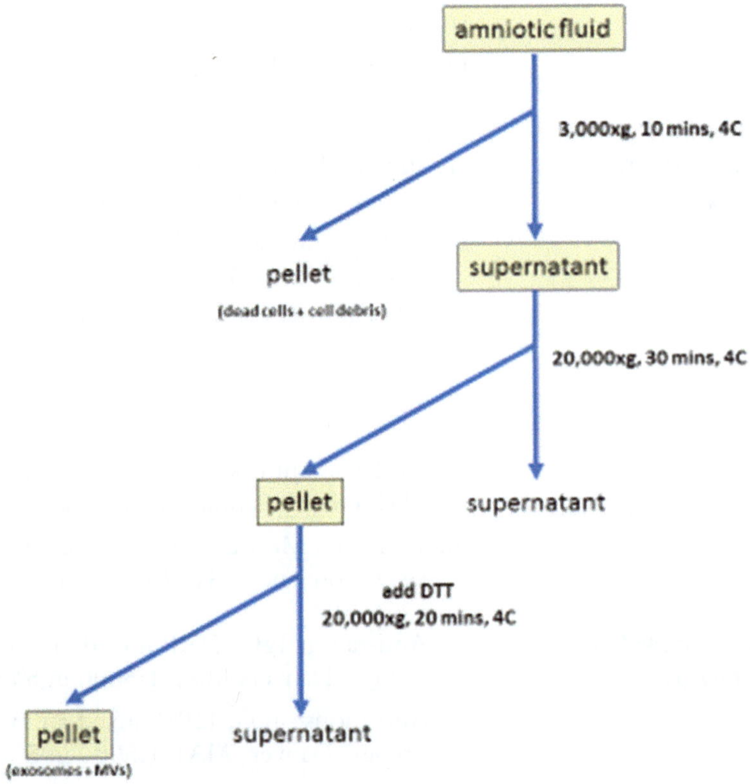

Fig. 1 Schematic diagram of ECV isolation from amniotic fluid. Starting material is subjected to two centrifugation spins. The pellet is subsequently treated with DTT and centrifuged again at 20,000 × *g*. The final pellet can then be subjected to downstream analyses

3.1 Purification of ECVs

1. Centrifuge amniotic fluid sample at 3000 × *g* for 10 min at 4 °C (*see* **Note 2**).
2. Transfer supernatant to fresh Eppendorf tubes.
3. Centrifuge sample at 20,000 × *g* for 20 min at 4 °C.
4. Decant and discard supernatant and add 50 μL D-Dithiothreitol (*see* **Notes 3** and **4**).
5. Pipette up and down to resuspend the pellet and centrifuge at 20,000 × *g* for 20 min at 4 °C.
6. Decant and discard supernatant. Store pellet at −80 °C until ready for further processing.

3.2 Preparation of ECVs and SDS-PAGE Analysis

1. Prepare fresh working 2× LDS-reducing agent sample buffer.
2. Resuspend pellet in 30 μL 2× LDS-reducing agent sample buffer.
3. Boil samples on heat block at 95 °C for 3 min.
4. Cool immediately on ice.
5. Load 15 μL of sample in 4–12% Bis-Tris gel secured in XCell Sure Lock electrophoresis cell, and run at 150 mV for 1 h or until dye front reaches the bottom of the gel.
6. Transfer gel to nitrocellulose membrane using the iBlot Transfer Device.

3.3 Western Blotting After Gel Electrophoresis

1. Incubate the nitrocellulose membrane in Ponceau S stain on the rocker for 5 min at room temperature.
2. Decant stain, rinse several times with dH_2O, and acquire an image of the stained blot.
3. De-stain in PBS-T on the rocker for 5 min at room temperature.
4. Prepare primary antibody in 5% milk/PBS-T at 1:1000 dilution (*see* **Note 5**).
5. Incubate membrane in primary antibody solution overnight at 4 °C.
6. Wash three times in PBS-T for 5 min each.
7. Prepare fresh HRP-conjugated secondary antibody in 5% milk/PBS-T at 1:5000 dilution.
8. Incubate membrane in secondary antibody solution for 45 min at room temperature.
9. Wash three times in PBS-T for 5 min each, on rocker.
10. Add 1 mL of each of the chemiluminescent substrates (SuperSignal west pico and luminol and peroxide chemiluminescence solutions), being careful to use separate pipette tips for each. The solution is activated immediately after mixing.
11. Process image on chemiluminescent developer. Representative western blot results are shown in Figs. 2 and 3.

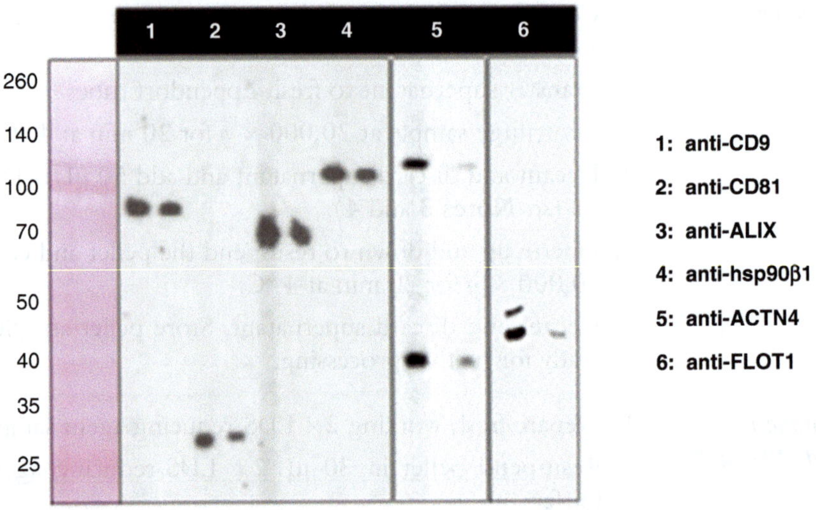

Fig. 2 Antibody optimization. Primary antibodies (Aviva Systems Biology, San Diego, CA) were tested at various dilutions using cultured melanoma cells (92.1) whole cell lysate. For each antibody, a 1:500 and 1:1000 dilution were tested (shown above); 1:1000 was deemed to be optimal

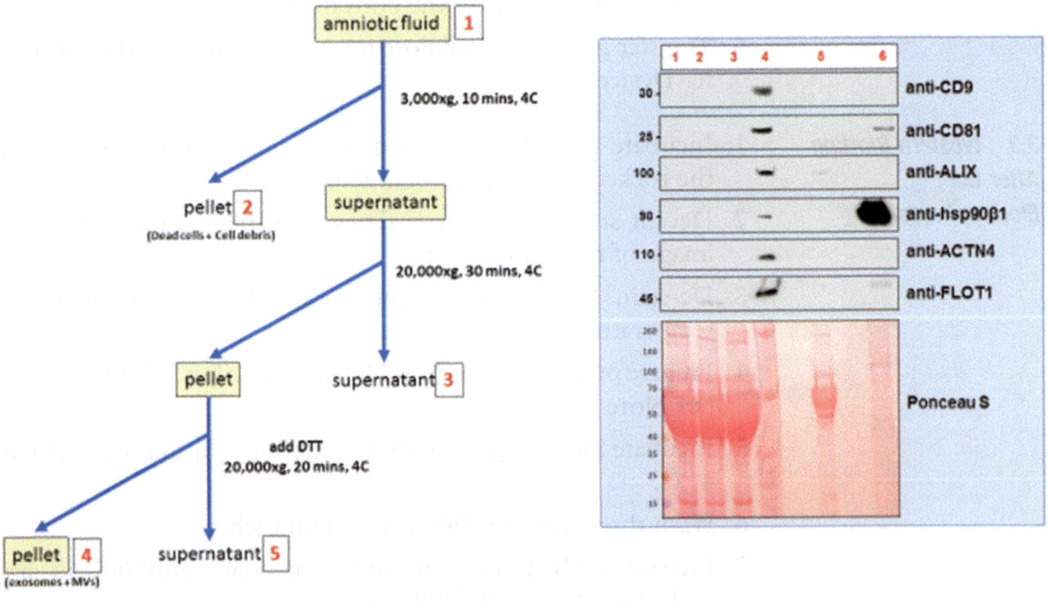

Fig. 3 Validation of ECV isolation procedure by western blotting using antibodies to canonical ECV protein markers, see panel on RIGHT. Multiple canonical protein markers for extracellular vesicles were detected in ECV fractions from AF including: CD9, CD81, ALIX, hsp90β1, ACTN4, and flotillin-1. Ponceau S staining reveals the requirement for DTT treatment to remove high-abundance proteins from the ECV pellet in order to visualize lower-abundance proteins and increase ECV yield (compare lanes 3, 4, and 5 in Ponceau S Stain). Lanes on gel correspond to steps from ECV isolation protocol, as denoted on left panel

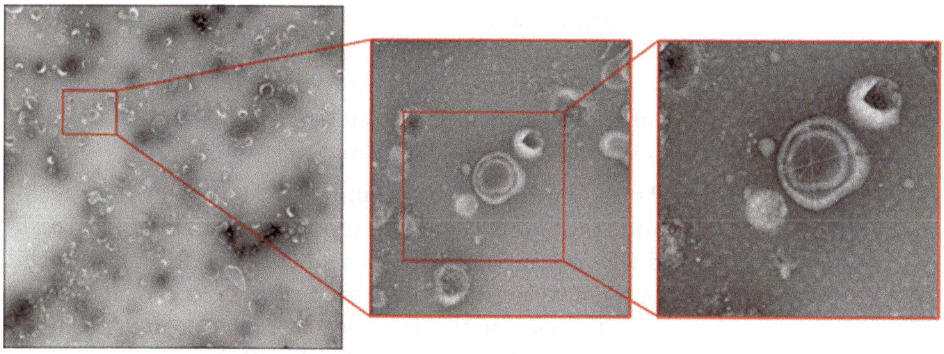

Fig. 4 Transmission electron microscopy imaging of amniotic fluid-derived ECVs. Samples were prepared for negative staining and were viewed at 25,000× magnification (left panel). We viewed an individual exosome and microvesicle at 200,000× magnification (right panel). The inner diameter of exosome is 123 nm in diameter and that of the microvesicle is 180 nm

3.4 Transmission Electron Microscopy

1. Resuspend ECV pellet in 2% PFA in 0.1 M sodium phosphate buffer.
2. Deposit 10 μL of sample onto Formvar-carbon-coated EM grids and let sit for 20 min at room temperature.
3. Blot off sample with filter paper, being careful to not completely dry out the grid.
4. Add 20 μL uranyl-oxalate solution and leave at room temperature for 5 min.
5. Remove stain with filter paper and let grids dry at room temperature.
6. Examine grids using transmission electron microscopy (*see* Fig. 4).

4 Notes

1. Any transmission electron microscope can be used. Our experience is with the JEM-1200 EXII transmission electron microscope.
2. We have used 1 mL starting volume of amniotic fluid sample for the exosome isolation and analysis, as described above (results shown in Fig. 3). However, we note that results can be obtained (and confirmed by western blotting and transmission electron microscopy) using <200 μL amniotic fluid sample, once conditions are optimized.
3. Pellets are usually light yellow in color, but some samples may not have visible pellets. We typically add 100 μL DTT to resuspend. For smaller pellets and/or smaller volumes, we suggest using lower volumes, e.g., 25–50 μL DTT, and test sample by western blotting.

4. If starting sample volume is high, sample may be split into multiple tubes for convenience (this may also be necessitated by rotor size and maximum volume/number of tubes). In such cases, final pellets from multiple tubes can be combined into one tube to increase ECV recovery.
5. Antibodies should be optimized by testing at various dilutions and conditions using the appropriate sample of interest. Routinely, we test all antibodies initially using cell lysate, and once optimal western blotting conditions are delineated, we subsequently test for the presence of target proteins using experimental samples of interest (*see* Fig. 2).

References

1. Palmas F, Fattuoni C, Noto A et al (2016) The choice of amniotic fluid in metabolomics for the monitoring of fetus health. Expert Rev Mol Diagn 16(4):473–486. https://doi.org/10.1586/14737159.2016.1139456
2. Kolialexi A, Tounta G, Mavrou A et al (2011) Proteomic analysis of amniotic fluid for the diagnosis of fetal aneuploidies. Expert Rev Proteomics 8(2):175–185. https://doi.org/10.1586/epr.10.112
3. Evans MI, Andriole S, Evans SM (2015) Genetics: update on prenatal screening and diagnosis. Obstet Gynecol Clin N Am 42(2):193–208. https://doi.org/10.1016/j.ogc.2015.01.011
4. Kamath-Rayne BD, Smith HC, Muglia LJ et al (2014) Amniotic fluid: the use of high-dimensional biology to understand fetal well-being. Reprod Sci 21(1):6–19. https://doi.org/10.1177/1933719113485292
5. Urbanelli L, Buratta S, Sagini K et al (2015) Exosome-based strategies for Diagnosis and Therapy. Recent Pat CNS Drug Discov 10 (1):10–27

Part IV

Non-Invasive Prenatal Testing

Chapter 20

Quad Screen Test, A Multiplexed Biomarker Assay for Prenatal Screening to Assess Birth Defects: The Columbia University Experience Using the Beckman Access2 Immunoassay Analyzer and Benetech PRA

Awet Tecleab, Alex K. Lyashchenko, and Alex J. Rai

Abstract

In the prenatal quad screen, the levels of four analytes in maternal serum are used to calculate the risk of serious birth defects. The Beckman Access2 Immunoassay System is an automated analyzer that enables rapid measurement of alpha-fetoprotein, unconjugated estriol, human chorionic gonadotropin, and dimeric inhibin A. The Benetech PRA software package is used to convert maternal serum analyte concentrations to multiples of the median (MoM) and calculates the risks of particular birth defects. The results from this simple and minimally invasive screen determine the need for more sensitive, specific, and usually riskier diagnostic procedures. We present herein some recent data from our experience at Columbia University Medical Center in New York, NY, using the Beckman Access2 immunoassay analyzer and Benetech PRA software package.

Key words Fetal defect markers, Prenatal diagnosis, Maternal screening, Quad screen

1 Introduction

Prenatal screening tests commonly use maternal blood or amniotic fluid for the detection of pregnancies with high risk of serious birth defects. The quad screen test measures the maternal serum levels of four biomarkers: alpha-fetoprotein (AFP), unconjugated estriol (uE3), human chorionic gonadotropin (β-hCG), and dimeric inhibin A (DIA). It is performed in the second trimester, with optimal sample collection time between 14 and 22 weeks [1], and is approved for screening of trisomy 18, trisomy 21 (Down syndrome), and open neural tube defects. It has a sensitivity of 80% for the detection of Down syndrome at a 5% false positive rate [2, 3].

Awet Tecleab and Alex K. Lyashchenko contributed equally to this work.

Brynn Levy (ed.), *Prenatal Diagnosis*, Methods in Molecular Biology, vol. 1885, https://doi.org/10.1007/978-1-4939-8889-1_20,

In order to accurately calculate the risks of birth defects using the quad screen, each laboratory must first establish the normal reference ranges of maternal serum AFP, uE3, β-hCG, and DIA levels using its own patient population to account for regional and demographic variation.

AFP is the most abundant fetal serum protein and is an important marker of open neural tube defects (ONTDs), which occur at a rate of 1–2 per 1000 live births in the United States [4]. It is synthesized by the fetal liver and the yolk sack, passes into the amniotic fluid in fetal urine, and reaches the maternal circulation through the placenta or by diffusion through the fetal membranes. In a fetus with an open neural tube defect such as anencephaly or spina bifida, the defective closure of the developing nervous system allows AFP to leak out and increases its concentration in the amniotic fluid and in the maternal serum [5].

In addition to ONTDs, AFP is also used as a marker for Down syndrome and trisomy 18, both of which are associated with decreased maternal serum AFP levels [6–9]. Prior to the development of this screening method, pregnant women aged 35 and above were routinely assessed for Down syndrome by the more invasive procedures of amniocentesis and karyotyping [6–8].

AFP is first detected in the maternal serum at about tenth week of gestation, its concentration starts to rise around week 16 and subsequently declines after about week 32 [ref. 10, and Table 1]. Thus, for prenatal screening, the maternal serum AFP concentration is typically measured in the second trimester, as the first trimester levels are too low to reliably differentiate between an affected and an unaffected fetus.

The Beckman Access2 Immunoassay System can quickly and accurately measure the levels of AFP and the other quad screen analytes as mass per unit volume of maternal serum (amniotic fluid can also be used for the measurement of AFP levels, but there are caveats- *see* **Notes 1–6**). However, in order to be able to interpret these results, each laboratory must establish its own normal reference AFP ranges in unaffected singleton pregnancies; this is routinely done using 50–100 maternal serum samples for each gestational week. In addition to gestational age, other factors such as maternal weight, race, and diabetes mellitus status also significantly affect maternal serum AFP concentration and must be taken into account [11, 12]. For this reason, each measured maternal serum AFP level is normalized to the appropriate median level in the reference population to derive the multiples of the median (MoM) value, which is then further adjusted for additional factors mentioned above. Table 1 shows the mean maternal serum AFP concentrations as well as the calculated MoMs for each gestational week 15–19 for 2359 samples analyzed at Columbia University Medical Center.

Estriol is the predominant form of estrogen in pregnant women. It is synthesized by the placenta, is made water soluble by

Table 1
Median maternal serum AFP levels by week of gestation

Week of Gestation	Number of samples	Median concentration (ng/mL)	Multiples of median concentration (ng/mL)		
			2.0	2.5	3.0
15	435	31.1	62.2	77.8	93.4
16	506	36.0	72.0	90.0	108.0
17	452	41.6	83.2	104.1	124.9
18	425	48.1	96.3	120.3	144.4
19	413	55.7	111.3	139.2	167.0
20	308	64.4	128.8	161.0	193.2

Table 2
The range in uE3 levels by gestational age week

GA week	Range of ue3 results (ng/mL)
13	0.42–0.50
14	0.52–0.62
15	0.64–0.76
16	0.79–0.94
17	0.97–1.17
18	1.20–1.44
19	1.49–1.78
20	1.84–2.20
21	2.27–2.72

conjugation with sulfate and glucuronate in the maternal liver, and is excreted by the kidney. However, approximately 10% of estriol circulates unconjugated [13]. Low maternal serum unconjugated estriol (uE3) levels are associated with Down syndrome and trisomy 18 [9, 14].

Table 2 shows the range in uE3 levels by gestational age week, derived from patients presenting at Columbia University Medical Center.

Human chorionic gonadotropin (hCG) is a glycoprotein hormone synthesized by the placenta that is used to screen for Down syndrome and trisomy 18. It is composed of alpha and beta subunits, with the beta subunit (β-hCG) being specific to hCG [12, 15]. The serum levels of β-hCG in non-pregnant women are very low, usually less than 5 IU/L, but soon after implantation of

Table 3
Median serum β-hCG levels in non-pregnant women

Reference population (non-pregnant females)	*N*	Median (mIU/mL)	Range (mIU/mL)	95th Percentile (mIU/mL), [95% CI]
$\geq$ 18 and < 40 years	132	0	0–0.6	0.3[0.2–0.4]
$\geq$ 40 years	141	0	0–3.1	1.5[1.1–2.9]
Post-menopausal	134	2.8	0.1–11.6	7.7[6.4–10.4]

the zygote, β-hCG levels increase rapidly and are used for early detection of pregnancy. The level of β-hCG doubles every 1.5 to 3 days for the first 6 weeks of gestation, continues to increase until the end of the first trimester, and then declines for the remainder of the pregnancy [16]. Maternal serum β-hCG levels are typically increased approximately two-fold in pregnancies with Down syndrome but much decreased in pregnancies with trisomy 18 [9].

The median, the range, and the 95th percentile values of maternal serum β-hCG concentrations in healthy non-pregnant women of several age groups measured at Columbia University Medical Center are shown in Table 3.

Inhibin A is a gonadal protein hormone secreted by the Sertoli cells of the testis or the granulosa cells of the ovary. It inhibits the secretion of follicle stimulating hormone (FSH) by the pituitary gland and regulates gamete production, as well as embryonic and fetal development [17]. Increased maternal serum dimeric inhibin A levels are associated with Down syndrome [18].

The median, the 2.5th, and the 97.5th percentiles of maternal serum dimeric inhibin A levels measured at Columbia University Medical Center in women at various stages of the menstrual cycle, as well as in postmenopausal women and normal men are shown in Table 4.

Once the appropriate reference ranges are established, the maternal serum concentrations for each analyte measured by the Beckman Access 2 Immunoassay System can be converted into multiples of the median by dividing the sample concentration by the median of the appropriate reference range, for that gestational age. The multiple of median (MoM) is further adjusted by the variables that are known to affect the MoM such as weight, race, prior pregnancies and deliveries, and age at the time of delivery.

The patient-specific risk for a specific abnormality is then calculated by multiplying the pretest probability, obtained from large epidemiological studies, by likelihood ratio based on the adjusted MoM.

Finally, the quad screen test results are reported as the maternal serum concentrations and the adjusted MoM values for each analyte, the risks for specific birth defects, and the overall interpretation.

Table 4
Median dimeric inhibin a levels

Population	*n*	Median (pg/mL)	2.5% Lower limit (pg/mL)	97.5% Upper limit (pg/mL)
Normal cycling females (days from LH surge)				
Early follicular phase (−14 to −10)	211	6.4	1.8	17.3
Mid follicular phase (−9 to −4)	264	11.7	3.5	31.7
Late follicular phase (−3 to −1)	121	29.0	9.8	90.3
Mid-cycle (day 0, LH surge)	96	41.8	16.9	91.8
Early luteal phase (1 to 3)	122	43.7	16.1	97.5
Mid luteal phase (4 to 11)	344	38.3	3.9	87.7
Late luteal phase (12 to 14)	138	12.5	2.7	47.1
Postmenopausal females	58	1.1	<1.0	2.1
Males	67	1.1	<1.0	2.0

1.1 Assay Principle

To measure AFP, β-hCG, and dimeric inhibin A levels, the Beckman Access2 instrument utilizes chemiluminescent noncompetitive two-site immunoassays. Briefly, the patient samples are incubated with two types of analyte-specific antibodies: (1) monoclonal antibodies immobilized on paramagnetic particles and (2) monoclonal antibodies conjugated to alkaline phosphatase (AP).

In the AFP immunoassay the sample is incubated with both the paramagnetic particle-immobilized antibodies and the AP-conjugated antibodies in one step. The reaction vessel is then washed in the presence of a magnetic field to remove the unbound reaction components, including any unbound AP-conjugated antibodies. Importantly, the paramagnetic particle-immobilized antibodies, the AFP, and the-AFP-bound AP-conjugated antibodies remain in the reaction vessel.

The β-hCG and inhibin A immunoassays use the same principle but are performed in two steps. The samples are first incubated with the analyte-specific paramagnetic particle-immobilized antibodies alone and the reaction vessel is then washed in the presence of a magnetic field to remove unbound reaction components. In the second step, the analyte-specific AP-conjugated antibodies are added and the wash step is repeated.

Following antibody incubation and washing, the reaction vessel is incubated with a chemiluminescent AP substrate (Lumi-Phos* 530). The light generated from the AP-substrate reaction, which is proportional to the analyte concentration, is detected using a luminometer. The serum levels of AFP, β-hCG, and inhibin A are determined from standard calibration curves.

To measure unconjugated estriol levels, the Beckman Access2 instrument uses a heterogenous competitive binding immunoassay. Briefly, the patient serum is added to a reaction vessel that contains AP-conjugated estriol, anti-estriol rabbit antibodies, and paramagnetic particles coated with goat anti-rabbit antibodies. The estriol from the sample competes with the AP-conjugated estriol for the binding sites of the anti-estriol rabbit antibodies. The resulting antigen-antibody complex is in turn bound by the anti-rabbit antibodies coating the magnetic particles. After incubation, the reaction vessel is washed in the presence of a magnetic field such that the substances not bound to the paramagnetic particles are washed away. As described above, Lumi-Phos* 530 is then added to the reaction mixture and the light generated by the reaction, which is inversely proportional to the estriol concentration, is detected using a luminometer. The serum level of the estriol is determined from a standard calibration curve.

1.2 Specimen

The recommended sample is maternal serum collected between 15 and 20 weeks of gestation (*see* **Note 2**). The samples must be accompanied by a requisition form that contains the complete patient demographics. This includes date of birth (not chronological age), expected day of delivery (based on measurement of fetal biparietal diameter or last menstrual period), specimen collection date, gestational age (number of completed weeks and additional days, *see* **Note 4**), weight at the time of sample collection, race, insulin dependent diabetes status prior to the pregnancy, whether it is a repeat sample, number of pregnancies and deliveries (para-gravida), and prior history of neural tube defects.

2 Materials

2.1 Common Material and Reagents

1. Benetech PRA—software package used to calculate the risk for a particular disorder based on MoM values (Benetech, Toronto, ON, Canada).
2. Beckman Access 2 automated analyzer and associated consumables, *see* below **items 3–10** (Beckman Coulter Inc., Brea, CA).
3. Reaction vessels.
4. Fiber-free applicator sticks.
5. Deionized water.
6. Citranox (cleaning solution).
7. Contrad 70 cleaning solution.
8. 2.0 mL sample cups.
9. Calibrated pipettes.
10. Pipette tips.

2.2 Reagents for AFP Measurement

Beckman Access AFP reagent and calibrator kit; this includes **items 1–6** listed below (Beckman Coulter Inc., Brea, CA).

1. R1: Access AFP reagent pack.
   (a) R1a—reagent pack containing mouse monoclonal anti-AFP antibody conjugated with paramagnetic particles.
   (b) R2a—reagent pack containing mouse monoclonal anti-AFP antibody conjugated with alkaline phosphatase.
2. AFP calibrators (S0 to S6)—calibrator material that corresponds to 0, 2.5, 5, 25, 100, 500, and 3000 ng/mL AFP. AFP assay requires calibration every 28 days. Calibrators should be run in duplicate to prepare calibration curve.
3. Calibration Card
4. Beckman access substrate: Lumi-phos*530.
5. Beckman access wash buffer II (R3 wash buffer II).
6. Beckman access AFP sample diluents—for dilution of samples with values outside of the analytical measurement range.
7. Level 1, 2, 3 controls, Lyphocheck maternal serum controls (BioRad, Hercules, CA, USA).
8. Control for amniotic fluid AFP (this is a pooled patient sample, and is prepared in our laboratory).

2.3 Reagents for Total β-hCG(Fifth IS) Quantitative Determination

Beckman Access β-hCG(fifth IS) reagent and calibrator kit, which includes the items listed below (Beckman Coulter Inc., Brea, CA).

1. R1: Access Total β-hCG(fifth IS) reagent pack.
   (a) R1a—reagent containing paramagnetic coated goat anti-mouse IgG: monoclonal mouse anti-βhCG.
   (b) R1b—protein (goat, murine, and recombinant).
   (c) R1c—reagent containing alkaline phosphatase conjugated rabbit anti-β-hCG.
2. Total β-hCG(fifth IS) calibrators.
   (a) S0: buffered bovine serum albumin (BSA) matrix with surfactant, <0.1% sodium azide, and 0.5% ProClin**300. Contains 0.0 IU/L hCG.
   (b) S1-S5: hCG at levels of approximate 6,35,195,620,1350 IU/L, respectively, in buffered BSA matrix with surfactant, <0.1% sodium azide, and 0.5% ProClin 300.
   (c) Calibration Card.
3. Beckman access substrate—Lumi-phos* 530.
4. Beckman access wash buffer II.
5. Level 1, 2, 3 controls, Liquicheck maternal serum (BioRad, Hercules, CA, USA).

6. The analytical range of the assay is 0.5–1000 IU/L. If β-hCG value is greater than 1000 IU/L, manual dilution can be performed by diluting 1 part of patient sample to 199 of wash buffer II. Result from manual dilution should then be multiplied by 200 to obtain sample result.

2.4 Reagents for Dimeric Inhibin A Quantitative Determination

Beckman Access inhibin A reagent and calibrator kit, which includes the following items (Beckman Coulter Inc., Brea, CA):

1. R1: Access Inhibin A reagent pack.
   (a) R1a—paramagnetic particles coated with mouse monoclonal anti-inhibin A.
   (b) R1b—mouse monoclonal anti-inhibin A alkaline phosphatase (bovine) conjugate.
   (c) R1c—Tris buffered saline, BSA, proteins (bovine, murine).
   (d) R1d—phosphate buffer, oxidizer.
   (e) R1e—Tris buffer, detergent.
2. Inhibin A calibrators.
   (a) S0: buffered bovine serum albumin (BSA) matrix with surfactant, <0.1% sodium azide, and 0.5% ProClin300. Contains 0.0 IU/L inhibin A.
   (b) S1–S6: Recombinant human inhibin A at levels of approximate 10, 50, 100, 500, 1000, 1500 pg/mL, respectively, in buffered BSA matrix with surfactant, <0.1% sodium azide, and 0.5% ProClin 300.
   (c) Calibration Card.
3. Beckman access substrate.
4. Beckman access wash buffer II.
5. Level 1, 2, 3 controls, Beckman Access inhibin A QC.
6. Beckman Access diluent buffer II.
7. The linearity for this assay is between 1 and 1500 pg/mL.

2.5 Reagents for Unconjugated Estriol (uE3) Measurement

Beckman Access unconjugated Estriol (uE3) reagent and calibrator kit, which includes the following items (Beckman Coulter Inc., Brea, CA).

1. R1: Access Total unconjugated Estriol reagent pack.
   (a) R1a—paramagnetic particle coated with goat anti-rabbit IgG.
   (b) R1b—Rabbit anti-estriol.
   (c) R1c—Estriol-alkaline phosphatase conjugate
2. Unconjugated Estriol calibrators.

(a) S0: buffered bovine serum albumin (BSA) matrix with surfactant, <0.1% sodium azide, and 0.5% ProClin300. Contains 0.0 IU/L unconjugated Estriol (uE3).

(b) S1–S6: Recombinant human unconjugated Estriol (uE3) at levels of approximate 0.07, 0.17, 0.34, 0.86, 3.4, 6.9 ng/mL, respectively, in buffered human serum matrix containing <0.1% NaN3 and 0.025% Cosmocil CQ.

3. Calibration Card.
4. Beckman access substrate Lumi-Phos 530.
5. Beckman access wash buffer II.
6. Level 1, 2, 3 controls, BioRad Liquicheck maternal serum (BioRad, Hercules, CA, USA).
7. For samples with uE3 concentration greater than 6.9 ng/mL, dilute sample with the zero calibrator and re-run the test. To obtain sample result, multiply by the appropriate dilution factor.

3 Methods

1. Mix the contents of unpunctured reagent packs by gently inverting several times until homogenous mix is observed.
2. Load reagents into the Beckman Access 2 instrument.
3. Calibrate the instrument. Follow the instruction provided by the vendor.
4. Confirm if the instrument calibration was successful.
5. Run controls and verify that the controls are within the acceptable limits.
6. Place patient samples on a rack and then load the rack in the instrument.
7. Select AFP, hCG5, inhibin or estriol free (for unconjugated estriol-3 assay) and run.
8. For samples with AFP concentration greater than 2550 ng/mL, order dilution (d-AFP).
9. Enter the result from this analysis into Benetech PRA, which will subsequently calculate MoM values and the risk of having open spina bifida, Down syndrome, and Trisomy 18. See also **Notes 4–5**.

3.1 Establishing and Implementing QC Range

1. Run QC in replicates, and on different days. Each clinical laboratory should have a defined standard operating procedure for this; we suggest a minimum of 20 replicates run over 20 days to capture all sources of variability.

2. Calculate mean, SD, and %CV. This should be reviewed and signed by clinical laboratory director, or appropriate designee.
3. Enter this QC range into the laboratory information system (LIS).
4. Run QC at the beginning of every shift and make sure that the controls are within acceptable limits, for each analyte.

4 Notes

1. Positive amniotic fluid-AFP results will trigger a reflex for additional testing (cholinesterase and fetal hemoglobin); we do not perform this testing in-house, it is sent to an outside reference laboratory.
2. Specimen for the measurement of AFP from maternal serum should be collected prior to amniocentesis.
3. Bloody amniotic fluid can have falsely elevated AFP level. In such circumstance, the amniotic fluid must be tested for the level of fetal hemoglobin using Kleihauer-Betke test, electrophoresis, or other appropriate tests.
4. Inaccurate gestational age is one of the most frequent causes of inaccurate screening test results. Results can be recalculated once accurate gestational age is obtained. For second trimester testing, recalculation should only be done when the difference in calculated and revised gestational age is >7 days.
5. Diagnosis of ONTD should not be made based on elevated AFP values only. Elevated AFP values have been found in other fetal abnormalities such as congenital nephrosis, omphalocele, Turner syndrome, or fetal demise [19, 20].
6. Amniotic fluids contain very high levels of AFP and hence when assaying for AFP from amniotic fluids, the sample should be pre-diluted. Dilute 1 part of amniotic fluid to 10 parts of Beckman Access sample diluents. This result should then be multiplied by 11 to obtain the final result.

References

1. Benn PA (2002) Advances in prenatal screening for Down syndrome: I. general principles and second trimester testing. Clin Chim Acta 323(1–2):1–16
2. Benn PA et al (2003) Incorporation of inhibin-A in second-trimester screening for Down syndrome. Obstet Gynecol 101(3):451–454
3. Wald NJ, Huttly WJ, Hackshaw AK (2003) Antenatal screening for Down's syndrome with the quadruple test. Lancet 361 (9360):835–836
4. Macri JN, Baker DA, Baim RS (1981) Diagnosis of neural tube defects by evaluation of amniotic fluid. Clin Obstet Gynecol 24 (4):1089–1102
5. Rose NC, Mennuti MT (1993) Maternal serum screening for neural tube defects and fetal chromosome abnormalities. West J Med 159(3):312–317

6. Combining maternal serum alpha-fetoprotein measurements and age to screen for Down syndrome in pregnant women under age 35 (1989) New England regional genetics group prenatal collaborative study of down syndrome screening. Am J Obstet Gynecol 160(3):575–581
7. Merkatz IR et al (1984) An association between low maternal serum alpha-fetoprotein and fetal chromosomal abnormalities. Am J Obstet Gynecol 148(7):886–894
8. Cuckle HS, Wald NJ, Lindenbaum RH (1984) Maternal serum alpha-fetoprotein measurement: a screening test for Down syndrome. Lancet 1(8383):926–929
9. Palomaki GE et al (1995) Risk-based prenatal screening for trisomy 18 using alpha-fetoprotein, unconjugated oestriol and human chorionic gonadotropin. Prenat Diagn 15 (8):713–723
10. Kjessler B, Johansson SG (1977) Monitoring of the development of early pregnancy by determination of alpha-fetoprotein in maternal serum and amniotic fluid samples. Acta Obstet Gynecol Scand Suppl 69:5–14
11. Brock DJ, Sutcliffe RG (1972) Alpha-fetoprotein in the antenatal diagnosis of anencephaly and spina bifida. Lancet 2 (7770):197–199
12. Wald NJ, Brock DJ, Bonnar J (1974) Prenatal diagnosis of spina bifida and anencephaly by maternal serum-alpha-fetoprotein measurement. A controlled study. Lancet 1 (7861):765–767
13. Penney LL, Klenke WJ (1980) Variability in unconjugated and total estriol in serum during normal third trimester pregnancy. Clin Chem 26(13):1800–1803
14. Bogart MH, Pandian MR, Jones OW (1987) Abnormal maternal serum chorionic gonadotropin levels in pregnancies with fetal chromosome abnormalities. Prenat Diagn 7 (9):623–630
15. Cole LA (2010) Biological functions of hCG and hCG-related molecules. Reprod Biol Endocrinol 8:102
16. Sturgeon CM, McAllister EJ (1998) Analysis of hCG: clinical applications and assay requirements. Ann Clin Biochem 35(Pt 4):460–491
17. van Zonneveld P et al (2003) Do cycle disturbances explain the age-related decline of female fertility? Cycle characteristics of women aged over 40 years compared with a reference population of young women. Hum Reprod 18 (3):495–501
18. Wald NJ et al (1997) Antenatal screening for Down's syndrome. J Med Screen 4 (4):181–246
19. Crandall BF (1981) Alpha-fetoprotein: the diagnosis of neural-tube defects. Pediatr Ann 10(2):38–48
20. Macri JN, Weiss RR (1977) The utilization of alpha-fetoprotein in prenatal diagnosis. Birth Defects Orig Artic Ser 13(3D):191–199

Chapter 21

Isolation of Cell-Free DNA from Maternal Plasma

James Stray and Bernhard Zimmermann

Abstract

Noninvasive prenatal genetic tests analyzing the cell-free fetal DNA in the circulation of expectant mothers are now performed routinely in clinical diagnostic laboratories. Leveraging the power of next generation sequencing (NGS), these tests can detect variation in chromosomal copy number or microdeletions early in gestation. All methods begin with blood collection followed by transport to the diagnostic lab, plasma separation, and purification of ccfDNA from the plasma to prepare it for molecular analysis. Preservation of ccfDNA in blood samples and highly efficient purification from plasma are paramount since the quality and quantity of target nucleic acids determine the sensitivity and therefore success of these assays. Maximizing quality and quantity and minimizing variation in extraction yield pose significant challenges for diagnostic labs, many of which use manual isolation methods for plasma volumes greater than 5 mL. One way to reduce variability is to automate the extraction processes and, to the extent possible, minimize hand-on operations. This chapter details two procedures for isolating ccfDNA from 10 mL plasma by manual and automated means using the QIAamp Circulating Nucleic Acid Kit and the QIAsymphony Circulating DNA Kit. The ccfDNA recovered is suitable for downstream processing in noninvasive prenatal tests for aneuploidy detection.

Key words Circulating cell-free DNA, Automation, Fetal, Noninvasive prenatal testing, QIAsymphony, QIAamp, Blood sample stabilization, Circulating DNA extraction, SNP-based aneuploidy detection

1 Introduction

Extracellular DNA detectable in the cell-free fraction of blood (plasma or serum; *see* **Note 1**) is defined as circulating cell-free DNA (ccfDNA). The half-life of naked DNA in blood and plasma is extremely short, on the order of minutes [1], kept so by active plasma nucleases including DNAse I, DNAse II, and phosphodiesterase I [2]. Circulating cell-free DNA (ccfDNA) survives slightly longer in the blood and avoids rapid degradation by remaining in complex with the histone octamer (2× (H2A, H2B, H3, H4)) as mono- and oligo-nucleosomes, with or without linker histones (chromatosomes), which act to protect 140 to 160 base pairs (bp) of DNA per histone core. Nucleosomes/chromatosomes and

Brynn Levy (ed.), *Prenatal Diagnosis*, Methods in Molecular Biology, vol. 1885, https://doi.org/10.1007/978-1-4939-8889-1_21,

poly-nucleosomes/poly-chromatosomes are shed into the bloodstream as part of normal physiology. The concentration of circulating cell-free DNA (ccfDNA) varies widely [3], in the ng/mL range, and reflects the rate at which chromatin fragments enter the bloodstream, less the rate of destruction by nucleases, and clearance by hepatic uptake and immune-depletion. Healthy individuals maintain an average steady state ccfDNA concentration of ~13 ng/mL, ranging between 0 and 100 ng/mL plasma [4, 5] (*see* **Note 2**). No one cell type or mechanism accounts for the accumulation of nuclear DNA in the blood, though the primary source is erythropoietic apoptosis, with variable contributions from general cell turnover, post engulfment macrophage secretion, and traumatic or necrotic cell death [6–8]. In addition to plasma ccfDNA in tight association with histones, cellular DNA and various RNAs survive plasma destruction protected within membrane microvesicles, exosomes, shed continually from many cell types through the normal process of exocytosis or blebbing [9].

Since the discovery that fetal ccfDNA is detectable and increases in concentration in the circulation of women throughout gestation [10], ccfDNA has become a key analyte for noninvasive prenatal diagnostics. Fetal DNA of placental origin is shed into maternal blood [11]. The properties of ccfDNA found in maternal plasma pose technical challenges: first among them is the extremely low total ccfDNA concentrations and the fact that the fetal ccfDNA is present on average at only 10%, but frequently less than 5%, in plasma samples [12]. In particular, the percentage of fetal DNA in the total ccfDNA is lowest during the first trimester of pregnancy. This issue is addressed by processing high sample volumes between 1 mL and 10 mL, depending on information content to be obtained from the sample. The second challenge is the high degree of ccfDNA fragmentation, which requires an efficient method for recovery of small DNA fragments. The length distribution of fragmented ccfDNA shows a predominant peak at approximately 165–175 bp, consistent with a majority of DNA-histone-protein complexes of a single nucleosome/chromatosome in size. The fetal fraction of ccfDNA is demonstrably shorter and only monosomal in length, with an average of ~145–150 bp protected [13–15]. If a sufficient volume of plasma is processed to give an increased concentration of ccfDNA in eluates, then secondary peaks migrating later relative to the predominant peak can be detected, consistent with oligonucleosomes/oligochromatosomes of 2 to 3 multinucleosomes in length (Fig. 1). Primarily, plasma input volumes of 2–4 mL are used for prenatal diagnostics [16]. But for a detailed analysis of NIPT samples (such as quantitative measurements of fetal chromosome dosage in, e.g., aneuploidy detection), even higher sample input volumes, up to 10 mL plasma, are preferred to ensure reliable detection in cases having low ccfDNA content and/or a low fraction of fetal ccfDNA.

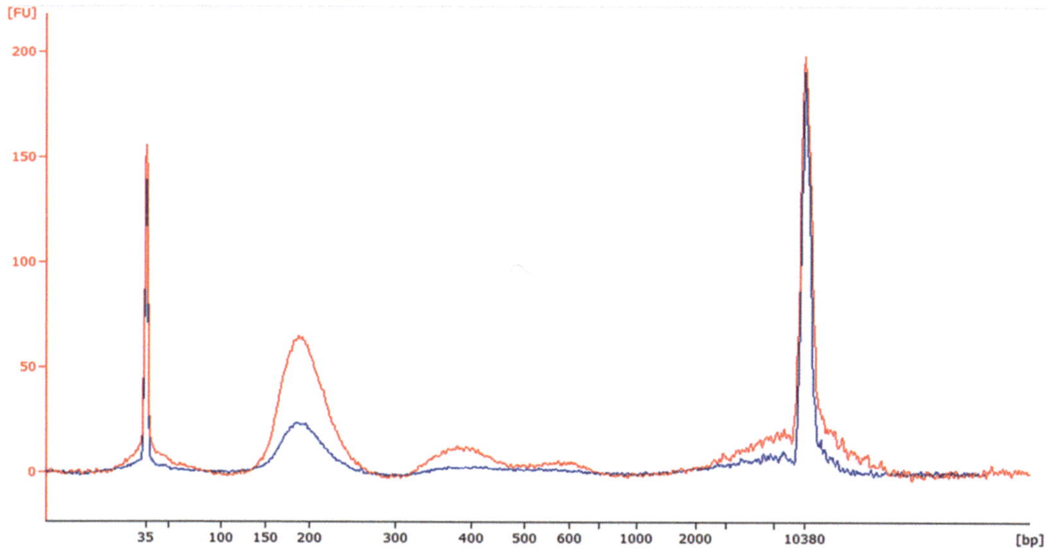

Fig. 1 Size distribution of extracted ccfDNA from 4 mL and 10 mL plasma. ccfDNA extracted from 4 mL plasma (blue) and 10 mL plasma (red) using the QIAsymphony Circulating DNA Kit. 1 μL eluate subjected to Agilent High Sensitivity DNA Chip. FU = fluorescent units, marker peak at 35 bp and 10,380 bp

In this chapter we will discuss the extraction of ccfDNA from large volumes of plasma (up to 10 mL), using the manual QIAamp Circulating Nucleic Acid Kit, used by Natera for plasma ccfDNA purification since offering the noninvasive prenatal test (Panorama™), and the newly developed QIAsymphony Circulating DNA Kit, an automated scalable method that operates on the QIAsymphony SP robotic platform.

In the last few years the rapid and widespread adoption of reliable NIPT screening has increased demand for an automated solution for large volume ccfDNA extraction methods. To meet demand and address this issue, a new chemistry dedicated for automated ccfDNA extraction with modified, scalable protocols for processing up to 10 mL was developed and compared to a manual ccfDNA extraction method also modified for a plasma input volume of 10 mL. Eluates from such extraction methods are used for prenatal diagnostics using Natera's Panorama™ V2 prenatal test (Fig. 2), detailed in [17, 18].

Developing an automated process for handling such high input volumes in parallel to drive extraction of 96 samples in one complete run in <2.5 h per batch of 24 samples is challenging, and required a new chemistry concept. The new chemistry is based on Anion-Exchange beads which require only a low volume of binding buffer added to samples which results in reduced overall processing volumes, and where sample volumes can be scaled with linear extraction efficiencies (Fig. 3a), allowing for parallel processing and higher throughput compared to chaotropic salt/silica-based

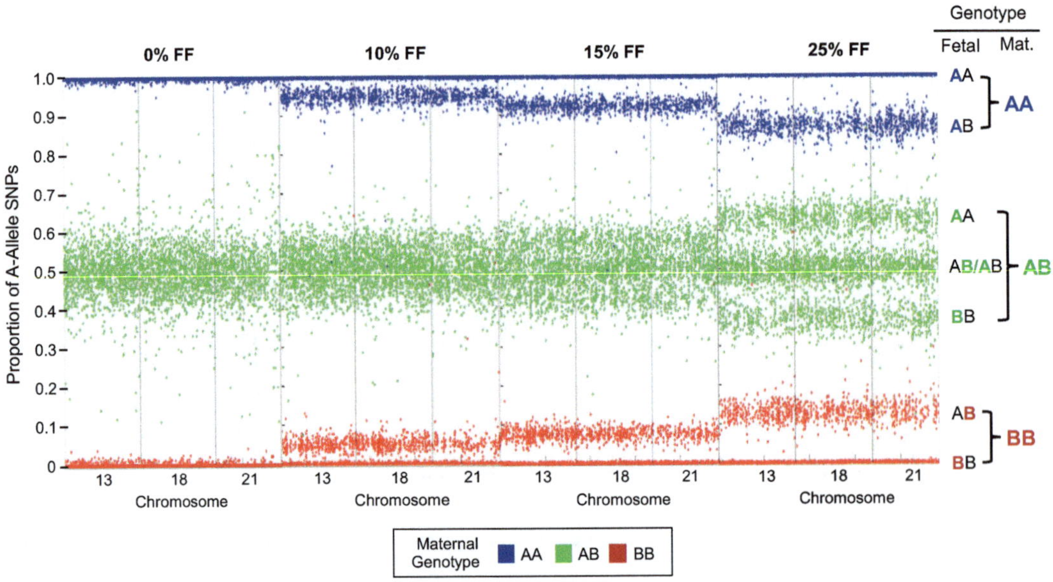

Fig. 2 Graphic representation of sequencing data. The Panorama SNP data are presented in a simplified fashion as the ratio of the two most likely alleles, labeled arbitrarily as A or B. This is not how the algorithm makes ploidy calls in practice, but is one way to visualize this very large data set. Y-axis: (A allele reads)/(Total allele reads). X-axis: Linear SNP position along each chromosome. Fetal and maternal genotypes are indicated to the right, **Red**: the homozygous maternal (AA) allele cluster, **Green**: the heterozygous maternal (AB) allele cluster, and **Blue**: the homozygous maternal (BB) allele cluster. Each spot represents the sum of maternal and fetal A allele read proportions from analysis of the ccfDNA, and depicts patterns typical for euploid autosomes at varying % fetal fraction (FF) of 0%, 10%, 15%, and 25%. The center triple green cluster, most evident at 25% fetal fraction, and the presence of blue and red peripheral clusters indicate the presence of two copies of chromosomes 13, 18, and 21 in these euploid examples

automated nucleic acid extraction methods with a comparable extraction efficiency (Fig. 3b).

The reason for failed laboratory diagnostic tests can often be attributed to the preanalytical sample processing [19] which emphasizes the importance of standardized workflows for ccfDNA applications: The ccfDNA extraction is embedded within this preanalytical process but the workflow starts at the sample collection, which includes blood collection, time until processing and stabilization. Since the transport of whole blood from the site of collection to the laboratory for processing can take up to several days, which determines the time span between blood collection and plasma separation, the choice of the blood collection tube (BCT) must not be undervalued. Next to the well-established anticoagulant preservatives EDTA and Citrate BCTs, several suppliers like Streck (Cell-free DNA BCT), PreAnalytiX (PAXgene Blood ccfDNA Tube) now offer tubes designed to prevent clotting, stabilize cells, and preserve ccfDNA using different stabilizing agents. Usage of these new BCTs has to be considered carefully because they can affect the quality and integrity of extracted ccfDNA and downstream assay compatibility (*see* **Note 3**).

A

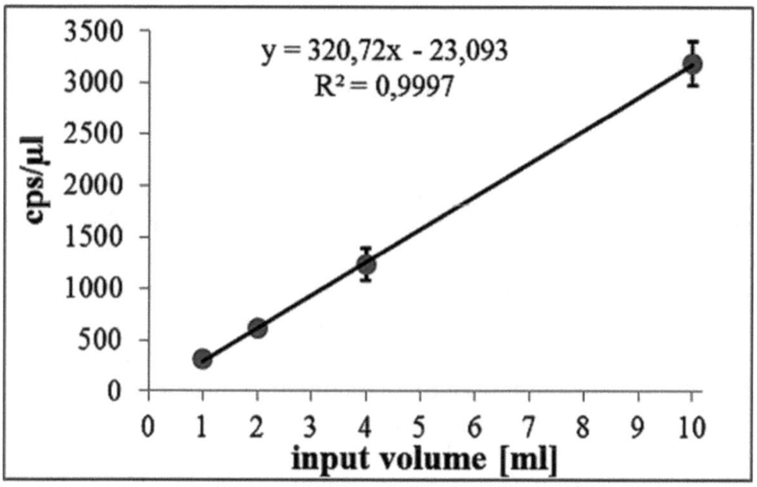

B

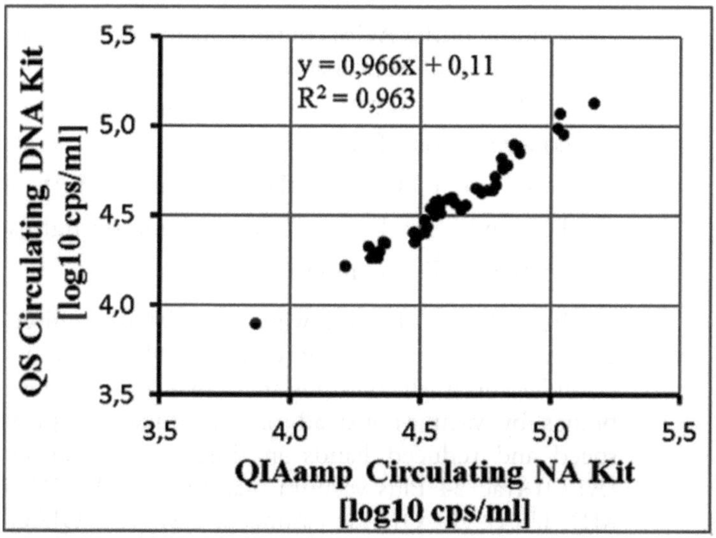

Fig. 3 Linearity of ccfDNA extraction from 1 to 10 mL plasma input for an automated ccfDNA extraction method (**a**) and performance comparison to a manual ccfDNA extraction method (**b**). (**a**) Pooled plasma generated from Cell-Free DNA BCT (Streck) was used. ccfDNA was extracted from 1 mL, 2 mL, 4 mL, and 10 mL plasma input on the QIAsymphony instrument using the QIAsymphony Circulating DNA Kit in combination with different protocols. ccfDNA yield was determined using an in-house real-time PCR assay for the 18S coding sequence (66 bp amplicon). Results were calculated as target copies (haploid genome copies) per µL eluate. (**b**) Blood draw from 48 single donors was performed in Cell-Free DNA BCT (Streck). ccfDNA was extracted from 4 mL plasma input using the QIAsymphony Circulating DNA Kit and the QIAamp Circulating Nucleic Acid Kit in comparison. ccfDNA yield was determined using an in-house real-time PCR assay for the 18S coding sequence (66 bp amplicon; ref. [20]). Results were calculated as target copies (haploid genome copies) per mL plasma input

2 Materials

2.1 Plasma Separation from Whole Blood

Venous maternal blood is collected into Streck Cell-free DNA BCT™ collection tubes and stored or shipped at ambient temperature prior to plasma isolation. The plasma separation is performed in the diagnostic laboratory as described in Subheading 3.1.

2.2 QIAamp Circulating Nucleic Acid Kit (QIAGEN, Germantown, MD, USA)

The QIAamp Circulating Nucleic Acid Kit provides reagents and components for manual extraction of ccfDNA. The extraction chemistry is based on using chaotropic salt, detergent, and proteinase K to release nucleic acids from membrane vesicles and bound proteins (such as nucleosome complexes) and to make these nucleic acid molecules available for binding to a silica membrane surface. The binding of these fragmented nucleic acids to the silica surface is then achieved by a combination of chaotropic salt and isopropanol, which make the binding of DNA and RNA to the hydrophilic surface thermodynamically favored. The kit contains the following reagents:

1. Lysis buffer ACL: contains guanidine thiocyanate, optional addition of 1 μg carrier RNA per sample.
2. Binding buffer ACB: contains guanidine thiocyanate, final concentration of isopropanol is 40%.
3. Wash buffer ACW1: contains guanidine hydrochloride, final concentration of ethanol is 56%.
4. Wash buffer ACW2: final concentration of ethanol is 70%.
5. Elution buffer: Buffer AVE (low ionic-strength solution).
6. Proteinase K, recombinant.

In addition, the following material is required for fast and efficient vacuum processing of up to 24 spin columns in parallel (samples and wash solutions are drawn through the column membranes by vacuum instead of centrifugation, providing greater speed and reduced hands-on time in purification procedures): (A) QIAvac 24 Plus vacuum manifold (QIAGEN, Germantown, MD, USA), (B) QIAvac Connecting System (QIAGEN, Germantown, MD, USA) and (C) Vacuum Pump capable of producing a vacuum of −800 to −900 mbar.

2.3 QIAsymphony Circulating DNA Kit (QIAGEN, Germantown, MD, USA)

The QIAsymphony Circulating DNA Kit provides reagents and components for automated extraction of ccfDNA using the QIAsymphony SP instrument (QIAGEN, Germantown, MD, USA). The extraction chemistry is based on using proteinase K to release nucleic acids from bound proteins (such as nucleosome complexes) and anion-exchange beads to bind the negatively charged ccfDNA to the positively charged bead surface under slightly acidic conditions. During three wash steps impurities (mainly proteins) are removed using a combination of increased pH of wash buffers and salt concentration. Elution takes place under slightly alkaline conditions to achieve a quantitative elution of bound ccfDNA while making sure that the eluted DNA is intact (e.g., double stranded).

In addition to the QIAsymphony SP instrument and QIAsymphony Circulating DNA Kit, the following QIAsymphony SP disposable plasticware is required:

1. Sample Prep Cartridges, 8-well cartridges (QIAGEN, Germantown, MD, USA).
2. 8-Rod Covers (QIAGEN, Germantown, MD, USA).

2.4 Panorama Prenatal Test (Version 2)

The Panorama prenatal test is a next generation genetic test that uses plasma ccfDNA from pregnant women early in gestation as an input to screen for genetic aneuploidies and microdeletions that affect child development. The assay begins by preserving ccfDNA in a library through a series of highly efficient matched molecular reactions designed to repair and amplify fragments in preparation for downstream processing. An aliquot of the library is used as input for a massively multiplex-specific target amplification reaction which reduces the complexity of the sequencing query space and greatly increases the sensitivity and specificity of the assay. Amplified targets are barcoded and readied for NGS sequencing. Sequence data is processed and an allele designation is assigned for each SNP to the mother and child. The plot in Fig. 2 depicts allele ratios obtained for SNPs arrayed linearly along a chromosome, and generated with input ccfDNA deriving from maternal blood having different estimated fetal fractions (FF). The higher the fetal fraction, the greater the proportion of fetal SNPs to the total SNPs (fetal + maternal) detected. This translates into a greater divergence between the fetal genotypes from the underlying maternal SNP genotypes (Figs. 2, 0% FF) where maternal AA, AB, and BB clusters are shown as red, green, and blue dots, respectively. The algorithm does not graphically interpret the results and can discern differences that are not obvious by visual inspection. However, this representation illustrates how the assay responds to fetal fraction and that signal to noise of Panorama, and similar assays, can benefit from efficient ccfDNA isolation methods that recover low abundant, short DNA fragments from large plasma volumes.

The Panorama V2 Sample Preparation Reagents were configured and optimized to generate a population of ccfDNA fragments in eight separate steps:

1. DNA End Repair, which converts 3′ or 5′ overhangs of ccfDNA fragments into blunt ends using a polymerase.
2. A-Tailing, to add a single 3′ A nucleotide to blunt-ended ccfDNA fragments to prepare ends for annealing and ligation to adapters.

3. Ligation, the covalent coupling of synthetic adapter sequences to both ends of A-tailed ccfDNA fragments.
4. Library Amplification, a PCR amplification of adapter-ligated ccfDNA fragments with forward and reverse primers complementary to adapters.
5. Library purification.
6. Specific target amplification, a massively multiplexed PCR reaction whose input is amplified ccfDNA library created in **steps 1–4**. The reaction amplifies a select set of 13,392 target loci across a subset of chromosomes, the information from which can be used to determine the presence or absence of certain aneuploidies.
7. Barcoding, final PCR reaction that appends a unique identifier to the end of each target amplicon and readies fragments for Illumina sequencing.
8. Pooling, quantification, and loading of flow cells for Illumina Sequencing. Individually barcoded PCR products are pooled with those originating from other cases and the concentration of the pool is determined and the pool diluted to a concentration that achieves the optimum cluster density for sequencing a given depth of read.

3 Methods

An overview of the complete ccfDNA workflow from blood collection to downstream analysis is depicted in a processing scheme (Fig. 4).

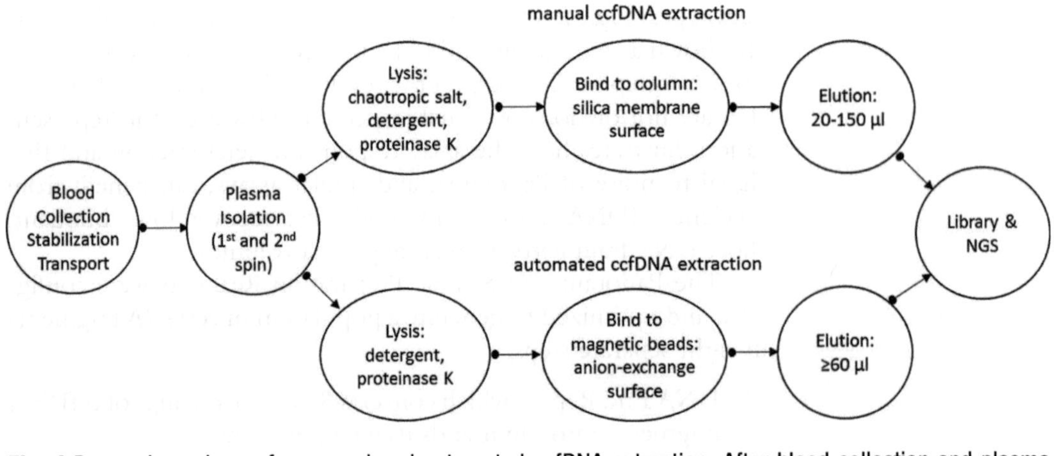

Fig. 4 Processing scheme for manual and automated ccfDNA extraction. After blood collection and plasma isolation two ccfDNA extraction methods are compared to each other: a manual extraction method based on denaturating agents in combination with a silica surface to bind DNA and a automated extraction method based on non-denaturating conditions using anion-exchange beads to bind DNA. Both methods result in different usable elution volumes before purified ccfDNA is subjected to downstream anlysis

3.1 Plasma Separation from Whole Blood

1. Obtain the blood samples to be processed. Visually check the sample IDs to ensure that there are two blood collection tubes (BCTs) per case.
2. For each pair of BCTs, label one 15 mL conical tube and one 50 mL conical tube with the corresponding sample ID.
3. Centrifuge the BCTs at 2000 rcf with maximum acceleration/deceleration for 20 min at 22 °C.
4. Use a 10 mL serological pipette to transfer the plasma from each pair of BCTs to the corresponding 15 mL conical tube (*see* **Note 4**).
5. Centrifuge the 15 mL conical tubes at 3220 rcf with maximum acceleration/deceleration for 30 min at 22 °C (*see* **Note 5**).
6. Transfer the plasma from the 15 mL conical tube to the corresponding 50 mL conical tube (*see* **Note 4**).
7. For each plasma sample, record the total plasma volumes and hemolysis grade:
   - Plasma Color (Hemolysis Grade): Yellow (None), Pink/Orange (Moderate), Red/Dark Red (Severe).
   - For none or moderately hemolyzed samples: continue to process for severely hemolyzed samples OR samples with a total volume of <6 mL: re-draw for a new sample.
8. For plasma samples with a volume 6 mL–9.9 mL that will be extracted immediately, add PBS to bring the total volume to 10 mL.
9. Discard the 15 mL conical tubes in a biohazard waste bin.
10. Store plasma samples that won't be extracted immediately at 4–8 °C or proceed to ccfDNA Extraction.

3.2 Manual DNA Isolation from Plasma Using a Modified QIAamp Circulating Nucleic Acid Kit

3.2.1 ccfDNA Preparation

1. Add 200 mL 100% isopropanol to 300 mL Buffer ACB concentrate to obtain 500 mL Buffer ACB. Mix well by inverting 10 times after adding isopropanol.
2. Add 25 mL 96–100% ethanol to 19 mL Buffer ACW1 concentrate to obtain 44 mL Buffer ACW1. Mix well by inverting 10 times after adding ethanol.
3. Add 30 mL 96–100% ethanol to 13 mL Buffer ACW2 concentrate to obtain 43 mL Buffer ACW2. Mix well by inverting 10 times after adding ethanol.

3.2.2 ccfDNA Extraction

1. For each 50 mL conical, label a LoBind 1.5 mL microcentrifuge tube with the corresponding sample ID.
2. For plasma samples with a volume of <10 mL that were stored at 4–8 °C, add PBS to bring the sample up to 10 mL.
3. Dispense 900 μL of Proteinase K into each plasma sample. Cap and invert each sample tube 5 times to mix the contents.

4. Dispense 8.8 mL of ACL to each plasma sample. Vortex each sample tube for 5 s.
5. Incubate the 50 mL plasma sample tubes in a 60 °C water bath for 45 min (*see* **Note 6**).
6. Dispense 18 mL of ACB to each plasma sample. Cap and invert each sample tube 10 times to mix the contents.
7. Incubate the plasma sample tubes in a wet ice bath for 10 min.
8. Label a QIAamp Mini spin column and column extender corresponding to the sample ID indicated on the 50 mL conical tubes.
9. Insert the column extenders into the corresponding spin columns.
10. Insert spin column/extender assemblies into VacConnectors on the QIAvac 24 Plus (*see* **Note 7**).
11. Connect the vacuum tubing to the QIAvac 24 Plus vacuum port.
12. Carefully pour each plasma sample lysate into the corresponding column extender. Take care not to overfill the extenders.
13. Engage the vacuum by turning on the compressor and adjusting the pressure to 800 mbar (*see* **Note 8**).
14. Refill the tube extenders as the plasma sample lysate volumes are drawn down.
15. Discard the 50 mL conical tubes and column extenders in a biohazard waste bin.
16. Turn on heat block and set to 56 °C (*see* **Note 9**).
17. Once the entire volume of the plasma sample lysates have been drawn through, dispense 600 μL of Buffer ACW1 into each column. Leave the lids open and allow to drain, with the vacuum compressor still running (*see* **Note 10**).
18. Dispense 750 μL of Buffer ACW2 into each column. Leave the lids open and allow to drain with the vacuum compressor still running.
19. Disengage the vacuum by lowering the pressure to 0 mbar and turning the power off.
20. Dispense 750 μL of 100% ethanol to each spin column, leaving lids open.
21. Engage the vacuum by turning on the compressor and adjusting the pressure to 800 mbar and allow columns to drain.
22. Turn off the vacuum by lowering the pressure to 0 and turning the power off.

23. Close the caps and remove the columns from the vacuum manifold. Place the columns into 2.0 mL collection tubes.
24. Discard the VacConnectors in a biohazard waste bin.
25. Place a pre-aliquoted tube of DNA Suspension Buffer in a heat block at 56 °C for at least 10 min.
26. Centrifuge the column/collection tube assemblies in a microfuge at 16,800 × *g* for 3 min.
27. Once the 3 min spin has finished, transfer the columns into new 2.0 mL collection tubes, open the lids and place in a heat block at 56 °C for 10 min.
28. Assemble the labeled 1.5 mL LoBind microcentrifuge tubes into a 96-well tube rack.
29. Dispense 50 μL of the preheated DNA Suspension Buffer into the center of each filter column (*see* **Notes 11 and 12**).
30. Transfer the filter columns from the 2.0 mL collection tubes to the corresponding 1.5 mL LoBind microcentrifuge tubes.
31. Close the column lids and incubate at room temperature (15 °C to 25 °C) for 7 min.
32. Centrifuge the spin column/microcentrifuge tube assemblies in a microfuge at 16,800 × *g* for 1 min. Check that the volumes appear consistent, and that no residual buffer is in the filter (*see* **Note 13**).
33. Discard the filter columns; cap the microcentrifuge tubes that now contain the DNA eluate and store at −30 °C to −10 °C in a pre-PCR room.
34. Pour the vacuum waste into a labeled chemical waste container.
35. Rinse the vacuum line twice with water.

3.3 Automated DNA Isolation from Plasma Using a Modified Protocol for the QIAsymphony Circulating DNA Kit

1. Turn on the instrument and log on after initialization.
2. Load the required elution rack into the "Eluate" drawer in "Elution slot 1."
3. Make sure the "Waste" drawer is properly prepared and perform an inventory scan of the "Waste" drawer, including the tip chute and liquid waste.
4. Load the required reagent cartridge(s) and consumables into the "Reagents and Consumables" drawer. Vortex the bead trough containing the magnetic particles vigorously for at least 3 min before first use. Make sure that the piercing lid is placed on the reagent cartridge and the lid of the magnetic-particle trough has been removed or, if using a partially used reagent cartridge, make sure the Reuse Seal Strips have been removed. Perform an inventory scan of the "Reagents and Consumables" drawer.

5. Aliquot the required plasma volume (*see* **Note 14**) into a sample tube and place the samples into the appropriate sample carrier, and load them into the "Sample" drawer. Plasma volumes from 1 mL to 10 mL can be used as sample input volume.
6. Using the touchscreen, enter the required information for each batch of samples and for Proteinase K to be processed which includes: sample information (depending on sample racks used), protocol to be run (1–10 mL) and elution volume and output position.
7. Place the Proteinase K into the appropriate sample carrier on positions 1 and 2, and load them into slot A of the "Sample" drawer. 11. Define the Proteinase K by pressing the IC button.
8. Press the Run button to start the purification procedure. All processing steps are fully automated. At the end of the protocol run, the status of the batch changes from RUNNING to COMPLETED.
9. Retrieve the elution rack containing the purified nucleic acids from the "Eluate" drawer (*see* **Note 15**). The DNA is ready to use or can be stored at 2–8 °C, −20 °C, or −80 °C.

4 Notes

1. CcfDNA is detectable in serum but due to the agglutination process when blood draw takes place in serum BCTs ccfDNA fraction in supernatant is strongly contaminated with fragmented genomic DNA. Therefore usage of serum BCT is not recommended for ccfDNA isolation.
2. Detection of ccfDNA in eluates: Due to the very low concentrations of ccfDNA in sample materials, measurement of DNA concentration by using a spectrophotometer is not recommended. For determination of concentration of circulating cell-free DNA, a sensitive and accurate fluorescence-based quantitation assay such as Quant-iT or PicoGreen-based assays (Thermo Fisher Scientific, Waltham, MA, USA), or a real-time PCR assay targeting single or multi-copy genes such as 18S RNA gene [20], or hRNaseP and hTERT, or hAlu and hrDNA repeats should be used. Because carrier RNA interferes with fluorescence-based assays, a real-time PCR assay is preferred for DNA quantification.
3. Blood Collection tubes offered for ccfDNA applications target two aims: Firstly, to stabilize the extracellular DNA (ccfDNA) in the plasma fraction of whole blood and secondly, the preservatives in such BCT tubes stabilize nucleated blood cells for extended times, thereby inhibiting the release of cellular

(nuclear) DNA, so that additional maternal genomic DNA is prevented from further diluting the fetal fraction [16]. Hence, these stabilizing BCTs allow for delaying the plasma separation up to several days after blood draw which makes it possible to ship the primary blood tube to a testing laboratory where the plasma is then separated. It is technically challenging to achieve such a stabilization effect for several days without affecting the integrity and purity of the ccfDNA fraction while ensuring, in parallel, the quantitative bioavailability of the ccfDNA for sensitive downstream applications after extraction from plasma. Therefore, the need for sample stabilization and the need for obtaining highly pure ccfDNA should be considered carefully because both aspects may have an impact on the reliability of results, making it necessary to compare the different tubes offered. The recently available PAXgene Blood ccfDNA Tube uses a non-crosslinking chemistry to stabilize whole blood while maintaining the quality and yield of ccfDNA.

4. Do not disrupt the blood cells.
5. After the first centrifugation step to separate the blood cell fraction from the plasma fraction and subsequent transfer of the plasma to a secondary tube, a second centrifugation step may be required due to the following considerations: (A) to ensure that remains of the buffy coat layer which are accidentally transferred after first centrifugation are completely removed from plasma to prevent genomic DNA contamination of ccfDNA fraction (low to medium speed centrifugation) and/or (B) to remove microvesicles (mainly exosomes) which also contain cell-free but membrane enclosed RNA and DNA which may also be extracted and measured in downstream analysis in parallel to the ccfDNA fraction (high speed centrifugation required).
6. Ensure that the isopropanol has been added to the Buffer ACB.
7. To avoid air leaks, make sure all connectors are firmly secure and close unused slots with plugs, or close the inserted VacValve.
8. Do not readjust the pressure, once the vacuum process has started.
9. Ensure that ethanol was added to the Buffer ACW1.
10. Ensure that ethanol was added to the Buffer ACW2.
11. Do not touch the filter membrane with the pipette tip.
12. DNA Suspension Buffer used alternatively to elution buffer AVE for elution of ccfDNA.
13. If residual buffer is present on the lip where the filter joins the column, or in the cap, pipet the buffer to the center of the filter

membrane and centrifuge in a microfuge at 16,800 × *g* for 1 min.

14. Automated DNA isolation: Make sure that correct sample volume including void volume is used to avoid sample flagging when using liquid-level detection mode (e.g., for 10 mL protocol 10.5 mL volume is required). If not sufficient sample is available fill up sample with PBS to obtain the required sample volume before loading onto the instrument. Alternatively, FIX labware has been designed to minimize dead volumes (e.g., for 10 mL protocol 10.1 mL volume is required). But it must be considered that FIX labware does not support liquid-level detection or clot detection. As further alternative the "Enable less sample" mode has been designed to use all available liquid in combination with liquid-level detection and clot detection in case less volume than required has been detected during sample transfer (e.g., for 10 mL protocol at least 9.4 mL volume is required). "Enable less sample" mode results in unclear flagged samples.

    Bubbles/foam in sample input tube may result in false liquid level detection and subsequent incomplete sample transfer. Remove bubbles in sample tube and avoid pipetting of sample on the inner wall of the vessel during sample loading.

15. Automated DNA isolation: It is recommended to remove the eluate plate from the "Eluate" drawer immediately after the run has finished. Depending on temperature and humidity, elution plates left in the QIAsymphony SP after the run is completed may experience condensation or evaporation.
    In general, magnetic particles are not carried over into eluates. If carryover does occur, magnetic particles in eluates will not affect most downstream applications. If magnetic particles need to be removed before performing downstream applications, tubes or plates containing eluates should first be placed in a suitable magnet and the eluates transferred to a clean tube.

Disclaimer

The scalable ccfDNA isolation methods presented here are for performance evaluations only.

References

1. Houk BE, Hochhaus G, Hughes JA (1999) Kinetic modeling of plasmid DNA degradation in rat plasma. AAPS PharmSci 1(3):E9
2. Tamkovich SN, Cherepanova AV, Kolesnikova EV, Rykova EY, Pyshnyi DV, Vlassov VV, Laktionov PP (2006) Circulating DNA and DNase activity in human blood. Ann N Y Acad Sci 1075:191–196. https://doi.org/10.1196/annals.1368.026
3. Steinman CR (1975) Free DNA in serum and plasma from normal adults. J Clin Invest 56

(2):512–515. https://doi.org/10.1172/JCI108118

4. Gormally E, Hainaut P, Caboux E, Airoldi L, Autrup H, Malaveille C, Dunning A, Garte S, Matullo G, Overvad K, Tjonneland A, Clavel-Chapelon F, Boffetta P, Boeing H, Trichopoulou A, Palli D, Krogh V, Tumino R, Panico S, Bueno-de-Mesquita HB, Peeters PH, Lund E, Gonzalez CA, Martinez C, Dorronsoro M, Barricarte A, Tormo MJ, Quiros JR, Berglund G, Hallmans G, Day NE, Key TJ, Veglia F, Peluso M, Norat T, Saracci R, Kaaks R, Riboli E, Vineis P (2004) Amount of DNA in plasma and cancer risk: a prospective study. Int J Cancer 111 (5):746–749. https://doi.org/10.1002/ijc.20327
5. Leon SA, Shapiro B, Sklaroff DM, Yaros MJ (1977) Free DNA in the serum of cancer patients and the effect of therapy. Cancer Res 37(3):646–650
6. Jahr S, Hentze H, Englisch S, Hardt D, Fackelmayer FO, Hesch RD, Knippers R (2001) DNA fragments in the blood plasma of cancer patients: quantitations and evidence for their origin from apoptotic and necrotic cells. Cancer Res 61(4):1659–1665
7. Raptis L, Menard HA (1980) Quantitation and characterization of plasma DNA in normals and patients with systemic lupus erythematosus. J Clin Invest 66(6):1391–1399. https://doi.org/10.1172/JCI109992
8. Zeerleder S (2006) The struggle to detect circulating DNA. Crit Care 10(3):142. https://doi.org/10.1186/cc4932
9. Thery C, Zitvogel L, Amigorena S (2002) Exosomes: composition, biogenesis and function. Nat Rev Immunol 2(8):569–579. https://doi.org/10.1038/nri855
10. Lo YM, Corbetta N, Chamberlain PF, Rai V, Sargent IL, Redman CW, Wainscoat JS (1997) Presence of fetal DNA in maternal plasma and serum. Lancet 350(9076):485–487
11. Sekizawa A, Yokokawa K, Sugito Y, Iwasaki M, Yukimoto Y, Ichizuka K, Saito H, Okai T (2003) Evaluation of bidirectional transfer of plasma DNA through placenta. Hum Genet 113(4):307–310. https://doi.org/10.1007/s00439-003-0987-4
12. Lo YM, Tein MS, Lau TK, Haines CJ, Leung TN, Poon PM, Wainscoat JS, Johnson PJ, Chang AM, Hjelm NM (1998) Quantitative analysis of fetal DNA in maternal plasma and serum: implications for noninvasive prenatal diagnosis. Am J Hum Genet 62(4):768–775
13. Chan KC, Zhang J, Hui AB, Wong N, Lau TK, Leung TN, Lo KW, Huang DW, Lo YM (2004) Size distributions of maternal and fetal DNA in maternal plasma. Clin Chem 50 (1):88–92. https://doi.org/10.1373/clinchem.2003.024893
14. Fan HC, Blumenfeld YJ, Chitkara U, Hudgins L, Quake SR (2010) Analysis of the size distributions of fetal and maternal cell-free DNA by paired-end sequencing. Clin Chem 56 (8):1279–1286. https://doi.org/10.1373/clinchem.2010.144188
15. Li Y, Zimmermann B, Rusterholz C, Kang A, Holzgreve W, Hahn S (2004) Size separation of circulatory DNA in maternal plasma permits ready detection of fetal DNA polymorphisms. Clin Chem 50(6):1002–1011. https://doi.org/10.1373/clinchem.2003.029835
16. Barrett AN, Zimmermann BG, Wang D, Holloway A, Chitty LS (2011) Implementing prenatal diagnosis based on cell-free fetal DNA: accurate identification of factors affecting fetal DNA yield. PLoS One 6(10):e25202. https://doi.org/10.1371/journal.pone.0025202
17. Hall MP, Hill M, Zimmermann B, Sigurjonsson S, Westemeyer M, Saucier J, Demko Z, Rabinowitz M (2014) Non-invasive prenatal detection of trisomy 13 using a single nucleotide polymorphism- and informatics-based approach. PLoS One 9 (5):e96677. https://doi.org/10.1371/journal.pone.0096677
18. Samango-Sprouse C, Banjevic M, Ryan A, Sigurjonsson S, Zimmermann B, Hill M, Hall MP, Westemeyer M, Saucier J, Demko Z, Rabinowitz M (2013) SNP-based non-invasive prenatal testing detects sex chromosome aneuploidies with high accuracy. Prenat Diagn 33(7):643–649. https://doi.org/10.1002/pd.4159
19. Lippi G, Chance JJ, Church S, Dazzi P, Fontana R, Giavarina D, Grankvist K, Huisman W, Kouri T, Palicka V, Plebani M, Puro V, Salvagno GL, Sandberg S, Sikaris K, Watson I, Stankovic AK, Simundic AM (2011) Preanalytical quality improvement: from dream to reality. Clin Chem Lab Med 49 (7):1113–1126. https://doi.org/10.1515/CCLM.2011.600
20. Horlitz M, Hartinger T, Graf S, Lucas A, Nocon A, Sprenger-Haussels M (2011) Yields of viral and circulating cell-free nucleic acids using the QIAamp (R) circulating nucleic acid kit. Circulating Nucleic Acids in Plasma and Serum:259–268. https://doi.org/10.1007/978-90-481-9382-0_35

Chapter 22

Noninvasive Detection of Fetal Aneuploidy Using Next Generation Sequencing

Kirsten J. Curnow, Rebecca K. Sanderson, and Sue Beruti

Abstract

Cell-free DNA (cfDNA)-based noninvasive prenatal testing (NIPT) utilizing next generation sequencing (NGS) is a highly sensitive and specific approach designed to screen for fetal aneuploidy. NIPT was first introduced in 2011 and has been rapidly adopted in a clinical setting because of the improved performance afforded compared with traditional prenatal serum screening options. We describe a PCR-free, paired-end sequencing-based NIPT, the VeriSeq NIPT Solution. This NIPT screens for fetal aneuploidy of chromosomes 21, 18, 13, X, and Y. Using the validated approach detailed here, users can achieve high sensitivities and specificities for trisomies 21, 18, and 13 as well as sex chromosome aneuploidies with low failure rates. The automated workflow can be completed in 1 day, with only 2 h of hands-on time from a single technician.

Key words Next generation sequencing, Paired-end sequencing, Noninvasive prenatal test, Cell-free DNA, PCR-free, Prenatal screening, Aneuploidy, Trisomy, Down syndrome

1 Introduction

Prenatal screening is currently used for the detection of common fetal aneuploidies. Traditional screening options include measurement of first and/or second trimester serum biomarkers and ultrasound examinations; these tests are primarily designed to screen for trisomy 21 (Down syndrome), with some tests also reporting a risk for trisomy 18 and trisomy 13. Although these tests have a sensitivity of around 80–90% for trisomy 21 [1], they have a false positive rate of around 5%. As a result, these tests have low positive predictive values (~5%), which means that only around 1 in 20 patients with a positive test have an affected pregnancy. Thus, there was a need for a more accurate approach with lower false positive rates thereby reducing the number of women undergoing unnecessary invasive procedures.

The discovery of cell-free DNA (cfDNA) in blood and determination that in pregnant women it is a mixture of maternal cfDNA

Brynn Levy (ed.), *Prenatal Diagnosis*, Methods in Molecular Biology, vol. 1885, https://doi.org/10.1007/978-1-4939-8889-1_22,

and fetal cfDNA (primarily placental origin) drove development of noninvasive prenatal testing (NIPT). Molecular analysis of cfDNA isolated from a maternal peripheral whole blood sample has proven to be a much more accurate and comprehensive method of screening for fetal aneuploidy [2]. With sensitivities above 90% and specificities of around 99.9%, NIPT has positive predictive values above 50%, which is around tenfold higher than biomarker-based tests [2]. A range of molecular technologies are used for NIPT: microarray, targeted sequencing, and whole-genome sequencing (WGS). Although test sensitivities and specificities are similar between the different methodologies, there are marked differences in the test failure rates. Whole-genome sequencing has several advantages: lower technical failure rates than targeted sequencing and microarray-based approaches [3–5]; data from non-test chromosomes can be used as a reference during analysis; comprehensive coverage information that can be useful in determining sample quality and fetal fraction estimation; relative ease of expanding the test menu, such as screening for other autosomal aneuploidies or select microdeletion syndromes.

Herein, we describe a validated WGS-based NIPT used to screen pregnant women of at least 10 weeks' gestation for fetal aneuploidy on chromosomes 21, 18, 13, X, and Y; the VeriSeq™ NIPT Solution [3] is available as an IVD in select countries and regions. This technology is also the basis for a commercially available NIPT offered in the CLIA-certified Illumina laboratory (Foster City, CA). The principles of the method are as follows: sample collection, plasma isolation, cfDNA extraction, library preparation, quantification, library pooling and sequencing, and analysis. Sample collection requires a minimum of 7 mL of maternal peripheral whole blood collected in a single Streck cell-free blood collection tube, which prevents cell lysis and genomic contamination and stabilizes the sample at room temperature. Subsequent sample preparation steps are part of an automated workflow utilizing a liquid handling system, and can be completed in just over a day with around 2 h of hands on time from a single technician. Plasma is isolated using standard centrifugation techniques. Cell-free DNA is extracted by adsorption onto a binding plate, washes, and then elution. The library preparation process is PCR-free, and involves end repair to convert 5′ and 3′ overhangs to blunt ends, addition of a single deoxyadenosine nucleotide at the 3′ end, then ligation of indexed adaptors to the cfDNA fragments. The adaptors serve two purposes: sample identification during sequencing; library capture on the solid surface of the sequencing flow cell for cluster generation and sequencing. After quantitation of library yield, 48-sample batch libraries are pooled; the amount of each library is adjusted to minimize variation in coverage. The library pool then undergoes paired-end sequencing on a next generation sequencer. Once sequencing is complete, the data is analyzed with nucleotide base calls made from the signal intensity measurements taken during sequencing. Paired-end read information is used to assess coverage and individual fragment size. As the size profiles of maternal and fetal cfDNA differ, fragment size information is useful in making fetal fraction estimates. Further, analysis is refined by binning fragment size, with a relative increase in the fetal signal achieved by focusing on shorter fragments. Next, secondary data analysis is performed: Reads are demultiplexed using the index sequences; sequence reads are mapped to the human genome; the number of unique reads is calculated within each 100 kb genomic bin; coverage is normalized on a subchromosomal level. The analysis software employs an algorithm based on multiple data inputs, including sequencing coverage, sequence read quality, and estimated fetal fraction, to determine under or over representation of chromosomes 21, 18, 13, X, and Y. The assay uses a dynamic threshold metric to determine whether the sample can be reported, obviating the need for an arbitrary fetal fraction cutoff. The NIPT protocol and reagents described herein result in the lowest failure rate among in-lab NIPT offerings with comparably high clinical performance.

2 Materials

2.1 Equipment

1. VeriSeq Onsite Server with preinstalled VeriSeq NIPT Assay Software (Illumina, Inc., San Diego, CA, USA).
2. VeriSeq NIPT Microlab STAR (Hamilton Company, Reno, NV; Hamilton Company, Bonaduz, Switzerland) with preinstalled VeriSeq NIPT Workflow Manager.
3. Next generation sequencing (NGS) system with the following capabilities: 2 × 36 bp paired-end sequencing; compatible with VeriSeq NIPT Sample Prep dual index adapters; automatic production of BCL files; two dye-based chemistry; 400 million paired-end reads per run; compatible with VeriSeq NIPT Assay Software.
4. Centrifuge and rotor assemblies for blood collection tubes with the following specifications: Refrigerated centrifuge capable of 1600 × *g* with no-brake option; swinging bucket rotor with buckets; bucket inserts, 48 or 96 tube capacity, 76 mm minimum depth; insert adapters to support 16 × 100 mm blood collection tubes. *Recommended*: Allegra 6 Series Centrifuge, 1600 × *g* (Beckman Coulter, Indianapolis, IN); Allegra Centrifuge GH-3.8 Rotor with buckets (Beckman Coulter, Indianapolis, IN); Allegra Centrifuge Bucket Covers, set of two (Beckman Coulter, Indianapolis, IN); Allegra Centrifuge Adapter Assembly, 16 mm, set of four (Beckman Coulter, Indianapolis, IN).

5. Centrifuge and rotor assemblies for microplates with the following specifications: Centrifuge capable of 5600 × *g*; swinging plate rotor with 96-well plate carriers, 76.5 mm minimum depth; support base for microplates. *Recommended*: Sorvall Legend XTR Centrifuge (Thermo Fisher Scientific, Waltham, MA); HIGHPlate 6000 Microplate Rotor (Thermo Fisher Scientific, Waltham, MA); either MicroAmp 96-Well Support Base (Thermo Fisher Scientific, Waltham, MA) or 96-Well PCR Plate Carrier (Thermo Fisher Scientific, Waltham, MA).
6. Gemini XPS or SpectraMax M2 Microplate reader (Molecular Devices, San Jose, CA).
7. SpectraMax High-Speed USB, Serial Adapter (Molecular Devices, San Jose, CA).
8. Thermal cycler with the following specifications: heated lid; 4 °C to 98 °C temperature range; ± 2 °C temperature accuracy; 2 °C per second minimum ramp rate; compatible with Twin.tec PCR Plate 96-well, full skirt.
9. 1000 μL Conductive Non-Sterile Filter Tips.
10. 300 μL Conductive Non-Sterile Filter Tips.
11. 50 μL Conductive Non-Sterile Filter Tips.
12. Deep-Well Reservoir (Corning Axygen, Tewksbury, MA).
13. MagNA Pure LC Medium Reagent Tubs 20 (Roche, Basel, Switzerland).
14. Deep-Well Plate 96 (Eppendorf, Hauppauge, NY).
15. Low Volume 384 Well Black Flat Bottom Polystyrene Microplate (Corning, Tewksbury, MA).
16. Twin.tec PCR Plate 96-well with a full-skirt (Eppendorf, Hauppauge, NY).
17. Microseal 'F' Foil (Biorad, Hercules, CA) or Foil seals (Beckman Coulter, Indianapolis, IN).
18. Cell-Free DNA Blood Collection Tube (BCT) CE (Streck, La Vista, NE).
19. Push Caps (Sarstedt, Numbrecht, Germany).

2.2 Reagents

1. VeriSeq NIPT Sample Prep Kit (Illumina, Inc., San Diego, CA, USA). The kit contains an Extraction Box, Library Prep Box, Accessory Box, and Workflow Tubes and Labels.
2. 100% Ethanol for molecular biology.
3. DNase/RNAse-free water.
4. Optional: Dulbecco's Phosphate-Buffered Saline (DPBS) for no template control (NTC).

2.3 Cell-Free DNA Extraction

For **steps 1** to **3** below, reagents to be prepared are supplied in the Extraction and Accessory Boxes of the VeriSeq NIPT Sample Prep Kit. Label the reservoir tubs and deep-well reservoirs with the name of the reagents.

1. Final Plasma deep-well plate. If previously refrigerated, let it stand for 30 min to bring to room temperature. Unseal plate before use.
2. Proteinase K: Prepare by slowly adding 3.75 mL Proteinase Buffer to each reagent vial, cap the vial and vortex until resuspended. For 48 samples, use 3 reagent vials. For 96 samples, use 4 reagent vials. Pool prepared reagent from all vials into a reagent tub.
3. Wash Buffer II: Add 100 mL 100% EtOH to each reagent bottle, inverting to mix. For 48 samples, prepare 1 bottle. For 96 samples, prepare 2 bottles. Mark checkbox on bottle/s.
4. 70% EtOH cleaning solution for cleaning vacuum system: 70% Ethanol, 30% DNase/RNAse-free water.

2.4 Library Preparation

For **steps 1** to **9** below, reagents to be prepared are supplied in the Library Prep and Accessory Boxes of the VeriSeq NIPT Sample Prep Kit. Label the reservoir tubs and deep-well reservoirs with the reagent names.

1. End Repair Mix: Thaw at room temperature and then vortex to mix.
2. A-Tailing Mix: Thaw at room temperature, vortex to mix, and then briefly centrifuge.
3. Ligation Mix: Thaw at room temperature, vortex to mix, and then briefly centrifuge.
4. Resuspension Buffer: Vortex to mix. Return to storage after use.
5. Hybridization Buffer: Thaw at room temperature and then vortex to mix. Return to storage after use.
6. VeriSeq NIPT DNA Adapter Plate: Thaw at room temperature, vortex to mix, and then centrifuge at 1000 × *g* for 20 s. Apply a plate barcode.
7. Sample Purification Beads: Let it stand for 30 min to bring to room temperature before mixing by vortexing or inversion until all beads are in suspension and the mixture is homogenous. Vortex vigorously before each use.
8. Combine A-Tailing Mix and Resuspension Buffer in a screw cap tube, vortex to mix, and then briefly centrifuge. For 48 samples: 900 μL A-Tailing Mix, 1200 μL Resuspension Buffer. For 96 samples: 1800 μL A-Tailing Mix, 2400 μL Resuspension Buffer.

9. Combine Ligation Mix and Resuspension Buffer in a screw cap tube, vortex to mix, and then briefly centrifuge. For 48 samples: 230 μL Ligation Mix, 1713 μL Resuspension Buffer. For 96 samples: 440 μL Ligation Mix, 3278 μL Resuspension Buffer.
10. cfDNA Elution Plate: If previously stored, thaw at room temperature, vortex for 1 min, and then centrifuge at 1000 × *g* for 20 s.
11. 80% Ethanol: 40 mL 100% Ethanol, 10 mL DNase/RNAse-free water.

2.5 Library Quantification

For **steps 1** to **3** below, reagents to be prepared are supplied in the Accessory Box of the VeriSeq NIPT Sample Prep Kit.

1. DNA Quantification Reagent: Thaw at room temperature. Vortex to mix, and then briefly centrifuge. Protect from light.
2. DNA Quantification Standard: Vortex to mix, and then briefly centrifuge.
3. Resuspension Buffer: Vortex to mix.
4. Libraries Plate: If previously stored, thaw at room temperature, vortex to mix, and centrifuge at 1000 × *g* for 20 s.

2.6 Library Pooling

For **step 1** below, the reagent to be prepared is supplied in the Library Prep Box of the VeriSeq NIPT Sample Prep Kit.

1. Hybridization Buffer: Thaw at room temperature, and then vortex to mix. Return to storage after use.
2. Libraries Plate: If previously stored, thaw at room temperature, vortex at 1500 rpm for 1 min, then centrifuge at 1000 × *g* for 20 s.

2.7 Preparing for Sequencing

1. Pool tubes: If previously stored, thaw at room temperature. Vortex briefly, then centrifuge briefly.

3 Methods

3.1 Process Blood Samples

1. Centrifuge barcoded blood samples at 1600 × *g* for 10 min at 4 °C (*see* **Note 1**). Begin plasma isolation (*see* Subheading 3.2) within 15 min of completing centrifugation. Repeat centrifugation if more than 15 min has elapsed.
2. Remove samples tubes from the centrifuge and visually inspect each tube to confirm that it contains at least 1.5 mL plasma above the buffy coat (*see* **Note 2**).
3. Uncap tubes and load all samples and any plasma controls into tube carriers (*see* **Note 3**).

The VeriSeq NIPT Solution utilizes a liquid handling system (VeriSeq NIPT Microlab STAR [ML STAR]) to minimize required hands-on time. Plasma Isolation (*see* Subheading 3.2), cell-free DNA extraction (*see* Subheading 3.3), and library preparation (*see* Subheading 3.4) steps are largely performed by the ML STAR (*see* **Notes 4, 5**).

3.2 Plasma Isolation

3.2.1 Preparation

1. Label 1 deep-well plate *Intermediate Plasma* and apply a barcode.
2. Label 1 deep-well plate *Final Plasma* and apply a barcode.

3.2.2 Procedure

1. On the ML STAR, open the AppLauncher, and then click *VeriSeq NIPT Method*.
2. Enter the Batch ID and username, and then click *OK*.
3. Click *New Batch*, and after initiation, click *OK* to begin plasma isolation.
4. Perform one of the following: To load an existing sample sheet, select the sample sheet associated with the batch, and then click *OK;* to proceed without selecting a sample sheet, click *No Sample Sheet*. The sample sheet is a comma-delimited file (SampleSheet.csv) that stores the information to set up and analyze a sequencing experiment. The file includes a list of samples and their index sequences, as well as the workflow to be employed.
5. Select the batch size, and then click *OK*. Select the number of no template controls (NTCs), and then click *OK*.
6. Confirm that all barcodes are affixed, and load the samples, tips, and plates onto the carrier (*see* Table 1). Click *OK* after each load prompt.
7. Make sure the carriers, labware, and reagents are loaded correctly, and then click *OK* in the Pre-Spin Deck Verification screen.
8. When alerted by the Workflow Manager, make sure that the ML STAR loading deck is free of any obstructions to allow the ML STAR to unload the carriers, and then click *Unload*.
9. Remove the Intermediate Plasma deep-well plate. Visually inspect the plate for consistent volumes in each well, the expected volume is 1000 μL. Make note of any inconsistencies and record at the end of the Plasma Isolation procedure. Seal the plate and centrifuge at 5600 × *g* for 10 min.
10. Click *Yes* to proceed to final Plasma Preparation.
11. Remove the plate seal and reload the plate as detailed in Table 1.
12. Select the *Intermediate Plasma plate has been spun* checkbox, and then click *OK*.

Table 1
ML STAR loading details for the plasma isolation procedure

Procedural step	Sample batch size	Carrier type	Track	Item	Site position
6	48	Tip	7–12	1000 μL tips	5
		Tube	15	Prepared blood samples tubes 1–24	1–24
		Tube	16	Prepared blood samples tubes 25–48	25–48
		Multiflex	19–24	Empty deep-well plate, Final Plasma - barcoded	4
		Multiflex	19–24	Empty deep-well plate, Intermediate Plasma – barcoded	5
		Reagent	47	[Optional] DPBS for no template control	5
	96	Tip	7–12	1000 μL tips	4, 5
		Tube	15	Prepared blood samples tubes 1–24	1–24
		Tube	16	Prepared blood samples tubes 25–48	24–48
		Tube	17	Prepared blood samples tubes 49–72	49–72
		Tube	18	Prepared blood samples tubes 73–96	73–96
		Multiflex	19–24	Empty deep-well plate, Final Plasma - barcoded	4
		Multiflex	19–24	Empty deep-well plate, Intermediate Plasma – barcoded	5
		Reagent	47	[Optional] DPBS for no template control	5
11	48, 96	Multiflex	19–24	Intermediate Plasma deep-well plate	5

DPBS Dulbecco's phosphate-buffered saline

13. When alerted by the Workflow Manager, make sure that the ML STAR loading deck is free of any obstructions to allow the ML STAR to unload the carriers, and then click *Unload*.
14. When prompted by the Workflow Manager, empty the carriers and deck.
15. Remove the Final Plasma deep-well plate. Visually inspect the plate for consistent volumes in each well (the expected volume is 900 μL), visible cell pellets, and excessive hemolysis. If you observe a visible cell pellet or excessive hemolysis, invalidate the affected sample at the end of the Plasma Isolation method or use Batch Manager.
16. When prompted by the Workflow Manager, click *OK*.
17. Enter comments about affected wells, and then click *OK*.
18. Perform 1 of the following: To continue to cfDNA Extraction, click *Yes*; To stop, click *Exit* (*see* **Note 6**).

3.3 Cell-Free DNA Extraction

3.3.1 Preparation

1. Label 1 new full-skirt plate *Intermediate*, and apply a plate barcode.
2. Label 1 new full-skirt plate *cfDNA Elution*, and apply a plate barcode.
3. Label 1 new deep-well plate *Extraction Intermediate*, and apply a deep-well plate barcode.
4. Apply a plate barcode to the DNA Binding plate.
5. Prepare the vacuum system: Remove the vacuum manifold and clean with 70% EtOH; empty the vacuum waste; ensure the ML STAR vacuum system is on.

3.3.2 Procedure

1. Click *OK* to start cfDNA Extraction. If the VeriSeq NIPT Method is not already open: Open the AppLauncher, and click *VeriSeq NIPT Method*; enter the Batch ID and username, and then click *OK*.
2. Load tips onto the tip carriers as detailed in Table 2, and then click *OK*.
3. Load counted tips onto the tip carriers as detailed in Table 2.
4. Enter the location of the first and last tips for each tip rack, and then click *OK*.
5. Scan Extraction Box barcodes. Enter the user name or reagent preparer initials, and then click *OK*.
6. Scan Accessory Box barcodes. Enter the user name or reagent preparer initials, and then click *OK*.
7. Confirm that barcodes are affixed, unseal the Final Plasma deep-well plate if necessary, and load plates onto the plate carrier as detailed in Table 2, and then click *OK*.
8. Confirm that the DNA Binding plate is barcoded, then click *OK*.
9. For a 48-sample batch size, cut a seal in half width-wise and apply over unused columns 7–12 of the plate before loading onto the vacuum manifold.
10. Load the DNA Binding plate onto the vacuum manifold with the barcode facing right, and then click *OK*.
11. Load reagent tubs onto the reagent carrier as detailed in Table 2, and then click *OK*.
12. Transfer the specified reagents into the deep-well reservoirs, and then load the reservoirs onto the deep-well carriers as detailed in Table 2, and then click *OK*.
13. Wait for the automated reagent volume check to complete.
14. Confirm that vacuum waste is not more than half full (empty recommended), and then click *OK*.

Table 2
ML STAR loading details for the cfDNA extraction procedure

Procedural step	Sample batch size	Carrier type	Track	Item	Site position
2	48	Tip	1–6	1000 μL tips	1, 2
			7–12	300 μL tips	1
	96	Tip	1–6	1000 μL tips	1, 2, 3, 4
			7–12	300 μL tips	1
3	48, 96	Tip	49–54	1000 μL tips	1
				300 μL tips	2
				50 μL tips	3
7	48, 96	Multiflex	19–24	New full-skirt plate, Intermediate - barcoded	1
				New full-skirt plate, cfDNA Elution - barcoded	2
				New deep-well plate, Extraction Intermediate - barcoded	4
				Final Plasma deep-well plate - barcoded	5
11	48	Reagent	47	16 mL Elution Buffer	1
				11 mL Proteinase K	2
	96	Reagent	47	16 mL Elution Buffer	1
				15 mL Proteinase K	2
12	48	Deep-well	39–44	125 mL Wash Buffer II	1
				125 mL Wash Buffer I	2
				60 mL 100% EtOH	3
				100 mL Lysis Buffer	4
				60 mL DNase/RNase-free water	5
	96	Deep-well	39–44	200 mL Wash Buffer II	1
				125 mL Wash Buffer I	2
				100 mL 100% EtOH	3
				100 mL Lysis Buffer	4
				100 mL DNase/RNase-free water	5

15. Confirm the placement of all carriers, labware, and reagents, and then click *OK* in the Extraction Deck Verification screen.
16. After the final vacuum step, centrifuge the DNA Binding plate, and then click *OK*: Remove the DNA Binding plate and clean the bottom surface with 70% EtOH; seal any uncovered wells on the DNA Binding plate and place it on the empty Final Plasma deep-well plate; centrifuge the DNA Binding plate/ Final Plasma plate assembly at 5600 × *g* for 10 min with the brake on.
17. During DNA Binding plate centrifugation, complete the vacuum cleaning: Wait for the automated waste disposal to complete; clean the vacuum manifold and inside the vacuum system with 70% EtOH, and then replace the vacuum manifold; select the *Manifold is on Vacuum* checkbox, and then click *OK*.

18. Remove vacuum manifold, and then click *OK*.
19. After centrifugation, unseal the wells containing samples on the DNA Binding plate and place it on the cfDNA Elution plate. The cfDNA Elution plate is on the vacuum manifold. Load the DNA Binding plate with the barcode to the right, and then click *OK*.
20. After the incubation step, select the *Plates are assembled as indicated* checkbox, confirming that the DNA Binding/ cfDNA Elution plate assembly is on a support base (if required by centrifuge).
21. Seal the uncovered wells on the DNA Binding plate and centrifuge at 5600 × *g* for 2 min with the brake on, and then click *OK*.
22. Visually inspect the cfDNA Elution plate for consistent volumes in each well. Expected volume is approximately 55 μL.
23. Seal and retain the cfDNA Elution plate for library preparation.
24. When alerted by the Workflow Manager, make sure that the ML STAR loading deck is free of any obstructions to allow the ML STAR to unload the carriers, and then click *Unload* to unload the deck.
25. Unload all carriers and clean the ML STAR deck, and then click *OK*.
26. Enter comments about affected wells, and then click *OK*.
27. Perform one of the following: To continue to Prepare Libraries, click *Yes*; to stop. Click *Exit* (*see* **Note 6**).

3.4 Library Preparation

3.4.1 Preparation

1. Label 1 new full-skirt plate *Libraries* and apply a plate barcode.
2. Make sure that the ML STAR thermal control is on.

3.4.2 Procedure

1. Click *OK* to start Library Preparation. If the VeriSeq NIPT Method is not already open: Open the AppLauncher, and click *VeriSeq NIPT Method*; enter the Batch ID and username, and then click *OK*.
2. Confirm that the following are prepared as indicated in the Reagent Preparation screen: A-Tailing Mix, Ligation Mix, and 80% EtOH; Sample Purification Beads, End Repair Mix, and VeriSeq NIPT DNA Adapter Plate.
3. Select the checkboxes, and then click *OK*.
4. Scan Library Prep Box barcodes. Enter the user name or reagent preparer initials, and then click *OK*.
5. Scan Accessory Box barcodes. Enter the user name or reagent preparer initials, and then click *OK*.

Table 3
ML STAR loading details for the library preparation procedure

Procedural step	Sample batch size	Carrier type	Track	Item	Site position
6	48	Tip	1–6	50 μL tips	1, 2
			7–12	300 μL tips	1, 2, 3, 5
	96	Tip	1–6	50 μL tips	1, 2, 3, 4
			7–12	300 μL tips	1, 2, 3, 4, 5
7	48, 96	Tip	49–54	1000 μL tips	1
				300 μL tips	2
				50 μL tips	3
9	48, 96	Multiflex	19–24	cfDNA Elution plate - barcoded	1
				DNA Adapter plate – barcoded	2
				New 96-well full-skirt plate, libraries - barcoded	3
				New 96-well full-skirt plates	4, 5
10	48, 96	Deep-well	39–44	50 mL 80% EtOH in a deep-well reservoir	1
				New 96-well full-skirt plates	2, 3, 4, 5
11	48, 96	Reagent	47	2.5 mL End Repair Mix	1
				Prepared A-Tailing Mix	2
				Prepared Ligation Mix	3
				10 mL Sample Purification Beads	4
				12 mL Hybridization Buffer	5

6. Load tips onto the tip carriers as detailed in Table 3, and then click *OK*.
7. If you stopped the protocol after the cfDNA Extraction procedure, load counted tips onto the tip carriers as detailed in Table 3.
8. Enter the location of the first tip for each tip rack, and then click *OK*.
9. Confirm that barcodes are affixed, and load plates (barcode facing right) onto the plate carrier as detailed in Table 3, and then click *OK*.
10. Load the deep-well carrier as detailed in Table 3, and then click *OK*.
11. Load reagent tubs onto the reagent carrier as detailed in Table 3, and then click *OK*.
12. Make sure that the carriers, labware, and reagents are loaded as indicated, and then click *OK* in the Library Deck Verification screen.

13. Wait for the automated reagent volume check to complete.
14. When alerted by the Workflow Manager, make sure that the ML STAR loading deck is free of any obstructions to allow the ML STAR to unload the carriers, and then click *Unload* to unload the deck.
15. Visually inspect the Libraries plate for consistent volumes in each well.
16. Seal and retain the Libraries plate.
17. Unload the carriers, clean the deck, and then click *OK*.
18. Enter comments about affected wells, and then click *OK*.
19. Perform one of the following: To continue to Quantify Libraries, click *Yes*; to stop, click *Exit* (*see* **Note 6**).

3.5 Library Quantification

3.5.1 Preparation

1. Turn on the fluorometer 10 min before use.
2. Apply a plate barcode to a new 384-well plate.
3. Apply a plate barcode to a new full-skirt plate.

3.5.2 Procedure

1. Click *OK* to start quantification. If the VeriSeq NIPT Method is not already open: Open the AppLauncher, and click *VeriSeq NIPT Method*; enter the Batch ID and username, and then click *OK*.
2. Scan Accessory Box barcodes. Enter the user name or reagent preparer initials, and then click *OK*.
3. Load tips onto the tip carrier as detailed in Table 4, and then click *OK*.
4. Confirm that barcodes are affixed, unseal the Libraries plate, and load plates (barcode facing right) onto the Multiflex carrier as detailed in Table 4, and then click *OK*.
5. Load reagent tubes without caps into the tube carrier as detailed in Table 4, and then click *OK*.
6. Load reagent tubs onto the reagent carrier as detailed in Table 4, and then click *OK*.
7. If you stopped the protocol after the Library Preparation procedure, load counted tips onto the tip carriers as detailed in Table 4.
8. Enter the location of the first tip for each tip rack, and then click *OK*.
9. Make sure that the carriers, labware, and reagents are loaded as indicated, and then click *OK* in the Quant Deck Verification screen.
10. Wait for the automated reagent volume check to complete.

Table 4
ML STAR loading details for the library quantification procedure

Procedural step	Sample batch size	Carrier type	Track	Item	Site position
3	48	Tip	1–6	300 μL tips rack	1
				50 μL tips rack	2
	96	Tip	1–6	300 μL tips rack	1
				50 μL tips rack	2, 3
4	48, 96	Multiflex	19–24	New full-skirt plates - barcoded	1
				New 384-well plate - barcoded	2
				Libraries plate – barcoded	3
				New 96-well full-skirt plates	4, 5
5	48, 96	Tube	46	DNA Quantification Standard	1
				DNA Quantification Reagent	2
6	48, 96	Reagent	47	New reagent tubs	1
				16 mL Resuspension Buffer	2
7	48, 96	Tip	49–54	1000 μL tips	1
				300 μL tips	2
				50 μL tips	3

11. When alerted by the Workflow Manager, make sure that the ML STAR loading deck is free of any obstructions to allow the ML STAR to unload the carriers, and then click *Unload* to unload the deck.
12. Unload the Libraries plate. Visually inspect the plate for consistent volumes in each well then seal the Libraries plate and store at room temperature until the fluorometric data analysis is complete.
13. Unload the remaining 96-well plates and visually inspect for consistent volumes in each well. Gross errors in volume can indicate an issue with pipetting steps.
14. Unload the 384-well plate and visually inspect for liquid in the appropriate wells. Seal the plate with a foil seal; centrifuge at 1000 × *g* for 20 s; then incubate at room temperature for 10 min, protected from light.
15. Unload all carriers and clean the ML STAR deck, and then click *OK*.
16. After incubation, remove the foil seal and load the 384-well plate onto the microplate reader. Make sure that A1 is in the top left corner, and click *Read*.
17. Export the data as an. XML file as follows: Right-click *Barcode*, select rename, scan the barcode of the Qualification plate, and

then click *OK*; at the upper-left corner, click the plate icon, and then select *Export* from the menu; select the *Expt1* checkbox, set the output format to XML, and click *OK*; Set the output file path and file name, and then click *Save*.

3.5.3 Analysis

1. On the ML STAR, in the Scanner Information screen, enter the fluorometer ID.
2. Enter comments about the fluorometer run, and then click *OK*.
3. Navigate to the. XML quantification file that contains the fluorometric data, and then click *OK*.
4. Review the standards curve and sample concentration analysis results, and then click *OK*.
5. If you need to rerun the plate, click *Rescan*. As samples are time and light sensitive, perform the Rescan immediately (when necessary).
6. Enter comments about affected wells, and then click *OK*.
7. Assess the results and proceed as follows: If the results pass specification, proceed to Pool Libraries; If the results fail specification, the system aborts the method and you must repeat the quantification procedures (*see* Subheading 3.5.2).
8. Perform one of the following: To continue to Pool Libraries, click *Yes*; to stop, click *Exit* (*see* **Note 6**).

3.6 Library Pooling

3.6.1 Preparation

1. Label an empty pooling tube Pool A. For 96 samples, label a second empty pooling tube Pool B.
2. Save the following denature program on a thermal cycler with a heated lid: Choose the preheated lid option and set to 102 °C; set the reaction volume to 50 μL; set the ramp rate to 4 °C per second; incubate at 96 °C for 10 min, and then 0 °C for 5 s; hold at 4 °C.

3.6.2 Procedure

1. Place the Libraries plate on the preprogrammed thermal cycler and run the denature program.
2. Click *OK* to start pool libraries. If the VeriSeq NIPT Method is not already open: Open the AppLauncher, and click VeriSeq NIPT Method; enter the Batch ID and username, and then click *OK*.
3. Select the pool concentration, and then click *OK*.
4. The target cluster density is 220–260 k/mm^2. If necessary, adjust the pooling concentration to achieve the target cluster density.
5. When prompted by the Workflow Manager, perform one of the following: To load a sample sheet, select the sample sheet

Table 5
ML STAR loading details for the library pooling procedure

Procedural step	Sample batch size	Carrier type	Track	Item	Site position
7	48, 96	Tip	7–12	50 μL filter tips	1
8	48, 96	Multiflex	19–24	Denatured Library plate	1
9	48	Tube	46	New 2 mL tube, Pool A	1
	96	Tube	46	New 2 mL tube, Pool A	1
				New 2 mL tube, Pool B	2
10	48	Reagent	47	3 mL Hybridization Buffer	1
	96	Reagent	47	3 mL Hybridization Buffer	1
11	48, 96	Tip	49–54	1000 μL tips	1
				300 μL tips	2
				50 μL tips	3

associated with the batch, and then click *Load*; to use system default values for remaining sample types or sex reporting, click *Use Default* for each setting.

6. Click *Start* to begin timer for denaturing plate.
7. Load tips onto the tip carriers as detailed in Table 5.
8. Load the Denatured Library plate (barcode facing right) onto the Multiflex carrier as detailed in Table 5, and then click *OK*.
9. Load pooling tubes onto the tube carrier as detailed in Table 5, and then click *OK*.
10. Load reagent tubs onto the reagent carrier as detailed in Table 5, and then click *OK*.
11. Load tips onto the tip carriers as detailed in Table 5. Enter the location of the first and last tips for each tip rack, and then click *OK*.
12. Make sure that the carriers, labware, and reagents are loaded as indicated, and then click *OK* in the Pooling Deck Verification screen.
13. When alerted by the Workflow Manager, make sure that the ML STAR loading deck is free of any obstructions to allow the ML STAR to unload the carriers, and then click *Unload* to unload the deck.
14. Unload the tube carrier. Cap each pooling tube, vortex, and then centrifuge briefly.
15. Sequence libraries as soon as possible after pooling. Store the Libraries plate at −25 °C to −15 °C for up to 7 days to enable repooling, if necessary. The Libraries plate is stable for up to 7 days cumulative storage at −25 °C to −15 °C.

16. Click *OK*.
17. Enter comments about affected wells, and then click *OK*.
18. Click OK at Pooling Complete screen (*see* **Note 6**).

3.7 Preparation for Sequencing

3.7.1 Preparation

1. Prepare the next-generation sequencing system with the following settings: Paired-end run with 36 x 36 cycle reads; dual indexing with 8-cycle index reads; run name the same as Pool Name.

3.7.2 Procedure

1. Add buffer and library pool directly to the sequencer sample cartridge as follows: 900 μL Hybridization Buffer; 450 μL Pool A; pipette to mix.
2. Proceed with sequencing using a next-generation sequencing system according to the manufacturer's instructions.
3. Confirm correct run configuration when prompted.
4. Repeat procedure for Pool B, if necessary.

3.8 Sequencing Data Analysis and Result Interpretation

1. After sequencing is complete, sequencing data is automatically sent to the VeriSeq NIPT Assay Software for analysis and sequencing report generation (please note, this is not a clinical report). The report includes classifications for each sample in the batch as well as an assessment of all run QC metrics. The analysis process takes approximately 4 h for a 48-sample batch.
2. The VeriSeq NIPT Solution employs an algorithm based on multiple data inputs, including sequencing coverage, sequence read quality, and estimated fetal fraction, to determine fetal chromosomal representation.
3. For samples that pass QC, the VeriSeq NIPT Assay Software automatically generates a result of ANEUPLOIDY DETECTED or NO ANEUPLOIDY DETECTED for chromosomes 21, 18, and 13 for each patient sample. A result of ANEUPLOIDY DETECTED indicates that the sample has screened positive for trisomy of the given chromosome.
4. Results on the fetal sex chromosome status are automatically generated and optionally reported. When no sex chromosomal aneuploidy is detected the report will state NO ANEUPLOIDY DETECTED appended with the sex classification: XX (female fetal sample) or XY (male fetal sample). Sex chromosome aneuploidies are reported as ANEUPLOIDY DETECTED appended with the particular aneuploidy detected: XXX, XXY, XYY, or XO (monosomy X). In rare cases, the sex chromosome values fall outside the reportable range and the system generates a result of SEX CHROMOSOMES NOT REPORTABLE; results for autosomal aneuploidy may still be reported for these samples.

5. The VeriSeq NIPT Assay Software uses statistics generated during sequencing to provide a fetal fraction estimation (FFE) for each sample. The FFE is the estimated fetal cfDNA component which is recovered by the assay and reported as a rounded percentage for each sample. The average standard deviation of this estimate across all samples is 1.3%. The FFE is not to be used in isolation to exclude samples when reporting results.
6. To make chromosomal representation calls, the VeriSeq NIPT Assay Software utilizes the individualized Fetal Aneuploidy Confidence Test (iFACT), a dynamic threshold metric that indicates whether the system has generated sufficient sequencing coverage, given the fetal fraction estimate for each sample. The system makes chromosomal representation calls only if a sample meets the iFACT threshold. If a sample fails to achieve this threshold, the QC assessment displays FAILED iFACT and the system does not generate a result. The iFACT assessment is applied to all samples.
7. In addition to iFACT, the VeriSeq NIPT Assay Software assesses several other QC metrics during analysis. The additional metrics include assessments of coverage uniformity on reference genomic regions and the distribution of cfDNA fragment lengths. The QC assessment displays either a QC flag or a QC failure for any metrics outside of the acceptable range (*see* Table 6). In the case of QC failure, the system does not generate a result for the sample. If a sample fails QC, a second plasma aliquot can be processed provided there is sufficient plasma volume in the blood collection tube.

Table 6
ML STAR loading details for the library pooling procedure

Failure mode	Possible result	Interpretation	Recommended action	Comments
Insufficient input plasma	Sample QC failure	Insufficient plasma volume	Redraw	Based on visual inspection of plasma volume.
Blood tube failure	No separation of blood into layers	Sample was not centrifuged	Make sure that the centrifuge started and the tube was spun at the correct force. Redraw sample.	
		Improper sample storage or transport	Redraw	Frozen samples will not separate.

(continued)

Table 6 (continued)

Failure mode	Possible result	Interpretation	Recommended action	Comments
Sample clog OR slow flow	Plasma contamination	Individual samples may clog the binding plate if there is significant contamination in the plasma sample	Inspect sample, if remaining plasma in tube is red or milky, cancel sample and request redraw. If sample appears normal, retest sample.	
	Hardware malfunction	Inadequate digestion of material during extraction	Retest sample.	
Individual Sample Analysis QC failure	Sequencing QC failure	Insufficient genetic input OR Mistransfer during sample handling	Check Sample Annotation. Check for similar performance on previous samples in relative plate position. Retest sample.	Indicates a bad sample input OR a mistransfer on the ML STAR. Insufficient genetic material can come from insufficient cfDNA in the plasma or cell-based DNA causing over-dilution of the sample for sequencing.
	Low FF or NES count	Insufficient data generated to make accurate reporting	Retest from plasma.	
Quantification QC failure	Failed quantification run—Batch median below minimum	Insufficient process yield	Repeat quantification.	Passing standards curve metrics indicates issue with library preparation.
	Failed quantification run	Standard curve failure due to bad quantification	Repeat quantification.	
Pooling Failure	Failure to complete sample pooling	Pooling Analysis is unable to calculate proper pool volumes	Reevaluate target pool concentration, rerun pooling analysis.	

4 Notes

1. Blood samples (7—10 mL whole blood) must be collected in Streck Cell-Free DNA BCT and must not be frozen. Blood collection tubes containing samples need to be stored at 4 °C within 5 days of collection, with plasma isolation completed within 10 days of sample collection.
2. Excessively hemolyzed blood samples should be cancelled. The ML STAR checks that wells are empty after vacuum steps, so blood samples that are too viscous will remain in the well; samples determined not to have been transferred are excluded from further analysis.
3. The Pluggo Decapper System (LGP Consulting) is useful for uncapping large numbers of BCTs.
4. The ML STAR should be observed during all automated steps.
5. Improper cleaning and maintenance of the ML STAR can lead to cross-contamination and poor assay performance.
6. There are several safe-stopping points: (1) After completion of plasma isolation, the Final Plasma plate can be sealed and stored at 2 °C to 8 °C for up to 7 days; (2) After completion of cfDNA extraction, the cfDNA Elution plate can be sealed and stored at −25 °C to −15 °C for up to 7 days; (3) After both the library preparation procedure and the library quantification procedure, the Libraries plate can be sealed and then stored at −25 °C to −15 °C for up to 7 days of cumulative storage; (4) After library pooling, the pooling tubes can be capped and stored at −25 °C to −15 °C for up to 7 days.

Acknowledgments

We thank the technical staff at the CLIA-certified Illumina laboratory (Foster City, CA) who developed these protocols for use in a clinical laboratory.

References

1. Malone FD, Canick JA, Ball RH, Nyberg DA, Comstock CH, Bukowski R, Berkowitz RL, Gross SJ, Dugoff L, Craigo SD, Timor-Tritsch IE, Carr SR, Wolfe HM, Dukes K, Bianchi DW, Rudnicka AR, Hackshaw AK, Lambert-Messerlian G, Wald NJ, D'Alton ME, First, Second-Trimester Evaluation of Risk Research C (2005) First-trimester or second-trimester screening, or both, for Down's syndrome. N Engl J Med 353(19):2001–2011. https://doi.org/10.1056/NEJMoa043693
2. Bianchi DW, Parker RL, Wentworth J, Madankumar R, Saffer C, Das AF, Craig JA, Chudova DI, Devers PL, Jones KW, Oliver K, Rava RP, Sehnert AJ (2014) DNA sequencing versus standard prenatal aneuploidy screening. N Engl J Med 370(9):799–808. https://doi.org/10.1056/NEJMoa1311037
3. Illumina Inc (2017) VeriSeq NIPT Solution Package Insert. https://support.illumina.com/content/dam/illumina-support/documents/

documentation/chemistry_documentation/dx/veriseq-nipt-solution/veriseq-nipt-solution-package-insert-1000000001856-02.pdf. Accessed 5 Feb 2018

4. Ryan A, Hunkapiller N, Banjevic M, Vankayalapati N, Fong N, Jinnett KN, Demko Z, Zimmermann B, Sigurjonsson S, Gross SJ, Hill M (2016) Validation of an enhanced version of a single-nucleotide polymorphism-based noninvasive prenatal test for detection of fetal aneuploidies. Fetal Diagn Ther 40(3):219–223. https://doi.org/10.1159/000442931
5. Jones KJ, Wang E, Bogard P, White K, Schmid M, Stokowski R, Nicolaides KH (2018) Targeted cell-free DNA analysis with microarray quantitation for assessment of fetal sex and sex chromosome aneuploidy risk. Ultrasound Obstet Gynecol 51(2):275–276. https://doi.org/10.1002/uog.18968

Chapter 23

Noninvasive Antenatal Screening for Fetal *RHD* in RhD Negative Women to Guide Targeted Anti-D Prophylaxis

Frederik Banch Clausen, Klaus Rieneck, Grethe Risum Krog, Birgitte Suhr Bundgaard, and Morten Hanefeld Dziegiel

Abstract

RhD negative pregnant women who carry an RhD positive fetus are at risk of immunization against the D antigen, which may result in hemolytic disease of the fetus and the newborn. Predicting the fetal RhD status by noninvasive antenatal screening for the fetal RhD gene (*RHD*) can guide targeted use of antenatal anti-D prophylaxis.

Cell-free fetal DNA is extracted from maternal plasma from RhD negative pregnant women at a gestational age of 25 weeks. A real-time PCR-based detection of two *RHD* exons enables reliable prediction of the fetal RhD status to determine the administration of antenatal prophylaxis, as well as postnatal prophylaxis.

Key words Noninvasive *RHD* typing, Cell-free fetal DNA, Anti-D, Antenatal prophylaxis, Hemolytic disease of the fetus and newborn, Real-time PCR

1 Introduction

1.1 Noninvasive Antenatal Screening for Fetal RHD

Immunization against the D antigen from the Rh blood group system is the major cause of hemolytic disease of the fetus and newborn (HDFN) and can cause fetal or neonatal death [1]. The introduction of postnatal immune prophylaxis in the 1960s drastically reduced the immunization incidents in pregnant, RhD negative women [2]. In several countries, antenatal prophylaxis is combined with postnatal prophylaxis to further minimize the immunization risk [1].

Noninvasive antenatal screening for the fetal RhD gene (*RHD*) enables antenatal prophylaxis to be targeted to only those women who carry an RhD positive fetus [3, 4]. A targeted antenatal prophylaxis thus avoids unnecessary treatment of pregnant women who carry an RhD negative fetus and are at no risk of immunization [5, 6]. In the European population, approximately 40% of the RhD

Brynn Levy (ed.), *Prenatal Diagnosis*, Methods in Molecular Biology, vol. 1885, https://doi.org/10.1007/978-1-4939-8889-1_23,

negative women are of no risk of immunization and should not be treated [5, 6].

Based on an analysis of cell-free fetal DNA from the plasma of pregnant women, a real-time PCR-based detection of the *RHD* predicts the fetal RhD status with high accuracy [3–6]. To target the antenatal prophylaxis by noninvasive antenatal *RHD* screening, it is essential that the assay has a high diagnostic sensitivity, thus avoiding false negative results that may result in immunizations and, consequently, HDFN. As a screening assay, the sensitivity is >99.3% from a gestational age of approximately 10–11 weeks and 99.6–100% from around 25 weeks [4].

1.2 Strategies for Gene Targeting

Due to the extensive polymorphism of the Rh blood group system and high degree of homology between the RhD and the RhCE gene, it is important to consider the most appropriate strategy to target the *RHD* gene in order to obtain an accurate and reliable prediction of the fetal RhD status in RhD negative pregnant women. Specifically, the choice and combination of exon targets is important. Genetic variants, such as silent genes, hybrid genes, or point mutations causing weak D types may complicate the prediction of the fetal RhD status [4, 7, 8]. As different *RHD* variants have different frequencies in different populations, the choice of gene targets may be based on the genetic composition of the population to be tested. Different combinations of *RHD* exons 5, 7, and 10 are usually applied [4, 6]. However, as false positive results are of minor clinical relevance, a simple setup will suffice for a screening assay for the large majority of populations. It is essential to obtain a high sensitivity as a false negative test result may lead to omission of anti-D administration, thus putting the woman in risk of immunization against D; the specificity is of secondary concern.

1.3 The Copenhagen Setup

According to the recommendations of the Danish Health and Medicines Authority, and as part of the RhD prophylaxis regime implemented in Denmark in January 2010, all non-immunized RhD negative pregnant women should be offered an antenatal screening for the fetal *RHD* at gestational age of 25 weeks [9]. The result of this test will guide antenatal anti-D prophylaxis administered at a gestational age of 29 weeks [9].

The Copenhagen setup is based on automated DNA extraction followed by a real-time PCR analysis of *RHD* exons 7 and 10 that are duplexed into one assay using the same reporting dye to increase sensitivity [10].

For the first 2 years of routine analysis, we have obtained a sensitivity of 99.97% [6]. During the last 4 years, we have encountered only one false negative result out of approximately 10,000 tested samples. Consequently, we have terminated the serological postnatal cord blood typing. Presently, both the antenatal and the postnatal anti-D prophylaxis are administered based on the recommendations from the antenatal *RHD* screening program in Denmark.

2 Materials

2.1 Blood Sample Processing

1. A standard blood sample centrifuge.
2. Sample racks for the QIAsymphony SP DNA extraction instrument (Qiagen Inc., Basel, Switzerland).

2.2 DNA Extraction

1. The QIAsymphony SP (Qiagen Inc., Basel, Switzerland).
2. The QIAsymphony DSP Virus/Pathogen Midi Kit using carrier RNA (Qiagen Inc., Basel, Switzerland) (*see* **Note 1**).
3. Sarstedt tubes without skirts (Sarstedt, Nümbrecht, Germany).
4. Reagent box, provided by the kit.
5. Plastic utensils for the QIAsymphony SP (Qiagen Inc., Basel, Switzerland), including pipetting tips.
6. AVE buffer, provided by the kit.
7. Sterile DNA free, RNase and DNase-free pipetting tips with filters for manual pipetting (MµltiGuard™ Barrier Tips, Sorensen BioScience, Inc., Salt Lake City, UT, USA).
8. Prepare the carrier RNA stock.
   (a) Add the provided 2 mL AVE buffer into the provided 1350 µg carrier RNA tube.
   (b) Vortex ×3 and centrifuge briefly to avoid liquid in the lid.
   (c) Make eight aliquots of 165 µL each (designated cRNA) and store at 4 °C.

2.3 Real-Time PCR

1. Instrument for automated PCR setup: QIAsymphony AS (Qiagen Inc., Basel, Switzerland).
2. Instrument for PCR: The real-time PCR ABI 7500 detection system (Applied BioSystems, Foster City, USA).
3. Software for PCR interpretation: 7500 System SDS software Version 1.4 (Applied BioSystems, Foster City, USA).
4. PCR plates: MicroAmp® Optical 96-Well Reaction Plates (Applied BioSystems, Foster City, USA).
5. PCR plate cover: MicroAmp™ Optical Adhesive Film (Applied BioSystems, Foster City, USA).
6. Sterile H_2O (Mini Plasco®, Braun Melsungen, Melsungen, Germany), store at 4 °C.
7. Sarstedt tubes with skirts for reagents to be inserted into the QIAsymphony AS, and Sarstedt tubes without skirts for storage or other purposes not involving the QIAsymphony AS.
8. Plastic utensils for the QIAsymphony AS, including pipetting tips.

Table 1
Primers and probes for real-time PCR detection of DNA in maternal plasma

Name	Sequence	Specificity
*RHD*ex7s	5′-CAGCTCCATCATGGGCTACAA-3′	*RHD*
*RHD*ex7a	5′-CCGGCTCCGACGGTATC-3′	*RHD*
*RHD*ex7p	5′-FAM-CAGCACAATGTAGATGATCTCTCCAAGCAG-TAMRA-3′	*RHD*
*RHD*ex10s	5′-CCTCTCACTGTTGCCTGCATT-3′	*RHD/RHCE*
*RHD*ex10a	5′-AGTGCCTGCGCGAACATT-3′	*RHD*
*RHD*ex10p	5′-FAM-TACGTGAGAAACGCTCATGACAGCAAAGTC-TAMRA-3′	*RHD/RHCE*
*GAPDH*s	5′-CCCCACACACATGCACTTACC-3′	*GAPDH*
*GAPDH*a	5′-CCTAGTCCCAGGGCTTTGATT-3′	*GAPDH*
*GAPDH*p	5′-FAM-AAAGAGCTAGGAAGGACAGGCAACTTGGC-TAMRA-3′	*GAPDH*

Ex exon, *s* sense, *a* antisense, *p* probe

9. Sterile DNA free, RNase and DNase-free pipetting tips with filters for manual pipetting (Sorensen BioScience, Inc., Salt Lake City, UT, USA)).
10. Primers and probes are listed in Table 1.
    (a) Reconstitute primers in sterile H_2O to a concentration of 90 μM and store at −20 °C.
    (b) Reconstitute the probes in sterile H_2O to a concentration of 40 μM and store at −20 °C (*see* **Note 2**).
    (c) Transfer 310 μL of each primer to a Sarstedt tube per primer to make up working solutions, store at −30 °C.
    (d) Transfer 100 μL of each probe to a Sarstedt tube per probe and add 300 μL sterile H_2O to each tube to make up 10 μM working solutions, store at −20 °C.
    (e) For each assay, transfer 100 μL each from the working solutions of sense primer, antisense primer, and the probe into one Sarstedt tube, named SAP, for example *RHD*ex7SAP (*see* **Note 3**).
11. TaqMan Universal PCR Master Mix 2× (Applied BioSystems) including uracil-*N*-glycosylase (UNG). Store at 4 °C.
12. Control DNA (prepared in-house from whole blood). DNA from an *RHD* negative woman is used as *RHD* negative control, and DNA from an *RHD* positive (*RHD* hemizygous) individual is used as *RHD* positive control.
    (a) Extract the DNA from whole blood using the QIAamp DNA Blood Mini Kit (Qiagen) (*see* **Note 4**).
    (b) Quantify eluted DNA using a spectrophotometer, and dilute with sterile H_2O to approximately 5 ng/μL, and store at −20 °C in 8 μL aliquots (*see* **Note 5**).

(c) The first time for each new donor, use the PCR assay for *RHD* to ensure that the DNA from an RhD negative donor is truly *RHD* negative, and that the RhD positive donor DNA is truly *RHD* positive, before using the DNA as control (*see* **Note 6**).

3 Methods

We receive a blood sample from the general practitioner (GP). Sample registration, processing, and DNA extraction is done in Area 1. Area 1 is a clean area, which is meticulously and constantly kept free of PCR products in order to preclude any risk of carry-over. Preparation of reagents and mastermix is done in a dedicated flow bench, also in Area 1.

Gloves are used all the time and changed frequently. Real-time PCR is done in Area 2. Areas 1 and 2 must be physically separated, and to avoid carry-over of PCR products, no transport is allowed from Area 2 to Area 1.

We test for glyceraldehyde 3-phosphate dehydrogenase (*GAPDH*) as a marker for total DNA. We do not use a control for fetal DNA; this is not necessary for a screening at a gestational age of 25 weeks.

3.1 Blood Sample Validation

A blood sample taken in 6 mL EDTA blood tubes from a pregnant RhD negative woman is received from the woman's GP. The blood sample must meet the following criteria to be included for further analysis:

1. The blood sample must be from a pregnant RhD negative woman.
2. The blood sample must be from a *non-immunized* pregnant RhD negative woman, thus without detectable anti-D (*see* **Note 7**).
3. Transportation time in days from venipuncture to centrifugation must not exceed 7 days (*see* **Note 8**).
4. The time of venipuncture must be at a gestational week of minimum 22 weeks (*see* **Note 9**).
5. The blood sample should appear undamaged.
6. The blood sample must not have been opened before arriving at the laboratory for analysis.
7. If one of the criteria from 1 or 3–6 is not met, a new sample is requested from the GP.

3.2 Blood Sample Processing

1. After arriving at the laboratory, store samples at room temperature until further analysis the same day. If a sample is stored overnight, place the sample at 4 °C.
2. Centrifuge the 6 mL EDTA blood tube at 1700 × *g* for 10 min (*see* **Note 10**).
3. From here, all handling of the sample is done using gloves.
4. Inspect the sample visually for appropriate approximate plasma volume (minimum 1.2 mL) and for hemolysis. If there is insufficient plasma material, or if the blood sample displays severe hemolysis, request a new blood sample from the general practitioner.
5. The centrifuged blood tube is then placed directly into a sample rack that can be inserted into the QIAsymphony SP.

3.3 DNA Extraction

1. Prepare the QIAsymphony SP instrument for DNA extraction (*see* **Note 11**).
2. Prepare and insert the reagent box.
3. Insert plastic utensils (*see* **Note 12**).
4. Insert the plate for DNA elution (*see* **Note 13**).
5. Prepare the carrier RNA.
   (a) Add 805 μL AVE buffer to each of two Sarstedt tubes without skirt.
   (b) Add 70 μL cRNA (from 2.2.6c) to each tube.
   (c) Vortex ×3 and centrifuge briefly.
6. Insert the carrier RNA, both tubes.
7. Insert the sample rack, containing the blood tube, into the QIAsymphony SP. A barcode reader in the QIAsymphony scans the tube for sample ID when inserting the sample rack.
8. Select the integrated run, which includes the programming of the QIAsymphony AS (*see* **Note 11**).
9. Select the "Cellfree 1000_V6_DSP default IC"-assay for DNA extraction.
10. Run the program.

3.4 Real-Time PCR

1. For the preparation of the *RHD* mastermix, we use a total PCR reaction volume of 25 μL consisting of 15 μL mastermix and 10 μL template-DNA. For the preparation of the *GAPDH* mastermix, we use a total PCR reaction volume of 25 μL consisting of 20 μL mastermix and 5 μL template-DNA (*see* **Note 14**).
2. Prepare the *RHD* mastermix.
   (a) Calculate the required volume of mastermix, according to number of samples tested (*see* **Note 15**).

   (b) Mark a Sarstedt tube *with* skirt "*RHD* mastermix."
   (c) Add 1 μL sterile H_2O per PCR well.
   (d) Add 12.5 μL Universal Master Mix (2×) per PCR well.
   (e) Add 0.75 μL *RHD*ex7SAP per PCR well.
   (f) Add 0.75 μL *RHD*ex10SAP per PCR well.
   (g) Vortex 3–5 times and centrifuge briefly.

3. Prepare the *GAPDH* mastermix.
   (a) Calculate the required volume of mastermix.
   (b) Mark a Sarstedt tube *with* skirt "*GAPDH* mastermix."
   (c) Add 6.75 μL sterile H_2O per PCR well.
   (d) Add 12.5 μL Universal Master Mix (2×) per PCR well.
   (e) Add 0.75 μL *GAPDH* SAP per PCR well.
   (f) Vortex 3-5 times and centrifuge briefly.

4. Prepare the control DNA.
   (a) Thaw the *RHD* negative control DNA aliquot (5 ng/μL), vortex, and centrifuge briefly.
   (b) Add 54 μL sterile H_2O each into three Sarstedt tubes with skirts.
   (c) Add 6 μL of the aliquot into the first tube, vortex, and centrifuge briefly.
   (d) Add 6 μL from the first tube into the second as well as into the third to obtain two tubes with 50 pg/μL each, vortex, and centrifuge briefly. These are the final *RHD* negative controls (*see* **Note 16**).
   (e) Thaw the *RHD* positive control DNA aliquot (5 ng/μL), vortex, and centrifuge briefly.
   (f) Add 54 μL sterile H_2O each to four Sarstedt tubes with skirts.
   (g) Add 6 μL of the aliquot into the first tube, vortex, and centrifuge briefly.
   (h) Add 6 μL from the first tube into the second tube, vortex, and centrifuge briefly.
   (i) Add 6 μL from the second tube into the third and fourth tubes to obtain two tubes with 5 pg/μL each, vortex, and centrifuge briefly. These are the final *RHD* positive controls (*see* **Note 17**).

5. Load the PCR reagents into the QIAsymphony AS, following a software protocol designed specifically as described above with triplicate analysis of *RHD* and a single analysis of *GAPDH* for each sample, non-template control samples, and *RHD* negative and *RHD* positive control samples.

6. Start the automated transfer of the elution plate from the QIAsymphony SP to the QIAsymphony AS.
7. Start the automated PCR pipetting setup.
8. When the PCR setup is completed, remove the plate and seal it with a cover (MicroAmp™ Optical Adhesive Film).
9. Insert the plate into the 7500 ABi PCR instrument; apply a template setup or follow the wizard instructions for setup (*see* **Note 18**).
10. Use the following thermal PCR profile: 2 min at 50 °C and 10 min at 95 °C, followed by 45 cycles of 95 °C for 15 s and 60 °C for 1 min.
11. To avoid carry-over of PCR products, it is essential to ensure a proper discarding of the PCR plates as well as to avoid returning to Area 1.

3.5 Interpretation of Results

1. For software analysis of the PCR results, use automated background and a fixed threshold of 2.0.
2. Consider a PCR reaction positive, if the cycle threshold (Ct) value is <42 (*see* **Note 19**).
3. General rules for the controls:
   (a) The non-template control can be positive in a maximum of two out of three (2/3) *RHD* PCR reactions (with a Ct-value <40).
   (b) The *RHD* positive control must be positive in minimum 2/3 PCR reactions ($Ct \leq 38$).
   (c) The *RHD* negative control can be positive in a maximum 1/3 PCR reactions ($Ct < 40$).
   (d) The non-template control must be negative for *GAPDH* ($Ct > 38$).
   (e) The *RHD* positive and *RHD* negative controls must be positive with *GAPDH*.
4. Interpretation rules for samples:
   (a) Consider a sample ***RHD* positive**, if all triplicate PCR reactions are positive (*see* **Note 20**).
   (b) Consider a sample ***RHD* negative**, if one or none PCR reactions are positive ($Ct > 40$), and if the *GAPDH* Ct-value is <35.
   (c) Consider a sample **Inconclusive**, if two PCR reactions are positive.
   (d) Consider a sample **Inconclusive**, if the *RHD* Ct-values are less than or equal to the Ct-values of *GAPDH*, which may indicate a possible *RHD* positive woman (*see* **Note 21**).

5. We recommend that all women with an ***RHD* positive** or **Inconclusive** sample result are offered antenatal anti-D prophylaxis.
6. If the criteria from 3a-e are not met, all the samples from the PCR run are retested using backup plasma, or a new blood sample is requested. If the *GAPDH* Ct-value is ≥35 for a seemingly *RHD* negative result, a new blood sample is requested, as a high Ct-value may indicate a poor DNA extraction with the risk of a false negative result. Overall, a result is only concluded and reported, when all the listed criteria are met (*see* **Note 22**).

4 Notes

1. We have not tested whether including the carrier RNA makes any difference as regards to the cffDNA yield, and it is possible that the maternal DNA fulfills the role of the carrier RNA. However, we have chosen to follow the manufacturer's recommendations.
2. We use our primers and probes quickly. If testing few samples, a higher concentration may be considered for the primer and probe stock solutions. We use HPLC purified primers. Primers can be purchased from, e.g., Eurofins MWG Operon, Edelsberg, Germany or TAG Copenhagen, Copenhagen, Denmark.
3. The SAP is named for Sense primer, Antisense primer, and Probe. We use this SAP solution containing all oligos of an assay simply to have fewer pipetting steps in the downstream analysis, thereby saving time and decreasing the risk of pipetting mistakes. In our experience, the SAP solution works well for about a year, and perhaps longer. However, as a consequence of the routine testing, we make a fresh SAP approximately every second week.
4. Other DNA extraction systems can be used.
5. We quantify the elution, then dilute to 10 ng/μL and quantify again, and then dilute to 5 ng/μL and re-quantify and note the estimated concentration. This procedure with two quantification steps ensures a more accurate final DNA concentration compared to a procedure with only a single quantification step. In principle, the *RHD* positive control DNA can be used as a reference DNA for a relative quantification of the cell-free fetal DNA, using the delta Ct-method. However, we find that using the control DNA for the delta Ct-method results in an inaccurate quantification, and we recommend using a universal standard curve, which does not need to be included on each PCR plate [11].

6. We use DNA from an *RHD* hemizygous individual to simulate the presumable hemizygous DNA from an *RHD* positive fetus. If necessary, the zygosity of the *RHD* positive control DNA can be assessed or confirmed by a zygosity test [12].
7. If the pregnant woman has a known anti-D, she is treated as an immunized woman. The sample is analyzed but with a different algorithm, where the minimum acceptable gestational week is 10 weeks.
8. Cell-free fetal DNA can remain stable even during prolonged transportation in EDTA-tubes. We have shown that the detection of cell-free fetal DNA, using the duplex *RHD* assay described in this method, is unchanged despite a transportation time of up to 9 days and despite an increase in the level of maternal DNA [11]. This finding is corroborated by others [13]. Consequently, we allow a sample to be 7 days old. However, we still require from the general practitioners that the anticipated transportation time must not exceed a maximum of 4 days, so that the transportation time does not exceed 7 days when samples are in transit over weekends or public holidays.
9. On a few occasions, samples from early pregnancy have been sent by mistake, such as gestational weeks 8, and this has been shown to result in false negative results [6]. We chose not to analyze samples before 22 gestational weeks, mainly because our validation was done with samples from 20 gestational weeks and onward, but also to help the general practitioners to comply with the request that the samples should be taken in gestational weeks 25. The overall system, however, is robust enough to analyze samples from earlier than gestational weeks 22.
10. We do not use a second centrifugation step to eliminate excess maternal DNA background. We have shown that this is not necessary for the detection of fetal *RHD* at gestational weeks 25 [11]. Avoiding a second centrifugation step also avoids further handling that can result in sample mixup or increased risk of contamination.
11. Preparing and running the QIAsymphony involves several steps in the QIAsymphony software. These have been left out here, as these steps will be incorporated into an analysis through a training program provided by Qiagen personnel. When the program is selected, one can select an integrated program that allows for a simultaneous setup of the QIAsymphony SP and AS. In this way, the program is initiated for both the DNA extraction as well as for the downstream PCR pipetting. However, the system allows you to prepare the QIAsymphony AS with utensils and reagents after starting the program.

12. It is important that the plastic utensils are inserted correctly; otherwise an instrument failure may occur.
13. It is also possible to use tubes for DNA elution.
14. When we extract DNA from 1 mL plasma, elute into 60 μL, and apply 10 μL for PCR testing, we are really testing an equivalent of 1/6 of 1 mL plasma (1000 μL × 10 μL/60 μL = 167 μL). This is also called the plasma-equivalent per PCR. A high plasma-equivalent per PCR is essential for a high sensitivity. Theoretically, if the plasma-equivalent is doubled, then the sensitivity is equally doubled; however, using a lower elution volume or a higher template volume may also increase the amount of PCR inhibitors in the PCR reaction. We use a PCR setup where we test three reactions for *RHD*. Using multiple reactions will increase the sensitivity, if one reaction is allowed to be negative.
15. The required mastermix volumes depend on the number of samples tested plus the controls, and some additional volume. We test the *RHD* positive and negative controls, as well as the non-template control as samples, thus accounting for three extra samples. In addition, a substantial dead volume is required. The QIAsymphony software will inform you of the number of reactions and estimate the required mastermix volume.
16. The reason for making two control tubes of each control is that the PCR setup program requires a set of reagents for each assay, *RHD* as well as *GAPDH*.
17. The difference of concentration in the two controls relates to their function. The *RHD* negative control serves as control to show that the *RHD* assay does not produce an unspecific PCR signal, which is shown at a higher concentration than the concentration to be expected from the maternal plasma. The *RHD* positive control with approximately 50 pg per PCR serves as control for a reliable detection of low-level DNA, yet kept at a concentration that results in positive amplifications in all triplicate reactions each time.
18. A txt.-file describing the sample IDs and the PCR setup can be exported from the QIAsymphony and imported to the PCR software, thus ensuring automated setup in the PCR instrument and sample ID tracking; the txt.-file carries the barcode of the PCR plate inserted into the QIAsymphony. The barcode of the plate can then be read upon inserting the plate into the PCR instrument, thus ensuring that the PCR setup and the sample IDs are connected to the correct plate.
19. If an amplification curve deviates from an expected curve shape, consult the raw data (e.g., "compliment" in the

software) to make a visual evaluation; use the data from the positive and negative controls to guide you.

20. An estimated 95%-limit of detection (LoD) for the *RHD* positive conclusion based on 3/3 positive PCR reactions is 9 copies per mL plasma. For the inconclusive results with 2/3 positive PCR reactions, the LoD is 6 copies per mL plasma.
21. Women that we suspect to be *RHD* positive are recommended anti-D prophylaxis. In addition, although without any clinical implications, we test the maternal blood (left from the DNA extraction) serologically for the RhD status using anti-D IgG LOR17 (reacting with most D variants including DVI) and GAN4B.5 (reacting with most D variants but not with DVI) as well as for RhC and RhE [6]. The results are kept to distinguish the outcomes: maternal weak D, DVI, and silent, nonfunctional *RHD* genes. During the first two years of routine testing, we also included further individual DNA testing of the maternal DNA for *RHD* exon 5, 7, and 10.
22. Additional comments that might be useful: In our laboratory we run approximately 80 samples per week, with a maximum of 20 samples per DNA extraction and PCR test. The full procedure can be done within a day and by one person. The DNA extraction step takes about 2 h and the PCR is about 1.5 h; registration, processing, and reporting take about 2 h. The current price, which covers reagents and personnel, is about 100 EUR per sample.

References

1. Urbaniak SJ, Greiss MA (2000) RhD haemolytic disease of the fetus and the newborn. Blood Rev 14(1):44–61. https://doi.org/10.1054/blre.1999.0123
2. Urbaniak SJ (1998) The scientific basis of antenatal prophylaxis. Br J Obstet Gynaecol 105 (Suppl 18):11–18
3. Clausen FB (2014) Integration of noninvasive prenatal prediction of fetal blood group into clinical prenatal care. Prenat Diagn 34 (5):409–415. https://doi.org/10.1002/pd.4326
4. Clausen FB, Damkjaer MB, Dziegiel MH (2014) Noninvasive fetal RhD genotyping. Transfus Apher Sci 50(2):154–162. https://doi.org/10.1016/j.transci.2014.02.008
5. Clausen FB, Christiansen M, Steffensen R, Jorgensen S, Nielsen C, Jakobsen MA, Madsen RD, Jensen K, Krog GR, Rieneck K, Sprogoe U, Homburg KM, Grunnet N, Dziegiel MH (2012) Report of the first nationally implemented clinical routine screening for fetal RHD in D- pregnant women to ascertain the requirement for antenatal RhD prophylaxis. Transfusion 52(4):752–758. https://doi.org/10.1111/j.1537-2995.2011.03362.x
6. Clausen FB, Steffensen R, Christiansen M, Rudby M, Jakobsen MA, Jakobsen TR, Krog GR, Madsen RD, Nielsen KR, Rieneck K, Sprogoe U, Homburg KM, Baech J, Dziegiel MH, Grunnet N (2014) Routine noninvasive prenatal screening for fetal RHD in plasma of RhD-negative pregnant women-2 years of screening experience from Denmark. Prenat Diagn 34(10):1000–1005. https://doi.org/10.1002/pd.4419
7. Daniels G (2009) The molecular genetics of blood group polymorphism. Hum Genet 126 (6):729–742. https://doi.org/10.1007/s00439-009-0738-2
8. Daniels G (2013) Variants of RhD--current testing and clinical consequences. Br J

Haematol 161(4):461–470. https://doi.org/10.1111/bjh.12275

9. Fagredaktion S, Poulsen A (eds) (2009) Anbefalinger for Svangreomsorgen [recommendations for pregnancy and birth], 1st edn. Danish National Board of Health, Copenhagen ISBN:978-87-7676-906-2
10. Clausen FB, Krog GR, Rieneck K, Rasmark EE, Dziegiel MH (2011) Evaluation of two real-time multiplex PCR screening assays detecting fetal RHD in plasma from RhD negative women to ascertain the requirement for antenatal RhD prophylaxis. Fetal Diagn Ther 29(2):155–163. https://doi.org/10.1159/000321347
11. Clausen FB, Jakobsen TR, Rieneck K, Krog GR, Nielsen LK, Tabor A, Dziegiel MH (2013) Pre-analytical conditions in non-invasive prenatal testing of cell-free fetal RHD. PLoS One 8(10):e76990. https://doi.org/10.1371/journal.pone.0076990
12. Krog GR, Clausen FB, Dziegiel MH (2007) Quantitation of RHD by real-time polymerase chain reaction for determination of RHD zygosity and RHD mosaicism/chimerism: an evaluation of four quantitative methods. Transfusion 47(4):715–722. https://doi.org/10.1111/j.1537-2995.2007.01175.x
13. Muller SP, Bartels I, Stein W, Emons G, Gutensohn K, Legler TJ (2011) Cell-free fetal DNA in specimen from pregnant women is stable up to 5 days. Prenat Diagn 31(13):1300–1304. https://doi.org/10.1002/pd.2889

INDEX

A

B

C

D

F

G

H

I

Brynn Levy (ed.), *Prenatal Diagnosis*, Methods in Molecular Biology, vol. 1885, https://doi.org/10.1007/978-1-4939-8889-1,

J

M

N

P

Q

R

S

T

U

W

MIX
Papier aus verantwortungsvollen Quellen
Paper from responsible sources
FSC® C105338

If you have any concerns about our products,
you can contact us on
ProductSafety@springernature.com

In case Publisher is established outside the EU,
the EU authorized representative is:
Springer Nature Customer Service Center GmbH
Europaplatz 3, 69115 Heidelberg, Germany

Printed by Libri Plureos GmbH
in Hamburg, Germany